RIBOFLAVIN

CONTRIBUTORS

CLARENCE P. ALFREY, Jr., Ph. D., M. D. – Professor of Medicine, Baylor College of Medicine, Houston, Texas.

HERMAN BAKER, Ph. D. – Professor of Medicine and Preventive Medicine, New Jersey Medical School, College of Medicine and Dentistry of New Jersey, Newark, New Jersey.

ARPAD G. FAZEKAS, M. D., Ph. D. – Research Assistant Professor of Medicine, University of Montreal, Montreal, Canada

OSCAR FRANK, Ph.D. – Associate Professor of Medicine, New Jersey Medical School, College of Medicine and Dentistry of New Jersey, Newark, New Jersey.

GRACE A. GOLDSMITH, M.D. – Professor and Director, Graduate Program in Nutrition, Tulane University, School of Public Health and Tropical Medicine, New Orleans, Louisiana.

SARA M. HUNT, Ph.D. – Chairman, Department of Community Health Nutrition, Georgia State University, Atlanta, Georgia.

WILLIAM J. JUSKO, Ph.D. – Associate Professor of Pharmaceutics, Director, Clinical Pharmacokinetics Laboratory, Millard Fillmore Hospital, State University of New York, at Buffalo, Buffalo, New York.

JOHN P. LAMBOOY, Ph.D. – Professor and Chairman, Department of Biochemistry, University of Maryland School of Dentistry, Baltimore, Maryland.

MONTAGUE LANE, M.D. – Head, Division of Clinical Oncology, Professor of Pharmacology and Medicine, Baylor College of Medicine, Houston, Texas.

GERHARD LEVY, PHARM. D. – Distinguished Professor, Department of Pharmaceutics, State University of New York at Buffalo, Buffalo, New York.

DONALD B. McCORMICK, Ph.D. – Professor, Section of Biochemistry, Molecular and Cell Biology; Division of Nutritional Sciences, Cornell University, Ithaca, New York.

ALLEN H. NEIMS, M.D., Ph.D. – Director, Roche Developmental Pharmacology Unit, Associate Professor of Pediatrics, Pharmacology and Therapeutics, McGill University, Montreal, Canada.

RICHARD S. RIVLIN, M.D. – Associate Professor of Medicine and Member, Institute of Human Nutrition, College of Physicians and Surgeons of Columbia University, New York, New York.

FRANK E. SMITH, M.D. – Associate Professor of Pharmacology and Medicine, Baylor College of Medicine, Houston, Texas.

JOSEF WARKANY, M.D., D.Sc. – Professor of Research Pediatrics, Children's Hospital Research Foundation, College of Medicine, University of Cincinnati, Cincinnati, Ohio.

WILLIAM R. WEIMAR – Graduate Student, Departments of Physiological Chemistry and Pediatrics, Johns Hopkins University, Baltimore, Maryland

RIBOFLAVIN

Edited by

Richard S. Rivlin, M.D.

Department of Medicine and
Institute of Human Nutrition
College of Physicians and Surgeons of Columbia University
New York, New York

PLENUM PRESS • *NEW YORK AND LONDON*

Library of Congress Cataloging in Publication Data

Rivlin, Richard S
  Riboflavin.

  Includes bibliographies and index.
  1. Riboflavin. I. Title. [DNLM: 1. Riboflavin. 2. Riboflavin deficiency. QU191 R625r]
  QP772.R5R58   574.1'926   74-31027

ISBN-13:978-1-4613-4421-6   e-ISBN-13: 978-1-4613-4419-3
DOI: 10.1007/978-1-4613-4419-3

© 1975 Plenum Press, New York
Softcover reprint of the hardcover 1st edition 1975
A Division of Plenum Publishing Corporation
227 West 17th Street, New York, N. Y. 10011

United Kingdom edition published by Plenum Press, London
A Division of Plenum Publishing Company, Ltd.
4a Lower John Street, London W1R 3PD, England

PREFACE

This volume represents an interdisciplinary approach to an understanding of the chemistry, physiology, and medical significance of the vitamin riboflavin. Information has been reviewed on the physiological role of the vitamin, the metabolic effects of riboflavin deficiency in animals and man, and the regulation of riboflavin metabolism. In each chapter early background material has been included, but the major emphasis has been on the many recent advances that have been made.

The early chapters of the book are concerned with the physical and chemical properties of riboflavin and its coenzyme derivatives and the nature of the interactions between flavoprotein apoenzymes and their coenzymes. The various methods currently available for measuring flavins in biological tissues, particularly in man, have been described in detail, together with newer procedures that appear to have certain advantages over existing techniques. Chapters dealing with the absorption, excretion, and metabolism of riboflavin provide basic data on the processes involved in vitamin uptake and in metabolic transformations.

The distribution of riboflavin in foodstuffs in the United States and abroad, and the consequences of riboflavin deficiency are presented largely in terms of their relation to human health. Timely questions such as the effects of organic farming and food processing upon riboflavin intake have been considered. The potential application of riboflavin deficiency as a chemotherapeutic agent is also discussed in terms of clinical significance. The important early observation that congenital malformations may be produced in animals as a result of maternal riboflavin deficiency has been amply confirmed by subsequent studies. Previously unpublished photographs have been used to illustrate an updated account of progress in this area.

An extended compilation of reports concerning various derivatives of riboflavin indicates which structural components of the molecule are essential for biological activity. It is noteworthy that several riboflavin derivatives have very significant ability to sustain growth and development of experimental animals.

The final two chapters of the book are concerned with specialized aspects of riboflavin—the relationship to cancer in animals and man and the control of vitamin metabolism by the endocrine system. These chapters indicate that endogenous factors such as hormones regulate the utilization of riboflavin in intermediary metabolism, particularly by governing conversion of the vitamin into its active coenzyme forms.

Knowledge in these fields has been accumulating rapidly. With the recent emphasis upon nutrition and health it is important to recognize which facts about vitamins can be regarded as established and which need to be elucidated by further inquiry. The rational administration of vitamins in health and in disease can be based only upon a firm scientific foundation.

The editor is indebted to each of the following colleagues for valuable assistance in the critical evaluation of submitted manuscripts: Carlos Menendez, Martha Osnos, Xavier Pi-Sunyer, Norton Rosensweig, David Rush, David Schacter, William Sebrell, and Arthur Wertheim, all of Columbia University; Arpad Fazekas, University of Montreal; Erich Hirschberg, New Jersey College of Medicine and Dentistry; F. Bacon Chow, Johns Hopkins University; Peter Hemmerich, University of Konstanz, Konstanz, Germany; and Donald McCormick, Cornell University. The assistance of Mrs. Phoebe Rosenwasser in the preparation and organization of the manuscripts has been most helpful.

New York   RICHARD S. RIVLIN

CONTENTS

Chapter 1
Physical and Chemical Properties of Flavins; Binding of Flavins to Protein and Conformational Effects; Biosynthesis of Riboflavin

WILLIAM R. WEIMAR AND ALLEN H. NEIMS

Chapter 4
Absorption, Protein Binding, and Elimination of Riboflavin

WILLIAM J. JUSKO AND GERHARD LEVY

Chapter 5
Metabolism of Riboflavin

DONALD B. MCCORMICK

Chapter 11
Riboflavin and Cancer

RICHARD S. RIVLIN

Chapter 12
Hormonal Regulation of Riboflavin Metabolism

RICHARD S. RIVLIN

PHYSICAL AND CHEMICAL PROPERTIES OF FLAVINS; BINDING OF FLAVINS TO PROTEIN AND CONFORMATIONAL EFFECTS; BIOSYNTHESIS OF RIBOFLAVIN

William R. Weimar and Allen H. Neims

It is our purpose to present in this chapter selected aspects of the chemical and physical properties of flavins, the influence of flavin binding on protein conformation, the modes of flavin-protein interaction, and the biosynthesis of riboflavin. Clearly, the diversity and extent of subject matter precludes comprehensive review. Rather, we choose to emphasize recent advances that seem to bear on future progress in flavoprotein biology and chemistry. Although some effort is made to establish historical perspective, it would be inappropriate and impossible to cite all the

WILLIAM R. WEIMAR—Departments of Physiological Chemistry and Pediatrics, John Hopkins University, Baltimore, Maryland. Supported by Graduate Training Grant GM-001841 from NIH. ALLEN H. NEIMS—Roche Developmental Pharmacology Unit, Department of Pharmacology and Therapeutics and Department of Pediatrics, McGill University, and the Montreal Childrens Hospital Research Institute, Montreal, Quebec, Canada. Joseph P. Kennedy, Jr., Scholar in Mental Retardation and Livingston Scholar in Epilepsy Research. Supported in part by USPHS Grant NS 09232 and MRC Grant MA 4769.

investigators whose studies have contributed to the advancements discussed here.

1. PHYSICAL AND CHEMICAL PROPERTIES OF FLAVINS

1.1. Nomenclature and General Properties

The physical and chemical properties of flavins have been studied extensively for many years. With the advent of sensitive spectroscopic instruments, fast reaction techniques, and such powerful tools as electron spin resonance (ESR) investigations of the past decade have focused on such subtleties as transient reaction intermediates, electronic properties of various redox states, and other physicochemical properties of mechanistic importance. It is our purpose to stress this recent physical organic and biophysical progress that has added new dimensions to flavin chemistry. Flavins are usually named as isoalloxazines (Fig. 1) although they can be designated also as benzopteridines. This option emphasizes the structural, biosynthetic, and probably evolutionary relationships between the flavins and pteridines. Biologically important isoalloxazines are substituted at C-7, C-8, and N-10. Hence 7,8-dimethyl-*N*-10 substituted isoalloxazines are often referred to as flavins, some of which are enumerated in Table I.

Certain general properties of the flavins are presented below; for greater detail, see Beinert.[9] Unless stated otherwise, the properties tabulated here refer to air-stable, oxidized flavoquinone forms.

1.1.1. Riboflavin

Molecular Weight (MW) 376.36: Melting points reported in the literature have ranged from 271° to 293°C. Part of this variation is

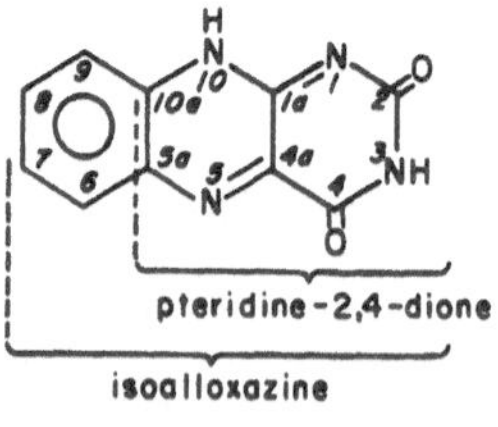

Fig. 1. Isoalloxazine.

TABLE I. *Structures of Common Flavins*

Flavin (7,8-dimethyl-N(10)-R-isoalloxazine)	R
Lumiflavin	$-CH_3$
Riboflavin	$-CH_2(CHOH)_3CH_2OH$
Flavin mononucleotide (FMN)	$-CH_2(CHOH)_3CH_2OPO_3^{-2}$
Flavin adenine dinucleotide (FAD)	$-CH_2(CHOH)_3CH_2O\overset{O}{\underset{O^{\ominus}}{\overset{\|}{P}}}O\overset{O}{\underset{O^{\ominus}}{\overset{\|}{P}}}O\text{-adenosine}$

due to polymorphism of riboflavin crystals with one common high-melting form (m.p., *ca.* 290°C) and either one or two low melting forms (m.p., *ca.* 280°C). Five milligrams of riboflavin can be dissolved in 100 ml water at 7°C. The lower melting form(s) of riboflavin is reported to be about ten times as soluble in water as the higher melting form. The fully reduced form (flavohydroquinone) is much less soluble. Riboflavin is very soluble, but unstable, in dilute alkali. Solutions of riboflavin are also sensitive to light. The solubility of riboflavin is increased by aromatic compounds such as nicotinamide, presumably because of intermolecular solvation "complexing." Practical use of this property is made in pharmaceutical preparations. Riboflavin is relatively stable in dry form under normal lighting. It is heat-stable in acid solutions, resistant to certain oxidizing agents, and reduced by dithionite, Zn/H^+, $TiCl_3$, or mild catalytic hydrogenation to yield the hydroquinone. There is no appreciable optical activity at 589 nm (Na D-line) except in alkaline solution.

1.1.2. Flavin Mononucleotide (FMN)

Molecular weight 456.4, m.p. 195°C, $[\alpha]_D^{28} + 44.5°C$ in water. FMN is very soluble in aqueous solutions. At alkaline pH, FMN, like riboflavin, is unstable; at acidic pH, the phosphate ester is hydrolyzed to give riboflavin. Thus, FMN is probably most stable at a pH of about 6.

1.1.3. Flavin Adenine Dinucleotide (FAD)

Molecular weight 785.6. Neutral aqueous solutions are very stable at 0-4°C. The rate of hydrolysis of FAD in acid is quite temperature-dependent. Like riboflavin and FMN, FAD is unstable in strong alkali.

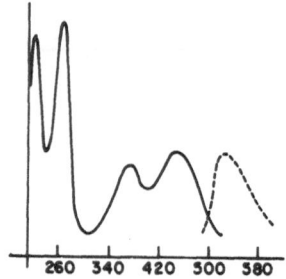

Fig. 2. Riboflavin spectra: — absorption, ---- fluorescence (from Penzer and Radda[105]).

It is destroyed by 365 nm light at a rate of about $\frac{1}{20}$ that of FMN or riboflavin. This stability of FAD is probably due to the same intramolecular complex formation that influences the absorption and fluorescence spectra (see below).

1.2. Electronic-Spectroscopic Properties: Flavoquinones (Fl_{ox})

1.2.1. Absorption

The u.v.-visible spectrum of riboflavin in aqueous solution consists of four major bands centered around 220, 266, 375, and 447 nm (Fig. 2, Table II). The spectrum of FMN is identical, but that of FAD differs in several respects. The positions of these bands and their extinction coefficients are dependent on the nature of the environment of the flavin chromophore, and electronic spectra do serve as probes of the microenvironment at the flavin molecule. The 375 nm band is affected most by solvent, generally shifting to shorter wavelengths (blue or hypsochro-

TABLE II. *Molar Extinction Coefficients for Riboflavin, FMN, and FAD in 0.1 M Phosphate, pH 7*

Extinction coefficient (10^3 cm^2 M^{-1})	Riboflavin	FMN	FAD
$\epsilon_{450\,(Fl_{ox})}$	12.2	12.2	11.3
$\epsilon_{375\,(FL_{ox})}$	10.6	10.4	9.0
$\epsilon_{260\,(FL_{ox})}$	27.7	27.1	36.9
$\epsilon_{450\,(FL_{red})}$	0.78	0.87	0.98

TABLE III. Solvent Effects on the Spectrum of Riboflavin

Solvent	Dielectric function [$Z(\epsilon)$]	Absorption band	
		Near u.v.	Visible
Water	94.6	375	445
Ethylene glycol	85.1	363	446
Ethanol	79.6	353	448
Acetic acid	79.2	355	445
Acetonitrile	71.3	344	445

mic shift) with decreasing solvent polarity (Table III). The position of the visible (445 nm) band is not strongly affected; it does split into several inflections in a hydrophobic environment because of the appearance of vibrational fine structure apparently within a single electronic transition as determined by fluorescence polarization. Both the 375 and 445 nm absorption bands in riboflavin have been assigned to $\pi \to \pi^*$ transitions, consistent with observed positions and high extinction coefficients. An excited state with polar character contributes to the 375 nm band, a fact which may account for the solvent-dependence of this absorption band. It is of interest that flavins in a hydrophobic environment have been postulated to be involved in phototropism in plants on the basis of similarity between the action spectrum for phototropism and the spectrum of riboflavin in castor oil.[36]

Isoalloxazine spectra are also affected by substituents. Methyl substituents at C-7 result in a shift to higher wavelengths (red or bathochromic shift) of the two long wavelength bands while methyl substituents at C-6 or C-8 affect only the 375 nm band.[104,105] Not surprisingly, substituents that affect the position of the 375 nm band also affect its solvent dependence. Substituents at N-10 and N-3 have only small influences on spectra. Substituents that extend conjugation in the system cause the expected bathochromic shifts since the transition energy is lowered. Ionization of the N-3 proton causes a small bathochromic shift. The monoprotonated form of riboflavin has a spectrum nearly identical to that of an N-1 substituted isoalloxazine, but it is different from those of isoalloxazines having no substituent at N-1. This suggests that in acidic media the proton is at N-1 in riboflavin, and hence that N-1 is the most basic position in the isoalloxazine nucleus.

1.2.2. Fluorescence

Flavoquinones show an intense fluorescence with λ_{max} *ca.* 530 nm for emission (see Fig. 2) and a fluorescence quantum yield $\phi_f = 0.25$

for riboflavin in water. Quenching of fluorescence occurs when the excited flavin loses sufficient electronic energy in nonradiative processes, such as collisional conversion of electronic energy to kinetic energy (I^-), heavy metal effects (Hg^{++}), magnetic perturbations (O_2), and electronic energy transfer $(^1Fl^* + Q \rightarrow Fl + Q^*)$. The latter mechanism has been implicated in recent studies of riboflavin fluorescence quenching by the transition metal ions, Fe^{+2} and Cr^{+3}.[133]

In cases where there are π–π interactions ("stacking") of the flavin and another aromatic species, energy can be transferred by the nonradiative process of exciton coupling, hence decreasing fluorescence. This type of interaction gives rise to hypochromicity of absorption bands and is responsible for both hypochromicity and fluorescence quenching observed in native ("stacked") DNA. Thus, due in part to their ability to form intermolecular complexes, aromatic compounds are good quenchers of flavin fluorescence. Indeed, such a complex, as distinct from charge transfer, has been confirmed by X-ray crystallography in the case of neutral lumiflavin and naphthalene-2,3-diol.[130]

FAD has a fluorescence only one-fifth that of FMN on a molar basis. In addition, there is hypochromicity of the 260-nm absorption band of FAD. These results are consistent with an intramolecular stacking interaction between the isoalloxazine and adenine rings. Unfortunately, the X-ray structure of FAD has not yet been determined due to inability to obtain suitable crystals. Such a structure of a 1:1 intermolecular complex of 5′-bromoadenosine with riboflavin has been reported by Voet and Rich.[138] When flavins are bound to proteins there is generally a dramatic quenching of fluorescence. Possible quenching groups include aromatic residues such as tyrosine, tryptophan, and phenylalanine; thiol groups; and metals in metalloflavoproteins. Recent studies of flavin analog binding and fluorescence[30] in Shethna flavoprotein suggest that the hydroxyl groups of the ribityl side chains play a role in fluorescence quenching (see also McCormick[84]). Thus protein may also facilitate quenching by binding the flavin in a conformation more favorable to intramolecular quenching mechanisms.

1.2.3. Optical Rotatory Dispersion (ORD) and Circular Dichroism (CD)

Under conditions where isoalloxazine-adenine interactions are indicated by fluorescence studies, the ORD of FAD exhibits a pronounced Cotton effect in the visible region,[37] a result consistent with the expected asymmetric perturbation. Dichroic bleaching experiments,[43] taken with other approaches, suggest that the oscillator vectors for the near-u.v.

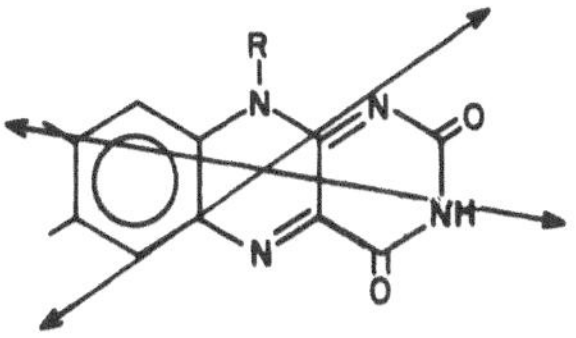

Fig. 3. Relative positions of the oscillator vectors giving rise to the near-u.v. and visible absorption bands in flavins. The double-headed arrows indicate that the absolute direction of the vectors is not determined (from Penzer et al.[107]).

(375 nm) and visible (447 nm) absorption bands are different. Molecular orbital treatments[67] suggest that visible wavelength transition is almost parallel to the long axis of the isoalloxazine nucleus, whereas the near-u.v. transition is at an angle of about 40° C to it (Fig. 3). Specific interactions (for example, substituents, binding to protein, and so forth) along one of the axes will exert predominant influence on the transition associated with that axis. Indeed, this information has been used to determine

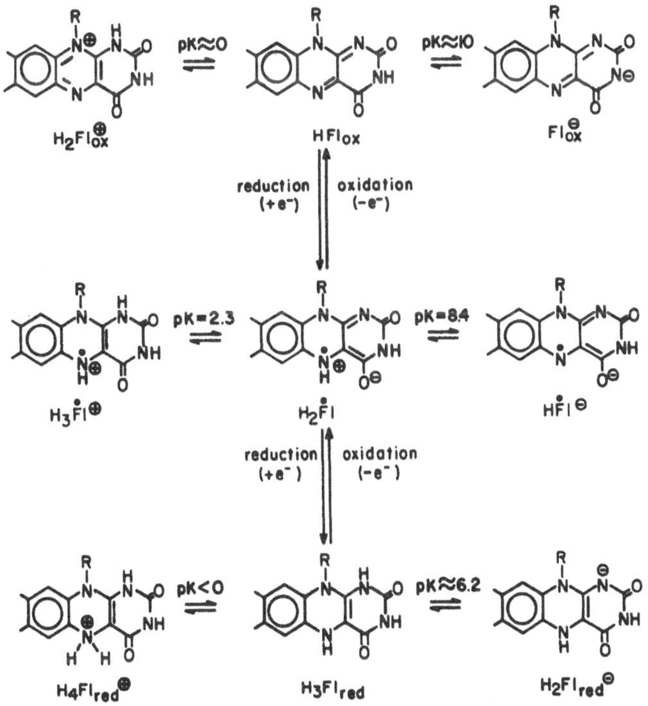

Fig. 4. Structural formulas of predominant tautomers of flavin redox species (after Müller et al.[96]; cf. Hemmerich and Spence[52]).

the relative orientations of prosthetic heme and FMN in cytochrome b_2.[113]

Circular dichroism promises to be an important tool in the study of flavoprotein chemistry. It has served as a probe of interactions at the flavin binding site.[29,30] Analyses of band positions and rotational strengths in the CD spectra of various redox forms of dehydrogenases and oxidases have revealed differences between these two classes of flavoproteins, but within each class the flavin environment was found to be similar (Fig. 4).

1.3. Electronic Spectroscopic Properties: Flavohydroquinones (Fl_{red})

Flavins are "bleached" upon reduction. This character of Fl_{red}, taken with its lack of fluorescence and sensitivity to oxygen, has tended to disguise the useful spectroscopic properties of the species. Recent studies at low temperature, however, do reveal useful fluorescent and optical information.[39a] Although the visible (450 nm) absorption band is decreased, a portion remains (Table I). There is also a significant shoulder at 390–400 nm $(\epsilon, 4000 \text{ M}^{-1} \text{ cm}^{-1})$, which Hemmerich and colleagues[27,50] state is due to noncoplanarity or folding along the N-5–N-10 axis in Fl_{red} compared with Fl_{ox}. This feature of trigonal nitrogen has been confirmed by X-ray crystallography.[62] The shoulder can be used with some confidence as an indication of the degree of noncoplanarity. Indeed, the influence of planarity on higher wavelength absorption is emphasized by the difference spectrum of $FADH_2$ and $FMNH_2$, in which isoalloxazine-adenine stacking in $FADH_2$ stabilizes the planar molecule.

From such spectra it has been concluded that $FADH^-$ is less planar than $FADH_2$. Substitution at N-5 and/or N-10 increases folding by steric factors and, in the cases of quarternary nitrogen derivatives, by electronic factors. 5,5-Disubstituted flavins including $FADH_3^+$ do not absorb above 330 nm; the u.v. spectra do, however, generate useful information about the symmetry of substitution at N-5. Moreover, 5,5-disubstituted and 4a,5-disubstituted flavins can be distinguished readily. 4a-Alkyl dihydroflavins are protonated at N-1, leading to a bathochromic shift of the near-u.v. band (*ca.* 360–390 nm), whereas N-5 alkyl flavins become protonated at N-5, producing a hypsochromic shift (*ca.* 340–305 nm; see Hemmerich,[50] p. 99).

1.4. Reactions of Flavoquinones

1.4.1. "Dark" Reactions

The reduction of Fl_{ox} is depicted classically as the combination of hydride addition and protonation. There is, however, no evidence to date that establishes this reaction sequence rather than alternative group transfer mechanism.

The hydride mechanism supposes that Fl_{ox} is reduced by nucleophilic attack by hydride with subsequent protonation, a process that would require initial polarization of the substrate X—H bond in the following manner:

$$Fl_{ox} + \overset{\delta^+}{X}{\underset{}{-}}\overset{\delta^-}{H} \rightarrow Fl^-_{red}\,H + X^+$$

Group transfer involves the nucleophilic attack of X^- with subsequent release of X^+ upon protonation or oxidation by oxygen. This process presumes initial polarization of the X—H bond in the opposite direction:

$$Fl_{ox} + \overset{\delta^-}{X}{\underset{}{-}}\overset{\delta^+}{H} \rightarrow Fl^-_{red}\,X + H^+$$

A series of elegant model reaction studies by Hemmerich and coworkers[48] demonstrate that the group-transfer mechanism simulates closely enzymatic dehydrogenations.

In either case, 1,5- and 4a,5-additions to Fl_{ox} are chemically feasible. The 1,5-reduction is thermodynamically reversible and follows the Nernst equation in polarographic studies. On the other hand, 4a,5-reduction is irreversible because of the slow cleavage of the C_{4a}—H(X) bond, as against disruption of the N—H bond in $1,5\text{-}H_2Fl_{red}$. There is some evidence for irreversible reduction in flavoproteins, a finding that casts some doubt on simple 1,5-reduction in biological reactions.[50] The stereochemistry of each of the two types of addition is distinct. Attack at C-4a would occur from above or below the plane of the ring, whereas nucleophilic addition to N-5 necessitates planar approach of the attacking species. Certain experiments shed light on the question of hydride *vs.* group transfer, as well as C-4a *vs.* N-5 addition. C-8,9 addition has also been described recently by Hemmerich *et al.*[49]

1.4.1A. BOROHYDRIDE REDUCTION. Borohydride reacts slowly with Fl_{ox}. The C-4 carbonyl is, however, slowly reduced to the corresponding alcohol. The finding that this well-established hydride reductant does not react readily with Fl_{ox} may be taken as some evidence against hydride transfer. Borohydride reduction does offer a means of modifying the flavin moiety of flavoproteins. Massey has found that reduction of the C-4 carbonyl of FAD in D-amino acid oxidase does not inhibit catalytic activity.[75,97]

1.4.1B. DITHIONITE REDUCTION. Dithionite interacts with flavin presumably through nucleophilic (SO_2^{-2} or $S_2O_4^{-2}$) substitution at N-5 (or C-4a). A two-electron mechanism is supported by the observation that the rate of comproportionation (see Section 1.4.1) of reduced and oxidized phytoflavin generates the blue semiquinone much faster than does dithionite reduction.[11] Furthermore, dithionite reduction of the semiquinone itself is slow.

1.4.1C. REACTIONS OF CARBANIONS, ENOLATE, AND OTHER ANIONS. Flavins carry out the dehydrogenation of dihydrophthalates; a carbanion-mediated reaction is suggested by the pH dependence of the reaction.[149,150] It was suggested that the dihydrophthalate carbanion transfers electrons to flavin without formation of a covalent intermediate, but other interpretations consistent with two-electron transfer can be envisaged. It has been noted that cyanide interacts with lumiflavin at pH 11 to generate a spectrum similar to that of Fl_{red}, a result that suggests nucleophilic addition. It is notable that a variety of carbanions and enolate anions in dimethylformamide reduce Fl_{ox}.[115] Recent work tends to rule out an N-5 covalent adduct in flavin-catalyzed reductions of carbonyls to carbinols.[115a]

Under alkaline conditions in dimethylformamide, the methyl esters of mandelic acid and phenylglycine are oxidized by flavin to the corresponding α-ketoacids.[14] Spectral data suggest additional oxygen-reversed reductions of flavins by 9-hydroxyfluorene and diethylaminomalonate. Since no spectral changes were seen with the methyl ester of phenylglycine, fluorene, and other selected substrates, the involvement of nucleophilic attack by a heteroatom substituent of substrate, as against carbanion attack, was favored:

$$\overset{H}{\underset{XH}{>\!C\!<}} \rightarrow \overset{H}{\underset{X^-}{>\!C\!<}} \overset{Fl_{ox}}{\rightarrow} \overset{H}{\underset{X\frown Fl_{red}}{>\!C\!\downarrow}} \rightarrow \;>\!C\!=\!X + Fl_{red}^-$$

A similar hypothesis has been proposed in the case of D-amino acid oxidase.[21]

1.4.1D. NADH. NADH reduces riboflavin in the absence of light.[123] A kinetic isotope effect (k_H / k_D) of 3.2 suggests a rate-determining character for C—H bond disruption. Dependence of the rate on ionic strength indicated a polar transition state ($C^- \ldots H^+$ or $C^+ \ldots H^-$). Hydride transfer was favored primarily on the basis of studies with four nonhomologous dihydronicotinamides. Although pyridine nucleotide-enzymatic reactions involve hydride transfers, there is no direct evidence for hydride transfer to Fl_{ox}. Data are consistent with the formation of a covalent pyridine nucleotide–flavin adduct.[50,76,77] A kinetically important complex of unknown nature between flavin and dihydronicotinamide has recently been observed.[16]

1.4.1E. MECHANISTIC STUDIES OF A FLAVOENZYME: D-AMINO ACID OXIDASE. A series of substituted phenylglycines have been studied as D-AAO substrates (100): Hammett plots showed that there was significant polarity in the rate-determining step and that electron-donating substituents decreased the reaction rate. Proton abstraction from the α-carbon of the substrate amino acid was proposed as involved in the rate determining step. More recent work (145) has shown that D-AAO can catalyze not only the oxidation of β-chloroalanine to form chloropyruvate, but also the nonoxidative elimination of HCl to give pyruvate. Under anerobic conditions, only pyruvate is obtained; intermediate ratios of [ClPyr]/[Pyr] are observed as a function of oxygen concentration. The rate of total ketoacid production is independent of $[O_2]$ suggesting a rate determining step independent of $[O_2]$. Kinetic isotope effects confirm that the α-CH bond is broken in the rate-determining step. An enzyme nucleophile presumably abstracts the α-proton regardless of the oxidation state of the flavin. When the amino acid cannot interact with flavin (fully reduced), this base catalyzes an E-2 type elimination. Data are consistent with a substrate heteroatom or carbanion adduct with flavin. Both studies are consistent with a two-electron transfer to the flavin and may relate to the inhibition of monoamine oxidase by 3-bromoallylamine.[112a]

1.4.2. Photoexcited Flavins

Many factors prompt presentation of a brief survey of flavin photochemistry. Certain photochemical reactions of flavins display striking analogy to enzymatic reactions. Although it is doubtful that they occur by the same mechanism, the photochemical processes do provide important model systems. Moreover, there is reason to suspect that the photoexcitation of flavins per se plays a role in certain biological

TABLE IV. *Photodegradation of Riboflavin (after Cairns and Metzler* [19])

		^{1}Fl*
Riboflavin	1. $h\nu$, anerobic 2. O_2	A. Lumichrome (16.8%) [a] B. 4′-ketoriboflavin ⎫ ^{3}Fl* ⎬ (17%) [a] C. 2′-ketoriboflavin ⎭ D. Formylmethylflavin (58%) [a] E. Unidentified minor products

[a] Percentages refer to relative yield after 50% photobleaching at pH 7.

systems—bacterial bioluminescence, the regulation of a wide variety of plant reactions, and possibly the mammalian visual apparatus. Finally, photochemical reactions have been used to advantage in modification of the flavin moiety of flavoproteins.

1.4.2A. INTRAMOLECULAR PHOTOREDUCTION (PHOTOLYSIS OF RIBOFLAVIN). In the absence of external reductant, the isoalloxazine portion of riboflavin undergoes extensive photoreduction with the ribityl side chain serving as electron donor. The photoproducts are oxidized spontaneously upon exposure to air. Many products of the overall reaction have been characterized, and some progress has been made with respect to the mechanism (Table IV [19]). Reactions A and B (Table IV) are rather insensitive to mM KI. This observation, taken with the finding that these pathways predominate at acidic pH, suggests intermediate involvement of a singlet state flavin (^{1}Fl*). The formation of lumichrome can be envisaged as a typical Norrish type II photoelimination with abstraction of "hydrogen" from the 2′-carbon as the crucial step. [82,83] Evidence for such a mechanism is based on the presence of a kinetic isotope effect with 2′-α-D flavin, but not with 2′-α-H, —OD flavin, [93] and the finding that flavins lacking a 2′-hydroxyl group still generate lumichrome upon photodegradation. [154] Reactions B and C seem likewise to involve α-"hydrogen" abstraction. [92] Reactions C and D probably involve the flavin triplet state (^{3}Fl*), since they are readily blocked by iodide (and low pH); the latter reaction may involve abstraction of hydrogen from the 2′-α-hydroxyl grouping.

1.4.2B. INTERMOLECULAR PHOTOREDUCTION. Flavins are reduced anerobically in the presence of light by a number of electron donors including amines, [18] amino acids, [106] NADH, [111] and dihydrophthalates. [149] Kinetic isotope effects indicate rate-determining disruption of a C—H bond in the electron donor, but do not distinguish between homolytic and heterolytic cleavage. Notably, semiquinone species are present transiently in photolysis of Fl_{ox} in the presence of EDTA and phenol.[131]

Hammett plots ($\rho = -1.1$) of the rates of photoreduction of substituted phenylglycines indicate that the flavin species is electrophilic, but there is little charge separation in the transition state.[106] Photoreductions are inhibited by low concentrations of collisional quenchers such as iodide and electron-rich compounds such as indoles and phenols under conditions where fluorescence ($^1F^*$) is not quenched. Estimates of the lifetime of the excited state indicate a minimum lifetime of 10^{-5} sec.[111] This would seem to rule out singlet flavin ($^1Fl^*$) as the reactive intermediate, since its lifetime is about 10^{-9} sec.[20,43] These results strongly suggest an electrophilic triplet state as the reactive flavin intermediate.

1.4.2c. Photoadditions to Fl_{ox}. α-Ketoacids[17,23] and β,γ-unsaturated carboxylic acids,[48,140] when irradiated with flavoquinones under anerobic conditions, undergo decarboxylation to yield stable acyl- or alkyldihydroflavins, respectively. Photoacylation with pyruvate yields two products: Fl_{red}, which is spontaneously reoxidized when exposed to oxygen, and 5-acetyl-Fl_{red}, which is reoxidized by oxygen only upon u.v. irradiation. Flavoproteins undergo a similar reaction[23]; the relative amounts of each photoproduct depends on the flavoprotein.

The photoalkylation of Fl_{ox} by phenylacetate yields 5-benzyl-Fl_{red} and 4a-benzyl-Fl_{red}; only the former is oxidized spontaneously by oxygen. Similar photoalkylation of xanthine oxidase does occur, with benzylation of FAD and inactivation of catalytic activity, 60% of which is recovered by irradiation in the presence of oxygen.[64]

Knappc and Hemmerich[63] have found that Fl_{ox} is photoalkylated by thiolane (Fig. 5) to give 5-thiolyl-Fl in high yield. The product exhibits two pK's, 7.4 (N-1) and 3.4 (N-5). There are pH optima for auto-oxidation at about 8 and 4. The relative planar character of species "A" (N-5 is sp²) may be responsible for the increased reactivity at pH 4 relative to $HFl_{red}X$. No stable radicals are detected due to the bulkiness of the thiolyl substituent, which does not readily achieve coplanarity. There is now evidence for an intermediate adduct in the EDTA-mediated photoreduction of flavins.[33a]

The potential significance of these model systems with respect to flavoenzyme mechanisms is apparent. For example, reduction-oxidation by group transfer is clearly feasible. Secondly, the mesoionic intermediate ("A," Fig. 5) could relate to the color observed in certain flavoenzyme-substrate complexes. Finally, the oxidation of $HFl_{red}X$ is slow with oxygen, but is rapid with one-electron acceptors [Fe $(CN)_6^{-3}$; Ce^{+4}],

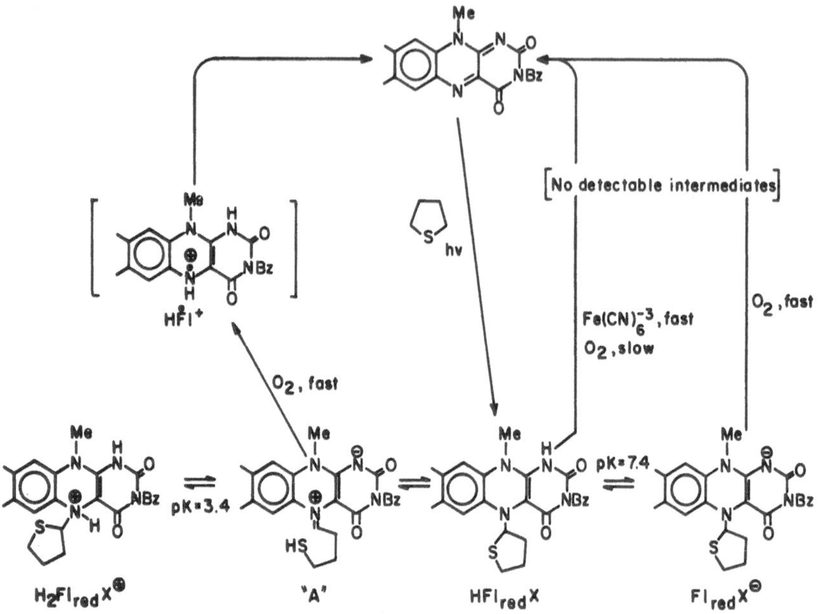

Fig. 5. Formation and oxidation of 3-ϕCH$_2$-5-(2-thiolyl)-1,5-dihydroflavin (HFl$_{red}$X) (from Knappe and Hemmerich[63]).

a characteristic of flavoprotein dehydrogenases. On the other hand, the rapid reaction of "A" with oxygen is reminiscent of flavoprotein oxidases.[77] One could speculate that the redox activity of the flavoprotein is regulated by protein-mediated stabilization of intermediates analogous to HFl$_{red}$S or "A."

1.4.2D. Aerobic Photoreductions. Flavins catalyze the aerobic photo-oxidation of a number of compounds. This can be accomplished via two routes: reversible photoreduction of Fl$_{ox}$ and photosensitization. In photosensitized reactions, triplet flavin transfers electronic energy to molecular oxygen to give singlet oxygen, a powerful oxidant. This route has been implicated in flavin-sensitized photo-oxidation of purines, aromatic amines, and phenols.[107] A simple technique has recently been described to ascertain the involvement of singlet oxygen in rate-determining steps.[91]

1.4.3. Oxidation of Flavohydroquinones

Kinetic studies show the reoxidation of free Fl$_{red}$ by oxygen is complicated.[40,77] From spectrophotometric studies, Fl$_{red}$ is shown to react directly with oxygen. Moreover, a $Fl_{red}\text{-}O_2$ compound(s) is suggested. Superoxide dismutase (erythrocuprein) dramatically slows down the oxidation suggesting that the superoxide anion (O_2^-) is produced in the reaction and plays a major role in subsequent oxidation (steps 5 and/or 6 below). The following reactions may be kinetically important in Fl_{red} oxidation:

1. $Fl_{red} \rightleftharpoons Fl_{red}\text{-}O_2$
2. $Fl_{red}\text{-}O_2 \rightarrow Fl\,\dot{H} + H^+ + O_2^-$
3. $2\,Fl\dot{H} \rightleftharpoons Fl_{ox} + Fl_{red}$
4. $(Fl\dot{H} + O_2 \rightarrow Fl_{ox}\,O_2^- + H^+)$
5. $Fl\dot{H} + O_2^- - H^+ \rightarrow Fl_{ox} + H_2O_2$
6. $Fl_{red} + O_2^- + H^+ \rightarrow Fl\dot{H} + H_2O_2$
7. $2\,O_2^- + 2H^+ \rightleftharpoons O_2 + H_2O_2$ (dismutation)

The nature of the oxygen-Fl_{red} adduct is unknown at present. Both 1a- and 4a-perhydroxyflavin(s) have been suggested.[48,49,51,77] It is suggested that the $Fl_{red}\text{-}O_2$ compound(s) may then decompose to H_2O_2, HO_2^- (O_2^- at pH 7), HO, and HO^+. The primary differences between the flavorprotein oxygenases, dehydrogenases, and hydroxylases may relate to the favored decomposition pathway. Oxidases yield H_2O_2 directly, dehydrogenases might yield O_2^- and the semiquinone, while the hydroxylases may react preferentially to give HO^+ or, possibly, $HO\cdot$ or HO_2^-, all of which are highly reactive hydroxylation agents.

As pointed out earlier in this chapter, free flavohydroquinone exists normally in a nonplanar conformation. Hemmerich[48,51] suggests that only the flattened Fl_{red} reacts vigorously with oxygen and that different classes of flavoproteins may preferentially stabilize different conformations of Fl_{red}.

1.4.3. Reactions of Flavin Semiquinones

Rate constants for disproportionation of flavin radicals have been studied by flash photolysis techniques.[132] Disproportionation designates the interaction between two radical moieties to yield oxidized and reduced species; comproportionation designates the reverse process. The following order of disproportionation rate constants was obtained: lumiflavin> FMN> FAD and neutral radicals> anionic radicals. Disproportionation occurs only very slowly in flavoproteins.[31]

$$2\,Fl\dot{H} \quad \underset{\text{Comproportionation}}{\overset{\text{Disproportionation}}{\rightleftarrows}} \quad Fl_{ox} + Fl_{red}$$

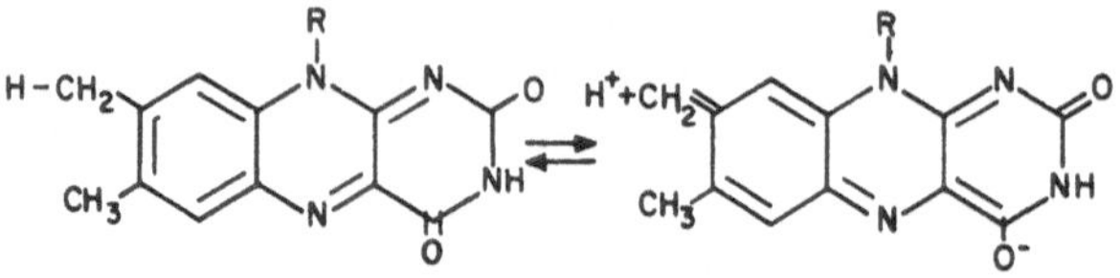

Fig. 6. Tautomeric form contributing to the reactivity of the C-8 methyl in flavins.

Neutral flavin radicals are oxidized by oxygen at a rate 10^4 times slower than the anionic forms.[132] The pK values for the neutral to anionic species are in the order FAD> FMN> riboflavin, lumiflavin. The rate of ferricyanide oxidation is essentially independent of pH.

1.4.3A. ELECTRON PAIR SPLITTING AND INTERFLAVIN CONTACT IN FLAVOPROTEINS. Flavin accepts redox equivalents as an electron pair plus a proton ("hydride" equivalent). Since subsequent electron acceptors in the electron transport chain are one-electron acceptors (Fe^{+++}/Fe^{++}), there may be a mechanism to "split" the electron pair at the same potential for transfer to cytochrome. Such splitting can occur if Fl_{red} comproportionated with another redox active group (X_{ox}) of equal potential to give two radicals, FlH and XH. If the X group is another flavin, then there may be interflavin contact either between flavin moieties within the same flavoprotein or between two flavoproteins intermolecularly.[51]

1.4.4. Reactivity of the C-8 Methyl Group

The C-8 methyl group of Fl_{ox} exhibits significant reactivity, presumably as the result of forms such as II (Fig. 6). Indeed, additional products are formed with aldehydes.[47] Notably, flavoproteins bearing covalently bound flavin are linked via the C-8 methyl group (see below).

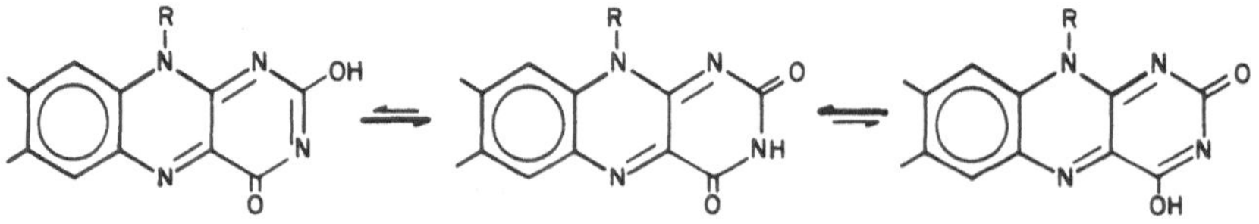

Fig. 7. Carboximide–iminol tautomeric forms of Fl_{ox}. The carboximide form is strongly favored at pH 7.

1.4.5. Carboximide-Iminol Tautomerization

The tautomerization of flavins is outlined in Fig. 7. Data on the formation and hydrolysis of iminol esters indicate a sizable increase in energy content of the iminol form coincident with the oxidation of Fl_{red}.[27] Iminol forms predominate in the flavosemiquinone species.

1.5. Flavin-Metal Interactions

1.5.1. Flavin Radical-Metal Chelates

Although there is great similarity between the strong chelator, 8-hydroxyquinoline, and tautomeric forms of flavins[1], fully oxidized or reduced flavins exhibit little capacity for this type of chelation.[52] The following reasons have been suggested: (a) for Fl_{ox}, the low basicity at N-5 and the limited concentration of iminol-form; and (b) for Fl_{red}, N-5 is also a poor σ electron donor at physiological pH, although there is significant iminol form. When metal ions with empty d-orbitals are added to a solution of half-reduced flavin at pH 7, the equilibrium is shifted toward flavin comproportionation because the metal forms a stable chelate with the flavin semiquinone.[94,95] Theoretical treatment[33] coupled with elegant ESR analyses by Ehrenberg and associates[32] reveals that electron spin from the radical is delocalized to the metal ion, which is coordinated to N-5. Partial double-bond character indicates back donation to the flavin via d-π overlap. The structure proposed for $H\dot{F}lZn^+$ is depicted in Fig. 8.

1.5.2. Flavoquinone-Metal Ion Charge Transfer Complexes

Selective affinity is exhibited by Fl_{ox} for metal species with filled d-orbitals that are capable of donating electrons to the lowest unoccupied π-orbital of HFl_{ox}. Only strong donor metals form reasonably stable charge transfer complexes. The spectra of such complexes exhibit broad red-brown absorption consistent with the d-π delocalization of charge transfer chelates.

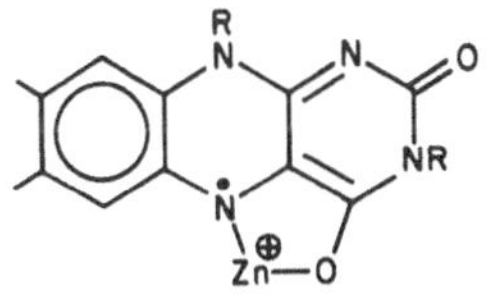

Fig. 8. Flavin radical-zinc (II) chelate (from Ehrenberg[32]).

1.52A. POSSIBILITY OF d-π "SANDWICH" OR FERROCENELIKE FLAVIN METAL INTERACTION. Although metal-flavin charge transfer complexes involving σ bonds between ligands are reasonably well described, the possibility of d-π sandwich-type interactions has not been excluded. Recent studies show that ferricyanide reacts with both the neutral and anionic radical at essentially the same rate, thus independently of the state of protonation of N-5.[132] These results suggest the possibility that ferricyanide might abstract an electron from the π-system of the aromatic (e.g., benzene) ring of the flavin via d-π overlap in a manner analogous to ferrocene systems. Indeed, ESR and MO studies have indicated appreciable unpaired spin density in the benzene ring of the isoalloxazine nucleus.[33,117]

1.5.2B. METALLOFLAVOPROTEINS. No flavin-metal chelate has yet been documented in proteins. Nonetheless, the finding that electron spin resonance relaxation occurs through the metal ligand does suggest flavin-metal interaction in metalloflavoproteins.[10] Interesting model reactions suggest an electron transfer between molybdenum and flavin mediated by cysteine-sulfhydrate.[66a]

2. EFFECTS OF FLAVIN COFACTORS ON NONPRIMARY PROTEIN STRUCTURE

2.1. General Considerations

The factors responsible for the generation of proteins with biologically active configurations are not simple even in the case of proteins without prosthetic groups or cofactors. With ribonuclease, there is evidence that the primary structure itself is the primary determinant.[3,151] With insulin, the primary sequence of a larger precursor protein seems most important for the orientation of stabilizing disulfide bonds.[120] With flavoproteins, it seems likely that the flavin cofactor itself, aside from functioning in an oxidation-reduction capacity, has significant influence on the achievement of an active configuration. Indeed, there do exist obligate flavoenzymes in which the direct catalytic participation of flavin is doubtful.[44] Nonetheless, even if one excludes from discussion those enzymes linked covalently with flavin, generalizations with respect to the effects of flavin cofactors on protein structure prove difficult.

The ease with which the flavin cofactor is separated from the protein component varies considerably among the flavoenzymes. The means by which the apoprotein is prepared could, per se, influence protein configuration and thus influence conclusions drawn from studies of reconstitution. For example, the apoprotein of NADH-dehydrogenase from beef heart can be obtained by mere dialysis against 20 mM phosphate buffer, pH 7.5, or by repeated precipitation with neutral ammonium sulfate[71]; the apoprotein of glycolic acid oxidase from spinach leaves has been prepared by treatment with neutral ammonium sulfate[155]; and D-amino acid oxidase from pig kidney dissociates into apoenzyme and FAD merely on dilution.[25] Other flavoproteins have required fairly drastic procedures for resolution: for example, flavodoxin with acidified potassium bromide[80,81]; D-amino acid oxidase with acidified ammonium sulfate[99] or neutral potassium bromide[74]; triphosphopyridine nucleotide-cytochrome c reductase,[55] glutathione reductase,[119] and glucose oxidase,[125] with acidified ammonium sulfate; microsomal cytochrome b$_5$ reductase[121] and glyoxylate carboligase[44] with acidified potassium bromide–ammonium sulfate; dihydroorotate dehydrogenase with methanol–ammonium sulfate[2]; xanthine oxidase with high concentrations of calcium chloride[12,65] or potassium iodide and reduced enzyme[112]; and *Azotobacter* free-radical flavoprotein with 3% trichloroacetic acid.[54]

In this volume, major consideration is given to the biological aspects of the flavin cofactors. As such, we must ask whether conclusions drawn with respect to the stability, conformation, and other properties of an apoprotein prepared by such methods are applicable to the newly synthesized apoenzyme as it leaves the template, or to the holoenzyme dissociating spontaneously within the cell. Although it seems likely that many experiments will prove relevant in this regard, the necessary caution is exemplified by the following quotation from Strittmatter[121] in discussing microsomal cytochrome b$_5$ reductase:

> . . . immediately after dissolving the protein precipitate [apoenzyme] after acid ammonium sulfate precipitation, the activity is low in the presence of FAD and gradually increases to a maximal level after 30 to 60 minutes of incubation at 0° in the absence of FAD. This suggests that during resolution at least a part of the apoprotein undergoes an apparent reversible alteration in structure to a form which cannot recombine with FAD to yield the original reductase structure. During the incubation the protein changes to a form which combines with FAD to yield an active enzyme. The apoenzyme is also more unstable immediately after acid precipitation.

Notwithstanding these considerations, it is noteworthy that the apoproteins derived from flavoenzymes exhibit marked differences among themselves in stability. The apoproteins derived from glycolic acid oxidase, soluble NADH dehydrogenase, and the *Azotobacter* free-radical flavoprotein are quite stable (references above), whereas the apoprotein from glyoxylate carboligase is similarly labile.[44] Most apoproteins exhibit a varying degree of lability compared to the holoenzyme—for example, D-amino acid oxidase, microsomal cytochrome b_5 reductase, glutathione reductase, glucose oxidase, and flavodoxin (references above). It may be noted that microsomal cytochrome b_5 reductase apoprotein becomes more labile at room temperature than when frozen,[121] whereas apoflavodoxin is less stable at $-20°C$ than at $0°C$.[80]

The process of reconstitution of holoenzyme from apoprotein and flavin has been studied in detail with respect to a limited number of flavoenzymes. In different cases, changes in secondary, tertiary, and/or quaternary protein structure have been observed. Various parameters of reconstitution have obeyed bimolecular kinetic equations, whereas others, with specific enzymes, have exhibited rate-limiting unimolecular conformational changes. At times, flavin analogs have substituted for, or inhibited, the binding of native cofactor in reconstitution. Indeed, with certain enzymes, the state of oxidation of the flavin cofactor has been found to influence protein structure. Finally, it is now apparent that the return of any single parameter on reconstitution—for example, catalytic activity—may not signify return to the native configuration of the enzyme-protein. Many of these conclusions seem best presented by a brief discussion of studies with glucose oxidase, lipoamide dehydrogenase, D-amino acid oxidase, flavodoxin, and glutathione reductase.

2.2. Specific Flavoproteins

2.2.1. Glucose Oxidase

The studies of Swoboda[125,126] with glucose oxidase from *Aspergillus niger* demonstrate many aspects of these considerations, as well as the techniques available for their exploration. The native oxidase contains

TABLE V. *Stability of Native Holoenzyme, Reconstituted Holoenzyme, and Apoenzyme of Glucose Oxidase (Modified from Swoboda[125])*

Experiment	Protein sample	Activity (%)
Heat denaturation	Native holoenzyme	98
50°C, 10 min	Apoenzyme	20
	Reconstituted holoenzyme	78
Pronase-P digestion	Native holoenzyme	98
1%, 0°C, 1.5 hr	Apoenzyme	21
	Reconstituted holoenzyme	100

TABLE VI. *Physical Constants Related to the Size and Shape of Glucose Oxidase Molecules (Modified from Swoboda*[125]*)*

Protein sample	Molecular weight (g)	Intrinsic viscosity (ml/g)	Sedimentation coefficient (S)	Molar frictional coefficient
Native holoen-zyme	153,000	4.2	8.0	1.2
Apoenzyme	153,000	10.3	Major component (80%) 4.5	2.2
			Minor component (20%) 8.0	1.2

two mole-equivalents of tightly, yet not covalently, bound FAD (dissociation constant less than 10^{-10} M); the FAD is not removed by dialysis at neutral pH. The apoenzyme has been prepared by a modification of the acidified-ammonium sulfate procedure of Warburg and Christian.[148] When stored for several weeks at 0°C, pH 6.1, and protein concentration of 10 mg/ml, the apoenzyme, upon treatment with excess FAD, reacquires 75% of its original activity. The FAD:apoenzyme stoichiometry is that which could be expected if 75% of the apoenzyme retained the capacity to be reactivated. The reconstituted holoenzyme, like the native oxidase, does not release FAD upon dialysis.

The relative lability of the apoenzyme, as against the native and reconstituted holoenzyme, to heat and pronase treatment is presented in Table V. The biophysical data presented in Table VI suggest that although the molecular weights of the native holoenzyme and apoenzyme are identical the native enzyme exists in a compact, nearly spherical form; whereas the major component of the apoenzyme is a loose, flexible coil. The reconstituted holoenzyme exists in the native configuration, at least by these criteria. The state of oxidation of flavin, even in the native holoenzyme, influences stability (Table VII), since the reduced holoenzyme is most resistant to heat.

Many facets of the process of recombination of apoenzyme and

TABLE VII. *Stability of Glucose Oxidase in Its Oxidized and Reduced Forms (Modified from Swoboda*[126]*)*

Sample	Activity (%), after 75°C, 3 min
Untreated enzyme	100
Heated oxidized enzyme	4
Heated enzyme reduced by glucose	36
Heated enzyme reduced by dithionite	33

FAD have been examined by Swoboda[125] in studies of the rates of recovery of enzymic activity, quenching of flavin fluorescence, enhancement of FAD absorbance, polarization of fluorescence, and the effect of cofactor analogs. In summary, it seems that the following series of reactions represent the minimum number of steps involved in the reconstitution of holoenzyme:

$$P_2 \overset{1}{\underset{}{\rightleftharpoons}} P_1$$

$$P_1 + FAD \overset{2}{\rightleftharpoons} P_1 - FAD \overset{3}{\rightarrow} P_1^1 - FAD \overset{4}{\rightarrow} P_2 - FAD$$

$$(P_2 + FAD \overset{5}{\rightarrow} P_2 - FAD)$$

where P_2 is apoenzyme in a configuration similar to or identical with native holoenzyme, and P_1 is the major component in the absence of FAD, the loose, flexible coil with increased lability. P_1^1 represents one of possibly many intermediate protein conformations.

Ultracentrifugation studies at varying protein concentrations provide evidence for the slow interconvertibility of P_1 and P_2. The rate of recovery of enzymatic activity depends on FAD concentration only when the concentration of FAD is low relative to apoenzyme. With limiting FAD, the rate of recovery of activity can be described by a second-order rate constant of $6.1 \cdot 10^6 \ M^{-1} \ min^{-1}$ (presumably reactions 2 and 5). In this case, the primary bimolecular reaction of apoenzyme and FAD is rate-limiting. The generally rapid reaction has been demonstrated also by the rapid increase in polarization of fluorescence of the FAD moiety upon admixture of limiting amounts of FAD with apoenzyme. The bimolecular event precedes a series of unimolecular reactions as measured by enhancement of FAD absorbance ($0.8 \ min^{-1}$, reaction 3) and quenching of the fluorescence of the dimethylisoalloxazine moiety ($0.18 \ min^{-1}$, reaction 4). Under conditions where FAD is four to five times more concentrated than apoenzyme, the rate of recovery of enzymatic activity is independent of [FAD] and exhibits an overall unimolecular rate constant of $0.16 \ min^{-1}$, similar to the quenching of fluorescence in reaction 4.

It should be noted that ADP and certain other analogs, but not riboflavin or FMN, can inhibit the reactivation of apoenzyme by FAD.[126] Indeed, ADP possesses the capacity to induce configuration alterations in the apoenzyme in the direction of reacquisition of the native, compact, nearly spherical form. If FAD is added before ADP, reconstitution occurs and prevents inhibition by ADP; if ADP is added before FAD, reactivation is prevented. If both are added simultaneously, a slower reactivation occurs, indicating that the initial primary bimolecular reaction between apoenzyme and ADP is reversible:

$$P_1 + ADP \rightleftharpoons P_1 - ADP \rightarrow P_2 - ADP$$

$$(P_2 + ADP \rightleftharpoons P_2 - ADP)$$

This overall process can be summarized by the following quotation from Swoboda[126]:

> When FAD is reacted with apoenzyme there is a rapid increase in polarization without much change in the intensity of flavin fluorescence. Subsequently the fluorescence is slowly quenched in a unimolecular reaction with approximately the same rate constant as that of the regeneration of enzyme activity. These changes can be explained in terms of the following mechanism. The initial polarization change is probably associated with the binding of FAD *via* its adenine, phosphate and ribose residues. If the protein does not initially have the right conformation, the dimethylisoalloxazine residue is left unattached until a unimolecular change in conformation allows it to interact with the protein. The interaction quenches the flavin fluorescence and is a compulsory step in the regeneration of enzyme activity.

2.2.2. Lipoamide Dehydrogenase

Lipoamide dehydrogenase from pig heart, like glucose oxidase, is tightly, but not covalently, linked to FAD; the cofactor is not removed by dialysis, and indeed it is only recently that a quantitatively successful preparation of the apoenzyme has been achieved.[57] The apoenzyme, prepared by a modification of the potassium bromide procedure of Strittmatter[121] is said by Kalse and Veeger[57] to be ". . . rather labile and easily denatures on freezing and thawing or on being kept at room temperature for a prolonged period." Aside from experiments similar to those described above with respect to glucose oxidase, the monomer–dimer interrelationship and diaphorase activity of lipoamide dehydrogenase provide the parameters that shed additional light on the potential effects of FAD on protein structure.

The apoenzyme of lipoamide dehydrogenase binds FAD in the ratio of 1 mol of cofactor/48,000 g protein in reversible fashion initially. With the use of two parameters—the stimulation of 2,6-dichlorophenol-indophenol diaphorase activity and the polarization of fluorescence—it was determined that this interaction between FAD and apoenzyme, itself complex with involvement of more than one protein conformation, exhibits a ΔH of -8300 cal/mol and a ΔS of -4 esu.[57] When constitution of the enzyme is carried out at 5°C, marked stimulation

(20 times greater than original holoenzyme) of diaphorase activity is observed, without return of lipoamide dehydrogenase activity. At 20°C there is a slow return of lipoamide dehydrogenase activity with slower loss of diaphorase activity. This conversion exhibits activation energy of 21,000 cal/mol, a second-order rate constant with respect to protein concentration and a small decline in the intensity of FAD fluorescence. These changes appear to be the result of a temperature-dependent dimerization of the reconstituted monomeric holoenzyme.[136,137]

After purification of the reconstituted lipoamide dehydrogenase, it exhibits the same heat stability and spectral and catalytic properties as the native holoenzyme. Although riboflavin and FMN do not combine with apoenzyme, other cofactor analogs do, with return of some catalytic activity.[136] It is pertinent to note that upon freezing and thawing, the diluted native holoenzyme, at low ionic strength, exhibits increased diaphorase activity, decreased lipoamide dehydrogenase activity, and a dissociable FAD (dissociation constant, 2 μM). These changes can be reversed by incubation of the enzyme at 20°C.[134] It is most significant to note that recovery of lipoamide dehydrogenase activity after dissociation at low protein concentration precedes recovery of original ORD, CD, and fluorescence properties; diaphorase activity; and sensitivity to inhibition by FMN.[135] In another vein—namely, the effect of protein on FAD conformation—Dekok *et al.*[22] have concluded that the complex between isoalloxazine and adenine nuclei is broken upon binding of FAD to lipoamide dehydrogenase; the fluorescence quenching is presumably due to interaction of isoalloxazine with protein.

2.2.3. D-Amino Acid Oxidase

The binding of FAD to D-amino acid oxidase is less tight than in the case of either glucose oxidase or lipoamide dehydrogenase. Under most assay conditions the binding seems to be freely reversible, and standard kinetic experiments generate an apparent K_m for FAD of about 0.1 μM.[139] Indeed, at low protein concentrations there is spontaneous dissociation of the native holoenzyme into FAD and apoenzyme.[25,35] At 25°C and pH 8.5 the rate constant for dissociation is 0.45 min^{-1} and for association $1.8 \cdot 10^6$ M^{-1}min^{-1}, for a deduced equilibrium constant of 0.25 μM. Massey and Curti[74] have prepared the apoenzyme in close to 100% yield by dialysis of the native holoenzyme against 1 M potassium bromide and 3 mM EDTA at pH 8.3. The apoprotein is relatively stable for weeks at 0°C and for months at −20°C. Although the yield is less, an apparently identical apoprotein can be prepared by the acidified ammonium sulfate procedure.

Massey and Curti[74] were able to separate the reconstitution process into at least two stages—a rapid binding of FAD and slower secondary conformational changes that correlate the appearance of catalytic activity with studies of the rates of enhancement of FAD absorbance at 493 mμ, the decrease in FAD fluorescence, and the decrease in protein fluorescence. The recovery of oxidase activity exhibited a rate constant of 0.044 min^{-1} at 1.4°C, a value that compares favorably with the enhancement of FAD absorbance at 493 nm (0.035 min^{-1} at 1.4°C). Adenine analogs such as AMP, ADP, and ADP-ribose inhibit the enzyme by competition with FAD, whereas isoalloxazine analogs inhibit by photoinactivation.[35] The effects of adenosine-replaced analogs of FAD had already been reported by McCormick et al.[87] The detailed studies of Yagi and collaborators[66] on the biophysical properties of the apoenzyme, holoenzyme, and benzoate complex provide additional important data bearing on the influence of cofactor upon protein structure.

The ready dissociation of FAD from the native holoenzyme provides, moreover, an interesting system in which the effects of FAD on protein structure can be studied without resorting to preparation of apoenzyme. With use of sulfhydryl-characterizing reagents, Hellerman et al.[46] described an interesting phenomenon now found applicable to other enzymes as well[21]:

> The evaluation of the catalytic activity of crystallized D-amino acid oxidase with respect to the action of any one of a variety of sulfhydryl-binding reagents provides in each case a linear correlation between the amount of inhibitor and the extent of inhibition. For individual enzyme molecules, inhibition is an all-or-none event. The observed activity of the flavoenzyme, at every stage of a titration, reflects accurately the relative amounts of fully active and inactive enzyme molecules present; the quantity of inactive enzyme is directly proportional to the amount of added inhibitor. The residual active enzyme, exhibiting an unaltered specific activity, remains soluble, but the inactive molecules precipitate spontaneously, thereby providing the means for a quantitative separation of the two fractions.

The most likely explanation of these phenomena relates to an increased exposure of sulfhydryl groups in the apoprotein.[25,46] The spontaneous equilibrium between holoenzyme and apoenzyme can be assumed to shift gradually toward apoenzyme as that fraction is depleted by reaction with sulfhydryl-characterizing reagent, thus allowing for an all-or-none inhibition and nonuniform distribution of inhibitor. It is emphasized, in light of earlier discussion, that these experiments do not necessarily suggest direct contact between enzyme–sulfhydryl and flavin but could merely indicate a more or less extensive conformational change in the apoprotein. Indeed, the presence of excess FAD does alter reactivity of the protein with respect to other functional group reagents—for example, 2,4,6-trinitrobenzenesulfonate.[152]

TABLE VIII. *Effect of Conditions of Incubation on Inhibition of* D-*Amino Acid Oxidase by Silver Nitrate (from Hellerman et al.* [46])

		AgNO₃ required for complete inhibition, moles/10⁵ g protein			
Conditions of incubation	Gas phase	°C = 0	23	38	46
D-Amino acid oxidase	Air	5.8	5.6	5.8	7.8
+FAD	Air		6.1	6.3	
+FAD	Oxygen			6.2	
+FAD	Nitrogen			6.3	
+FAD + D-alanine	Air	5.9	6.0	8.5	9.3
+FAD + D-alanine	Oxygen	5.9	7.0	9.3	9.3
+FAD + D-alanine	Nitrogen	6.8	7.4	9.7	11.7

Although the oxidase contains six sulfhydryl groups per mole of monomer (about 50,000 g), only three thiols react with inhibitor—for example, silver ion. This fraction of reactive thiol varies as a function of the presence of excess FAD, the state of oxidation of FAD, and the temperature (Table VIII). Indeed, the sensitivity of the enzyme to inhibition by sulfhydryl-characterizing reagents of varying reactivity is dramatically a function of the aforementioned conditions (Table IX). Compare cytochrome b_5 reductase.[122]

2.2.4. Flavodoxin

Mayhew[80,81] has successfully prepared stable apoproteins from flavodoxins from *Peptostreptococcus elsdenii, C. pasteurianum,* and *Clostridium* MP by dialysis against 2 M potassium bromide at pH 3.9. Reconstitution of the holoenzyme with FMN yields a complex with "the same light absorption and fluorescence properties, catalytic activity, and oxidation-reduction behavior as the native flavodoxin." The dissociation constant at pH 6.55 and 20°C was assessed to be 4.26×10^{-10} M. Of interest, particularly with respect to comparisons with glucose oxidase, lipoamide dehydrogenase, and D-amino acid oxidase, is the observation that reconstitution, as evaluated by the quenching of flavin fluorescence, can be characterized by a second-order rate constant of 2.6×10^5 M^{-1}sec^{-1}. Additional first-order changes were not observed. In addition, iso-FMN and 3,4-dihydro-FMN formed tight complexes with apoflavodoxin, the former possessing catalytic activity. Ludwig et al.[70] have initiated interesting crystallographic studies with flavodoxin. "The results suggest that there may be structural differences between the oxidized and semiquinone forms of the protein; on the other hand,

TABLE IX. Effect of Incubation Conditions on Degree of Inhibition Produced by Various Reagents Acting for 30 min (from Hellerman et al.[46])

Conditions of incubation	Gas phase	Percentage of residual enzymatic activity					
		Silver nitrate, 10^{-6} M	γ-(p-arsenoso phenyl)-n-butyrate, 10^{-3} M	Mercuric acetate, 10^{-4} M	p-chloromer-curibenzoate, 10^{-4} M	Cadmium chloride, 10^{-4} M	Sodium arsenite, 3×10^{-3} M
D-Amino acid oxidase	Air	0	0	0	0	0	91
+D-alanine	Air	0		0	0	30	98
+FAD	Air	0	0	0	0	97	95
+FAD + D-alanine	Oxygen	0	0	0	0	95	92
+FAD + D-alanine	Air	0	0	25	39	98	99
+FAD + D-alanine	Nitrogen	0	0	81	92	105	99

structural changes accompanying reduction of the semiquinone appear to be small.''

2.2.5. Glutathione Reductase

The biological significance that can be related to the interaction between apoenzyme and flavin cofactor is exemplified by the work of Staal *et al.*[118] with erythrocyte glutathione reductase (see Chapter 9). Glutathione reductase was purified extensively from the erythrocytes of a patient with nonspherocytic hemolytic anemia related to glutathione reductase deficiency. Although the apparent K_m values for GSSG and NADPH differed only slightly from those exhibited by enzyme prepared from normal human erythrocytes, the enzyme from diseased erythrocytes was significantly more heat-labile. This lability was eliminated by the addition of 10 μM FAD. After preparation of the apoenzyme by the acid–ammonium sulfate procedure, the normal and abnormal enzymes exhibited apparent K_m values for FAD of 0.55 μM and 3.7 μM, respectively. The reduced affinity for FAD by the abnormal reductase is supported by the observation that FMN inhibits the abnormal holoenzyme, whereas the normal reductase exhibits no loss of activity at identical FMN concentrations. It can be hypothesized that the decreased stability of abnormal glutathione reductase relates to the decreased affinity for FAD. If this proposal proves correct, it provides an exciting correlation between the *in vitro* and *in vivo* situation. Indeed, as a consequence of *in vitro* studies, Staal *et al.*[118] state ". . . we administered a flavin preparation as a 'therapeutic' agent to the patient (10 mg FMN/day). After a few weeks the enzyme activity had increased to an almost normal level. When this treatment was stopped, the glutathione reductase activity started to decline again.''

2.3. Summary

The effects of flavin cofactor binding on nonprimary protein structure are complex and diverse. Generally, however, union with flavin tends to stabilize the enzyme-protein with respect to thermal, proteolytic, and functional-group reagent inactivation. The quantitative significance of the stabilization varies considerably from enzyme to enzyme. Attention must be directed toward the means by which apoenzyme is prepared; appropriate caution is required in the extension of *in vitro* data to *in vivo* speculation.

3. BINDING OF FLAVIN COFACTORS

3.1. General Considerations

It is apparent from the foregoing discussion that FMN and FAD are not bound in uniform fashion to the protein component of the various flavoproteins. Although affixation is occasionally covalent, as in the cases of succinate dehydrogenase[60] and monoamine oxidase,[59] most flavoproteins dissociate under conditions that do not disrupt covalent bonds. Many noncovalently linked flavoproteins exhibit apparent dissociation constants in the range of 10^{-10} to 10^{-8} M. The apparent dissociation constant of D-amino acid oxidase, one of the more readily dissociable flavoenzymes, is about 2.5×10^{-7} M; at the other extreme, the dissociation of certain flavoproteins is not detectable under physiological conditions. A recent tabulation of some flavoproteins and their characteristics is available.[24] In each case it seems reasonable to conclude that the flavin cofactor interacts with protein at multiple sites, the natures of which have remained somewhat elusive. Much of the difficulty can be attributed to the marked heterogeneity amongst the flavoproteins. Indeed, for example, the degree of quenching of flavin fluorescence varies considerably from system to system. Moreover, some flavoenzymes exhibit marked specificity for FMN or FAD; others bind and function with either, as well as with a variety of nonphysiological analogs.

3.2. Covalent Binding

The early studies of Kearney and Singer,[60] Wang *et al.*,[146] and other revealed that FAD was covalently affixed to the mammalian succinate dehydrogenase-protein. Since then, particularly within the last few years, much progress has been made with respect to elucidation of the structural characteristics of this bonding. The isolation of flavin-peptides obtained after the proteolytic digestion of succinate

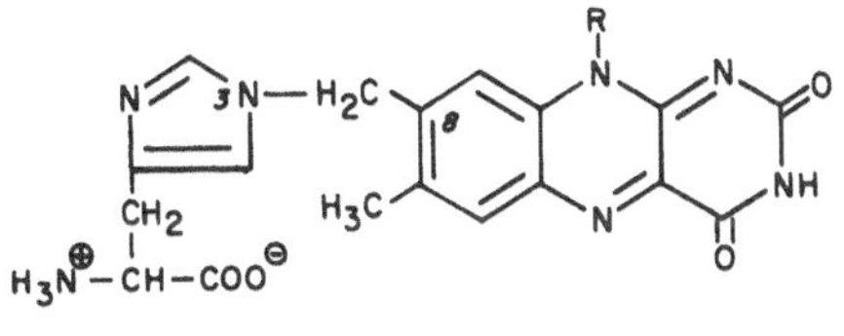

Fig. 9. Histidylriboflavin.

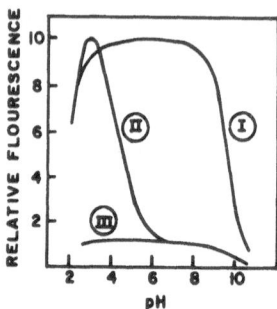

Fig. 10. pH-fluorescence curves of flavins and flavin peptides. (I) riboflavin; (II) histidyl-8α-riboflavin; (III) pure monoamine oxidase flavin pentapeptide (from Kearney *et al.*[59]).

dehydrogenase[58,147] provided the impetus for much subsequent investigation. The elegant applications of techniques such as ESR and NMR (nuclear magnetic resonance),[142,116] amino acid sequence analyses,[61,143] and the synthesis and characterization of appropriate analogs[38,86] have clarified the mode of cofactor binding in succinate dehydrogenase. Flavin is affixed to protein via a linkage between the 8α-methyl group of the isoalloxazine moiety and N(3) of the side chain of a histidyl residue of the protein (Fig. 9).[144] The fluorescent intensities of the flavin-peptide from succinate dehydrogenase and the synthetic histidyl riboflavin are pH dependent, with a pK of 4.5 (Fig. 10). On the basis of similar characteristics, it seems likely that comparable binding occurs in the cases of mammalian sarcosine dehydrogenase[34,101] and 6-hydroxy-D-nicotine oxidase from *Arthrobacter oxidans*.[15]

On the other hand, the fluorescence-quenching of flavin-peptide isolated from mammalian monoamine oxidase does not exhibit this type of pH dependence (Fig. 10).[59] The application of techniques similar to those enumerated above has revealed that the FAD in monoamine oxidase is bound to protein via linkage between the 8α-methyl group of the isoalloxazine moiety and the sulfur atom of a cysteinyl residue of the polypeptide (Fig. 11).[39,141] A similar linkage seems likely also

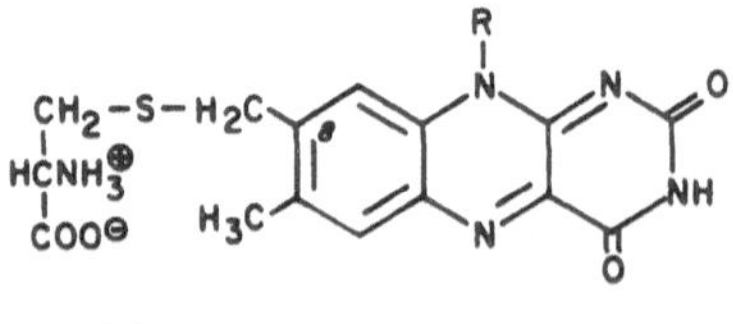

Fig. 11. Cysteinylriboflavin.

in the case of a flavocytochrome from *Chromatium*.[53] It seems reasonable to expect continued rapid progress in this area and the related studies of biosynthetic mechanism.

3.3. Noncovalent Binding

Assessment of cofactor binding and/or function has depended on determinations of catalytic activity, difference spectra, equilibrium dialysis, fluorescence characteristics, and/or circular dichroism. With use of one or more of these assays, most investigations of the mode of cofactor binding have focused on (1) the action of cofactor analogs; (2) the effect of functional group reagents; and (3) the influence of pH, temperature, ionic strength, and so forth, on binding. The conclusions derived from each approach have significant shortcomings, usually because of the dependence of protein conformation on cofactor binding and the equally important dependence of cofactor binding on protein conformation. These functions have been discussed above. Suffice it to say here that the apoenzyme differs from holoenzyme in more ways than the mere absence of flavin cofactor; these differences seem also to be a function of conditions and time.

Before discussion of selected investigations we emphasize the importance of the foregoing considerations by a few examples. FMN does not inhibit the catalytic activity of native, FAD-linked glutathione reductase; however, FMN does compete with and retard the binding of FAD by the resolved apoprotein.[119] Similar comments apply to studies with functional group reagents. It is not valid to conclude that sulfhydryl groups are important in flavin binding just because treatment with organic mercurial or an alkylating agent evokes release of cofactor (or prevents its binding by apoenzyme). The conformational dependence on cofactor binding could also explain other evidence such as the protection of one or more functional groups by flavin; it is not necessary to invoke direct "covering" of the functional group by cofactor.

3.3.1. FMN-Linked Flavoproteins

The apoproteins of flavodoxin,[80,81] old yellow enzyme,[127,128] and Shethna flavoprotein from *Azotobacter*[54,129] have been isolated and are relatively stable. Each reassociates with FMN with almost complete quenching of cofactor fluorescence. The dissociation constants of the three proteins, under slightly different conditions, are 4.3×10^{-10} M,

7.5×10^{-9} M, and 1.3×10^{-9} M, respectively. The rate constants of association of apoprotein and FMN are similar: 2.6×10^5 M^{-1}sec^{-1}, 1.7×10^5 M^{-1}sec^{-1}, and 7.9×10^5 M^{-1}sec^{-1}, respectively. The optimal pH for association of FMN with flavodoxin and Shethna flavoprotein is between 4 and 5, whereas old yellow enzyme combines with FMN most rapidly at a pH of about 9. It has been suggested therefore that ionization of only one of the phosphate hydroxyl groups is preferred with the former proteins, while binding of FMN to old yellow enzyme is optimal when both hydroxyl groups are ionized. More recent studies reopen the question.[71a]

Investigations with FMN analogs are abundant. With flavodoxin from *P. elsdenii*[80,81] the binding of FAD, riboflavin, and lumiflavin is negligible, with minimum dissociation constants of 10^{-3} M; flavodoxin from *D. gigas*, however, binds and functions with FAD.[26] Flavodoxin[80,81] does bind iso-FMN (methyl groups in the 6 and 7 positions) and 3,4-dihydro-FMN effectively and functions catalytically with the former in spite of possible protein conformational alteration.[70] These data suggest that positions 4, 6, and 8 of isoalloxazine are not of selective significance in cofactor binding. Riboflavin binds weakly to old yellow enzyme.[128]

The elegant studies of Tollin and Edmondson[129] have utilized fluorescence quenching, difference spectra, and circular dichroism (CD) to evaluate the binding of flavin analogs to Shethna flavoprotein. Since the isoalloxazine moiety is optically inactive, CD changes in the visible range indicate interaction with the optically active side-chain ribityl

TABLE X. *Association Constants of Flavin Analogs and Shethna Flavoprotein (from Tollin and Edmondson*[129]*)*

Flavin	K_a (M^{-1})
FMN	$2 \cdot 10^8$
3-Me-FMN	$4 \cdot 10^7$
2-thio-FMN	—
isoFMN	$5 \cdot 10^7$
FAD	$9 \cdot 10^5$
Riboflavin	$2 \cdot 10^6$
Isoriboflavin	$2 \cdot 10^6$
N-10-ω-carboxybutylisoalloxazine	$3 \cdot 10^6$
N-10-ω-hydroxylpentylisoalloxazine	$2 \cdot 10^6$
Lumiflavin	$1 \cdot 10^5$
3-Me-riboflavin	Not bound
Tetra-O-acetylriboflavin	Not bound

hydroxyl groups and/or protein. The study of analogs that lack nonterminal hydroxyl groups (for example, N-10-ω-hydroxypentyl isoalloxazine) permits further clarification. Association constants are presented in Table X. These and other data are summarized by Tollin and Edmondson[129]:

> The association constants for the FMN derivatives are quite high, indicating a strong interaction. . . . Removal of the terminal phosphate reduces the association constant by about two orders of magnitude as seen from a comparison of FMN and isoFMN with riboflavin and isoriboflavin. Most striking is that 3-Me-FMN is bound quite strongly while 3-Me-riboflavin is not bound at all . . . . This suggests the following: (1) interactions at the N(3) position and the phosphate are quite important in binding; (2) the conformation of the protein about the binding site is different when FMN is bound than when riboflavin is bound; (3) this difference in conformation is elicited by a phosphate-protein interaction.

Turning attention now to the relevant protein groupings, the side chains of tyrosine, lysine, cysteine, and tryptophan have been implicated more or less strongly as participants in the binding process. Tyrosyl side-chain involvement has been suggested in all three of these flavoproteins. Evidence is based on interference with binding by the action of tetranitromethane and iodine, and reciprocal protection of tyrosine against the action of these agents by FMN[54,80,81,121,128]; pH titration data are supportive.[129]

Sulfhydryl-characterizing reagents interfere with the binding of FMN in the case of flavodoxins[80,81] but not Shethna flavoprotein.[54] Titration data implicate primary amino groups,[128] whereas tryptophan has been suggested in studies with N-bromosuccinamide and flavodoxin.[85] Recent work tends also to implicate the involvement of tryptophanyl residues; for example, Ryan and Tollin[114a] and references quoted therein. We re-emphasize our opinion of the difficulties encountered in interpretation of such studies with functional group reagents.

3.3.2. FAD-Linked Flavoproteins

Many of the data discussed in the earlier sections of this chapter (glucose oxidase, D-amino acid oxidase, lipoamide dehydrogenase) have bearing on the present discussion and will not be repeated. We call attention, however, to the aforementioned importance of adenosine and phosphate moieties for binding and induction of protein conformation changes. It is notable also that although most FAD-linked enzymes specifically require FAD, some do not. Cytochrome b_5 reductase exhibits catalytic activity with FAD, FMN, and riboflavin; the flavins herein reveal apparent dissociation constants of $<10^{-9}$ M, 0.8×10^{-8} M, and about 2×10^{-6} M, respectively.[121]

3.4. Summary

Flavin cofactors are found noncovalently and covalently affixed to protein. Elucidation of the structures of covalently affixed flavins progresses rapidly with recognition of the importance of the linkage between the 8α-methyl group of isoalloxazine and enzyme–histidyl or cysteinyl residues. The biosynthetic mechanisms, however, remain unclarified. Many facets of the noncovalent linkage have been discussed briefly. Once again, there is reason to suspect significant diversity among the flavoproteins.

4. BIOSYNTHESIS OF RIBOFLAVIN

4.1. General Considerations

Many microorganisms and plants synthesize riboflavin from simple precursors. Indeed, certain organisms, such as *Eremothecium ashbyii*, *Ashbya gossypii*, and *Candida* sp., produce unusually large quantities of the vitamin; these organisms have served frequently in studies concerned with elucidation of the biosynthetic process. Although detailed reviews of the extensive studies are available,[13,28,42,69,109] we present here a brief resume with the purpose of emphasizing two important aspects of the biosynthetic scheme: (1) the metabolic relationship between purines, pteridines, and riboflavin, and (2) the involvement of 6,7-dimethyl-8-ribityllumazine. It must be noted at the outset that the pathways to be presented have been deduced from data derived from experiments involving many different organisms. It seems reasonable to expect that some variation, trivial or important, between synthetic processes in the different organisms will be found.

4.2. Purines as the Precursor of 6,7-Dimethyl-8-ribityllumazine and Riboflavin

Much evidence supports the supposition that a purine serves as the obligatory precursor of riboflavin. Early studies by MacLaren[72] and Giri and Krishnaswamy[41] revealed that purine supplements stimulated flavogenesis without stimulating growth in certain microorganisms. Plaut[108] determined the pattern of incorporation of radiocarbon from formate, bicarbonate, and glycine into riboflavin by *Ashbya gossypii*.

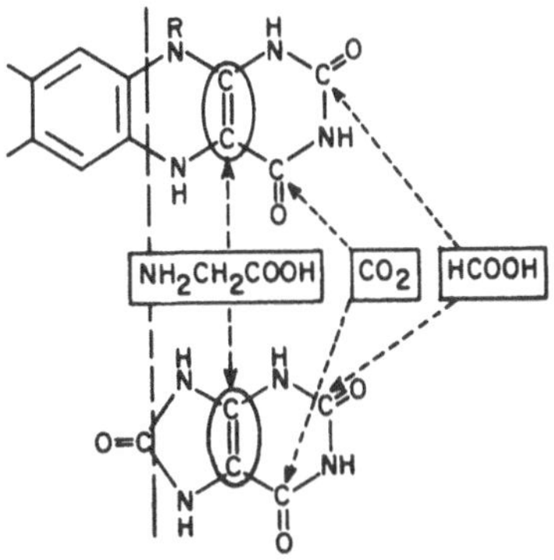

Fig. 12. Comparison of the site of incorporation of radioactive compounds into a purine (lower structure) and into riboflavin (upper structure) (from Plaut[108]).

The analogous incorporations into rings B and C of isoalloxazine, on the one hand, and a purine, uric acid, on the other are seen in Fig. 12. A similar pattern is observed also in the case of pteridine biosynthesis.[109] The experiments of McNutt[88-90] using variously labeled adenines provided evidence for the essentially direct conversion of purines to precursors of riboflavin. The process was found to involve cleavage of the imidazole portion of the purine with loss of carbon in position 8 before incorporation of the remaining diaminopyrimidine. Indeed, the precursor role of the diaminopyrimidine (or a derivative thereof) was documented by McNutt[90] using xanthine labeled with ^{14}C and ^{15}N.

Although these investigations established the precursor character of purines with respect to riboflavin biosynthesis, it remained for Howells and Plaut[56] to establish the obligatory nature of this relationship. They observed that a purine-requiring mutant of *E.coli* could incorporate radiocarbon from guanine, but not from glycine, into the isoalloxaine moiety. The results of Nagatsu *et al.*[98] corroborate some of these conclusions in an interesting fashion. *Eremothecium ashbyii* synthesizes riboflavin and FAD, but not FMN.[153] When the microorganism was grown in the presence of ^{14}C-formate, one-third of the label of FAD was found in position two of the isoalloxazine moiety; the remainder, twice as much label, was located in the adenine portion of the molecule, presumably in positions 2 and 8.

Recent studies, primarily with use of mutants of *Saccharomyces cerevisiae,* indicate that guanine or a derivative thereof is the specific purine precursor of riboflavin (Fig. 13). Bacher and Lingrens[4,6] have observed the accumulation of 6-hydroxy-2,4,5-triaminopyrimidine and

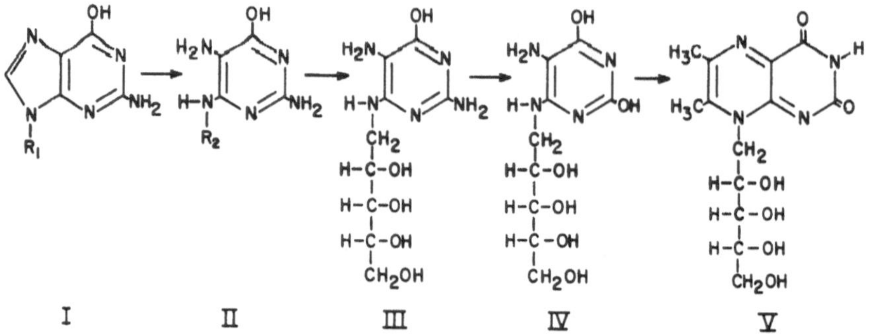

Fig. 13. Proposed scheme of riboflavin biosynthesis (modified from Bacher and Lingens [6]). The structures of R_1 and R_2 remain unknown.

2,5-diamino-6-hydroxy-4-ribitylaminopyrimidine (III, Fig. 13) by the riboflavin-deficient mutants. This derivative is presumably deaminated to 5-amino-2,6-dehydroxy-4-ribitylaminopyrimidine (IV, Fig. 13), isolated from a distinct mutant by Lingrens et al.,[68] itself the precursor of 6,7-dimethyl-8-ribityllumazine (V, Fig. 13). The conversion of IV to V presumably also involves a compound related to acetoin or its oxidation product, diacetyl.[79] This role for a guanine derivative is supported by the studies of Bacher and Lingrens [5] in which a mutant of *Aerobacter aerogenes*, which could not synthesize or interconvert purines, was found to incorporate label from guanine, but not xanthine, into riboflavin. Baugh and Krumdieck [7] obtained similar results using decoyinine, an antibiotic that blocks the conversion of XMP to GMP. These investigators point out the known precursor role of GTP in folate biosynthesis (pteridine moiety) and suggest the possibility of common intermediates in the biosynthesis of the two vitamins.

4.3. Conversion of 6,7-Dimethyl-8-ribityllumazine to Riboflavin

The precursor role of 6,7-dimethyl-8-ribityllumazine in riboflavin biosynthesis seems established.[73,78] Studies on the mechanism of riboflavin synthesis from the lumazine (V, Fig. 13) provide an exciting demonstration of the convergence of the enzymatic experiments of Plaut and colleagues [109,110] and the chemical investigations of Wood and collaborators.[102,103,114] Early enzymatic studies (for review, see Introduction, Harvey and Plaut [45]) revealed the stoichiometry of the reaction

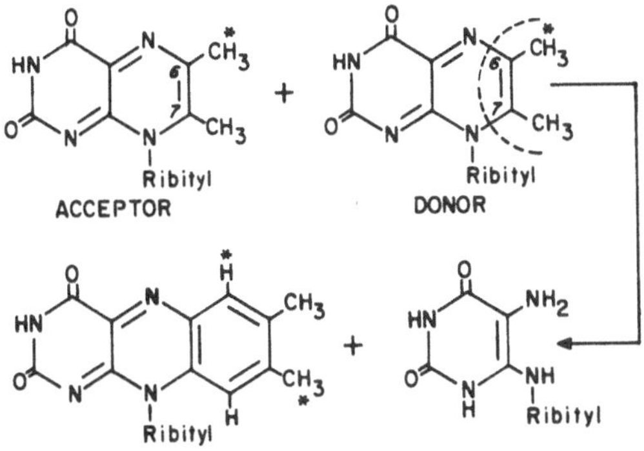

Fig. 14. Stereospecific transfer of the 4-carbon fragment (from Beach and Plaut[8]).

catalyzed by riboflavin synthetase to be

2(6,7-dimethyl-8-ribityllumazine) → riboflavin

+ 4-ribitylamino-5-amino-2,6-dihydroxypyrimidine

A similar reaction with good yield occurs nonenzymatically, albeit slowly.[114] Investigations with radiocarbon revealed that carbon atoms 6 and 7 (and their respective methyl substituents) of donor lumazine are incorporated at the hand of riboflavin synthetase into acceptor lumazine to form the o-xylene moiety of riboflavin (Fig. 14). Riboflavin synthetase, the enzyme that catalyzes this reaction, has been detected in many plants and flavogenic microorganisms and has been purified highly from yeast.[45] A series of elegant substrate and inhibitor analog studies[45] served to establish clearly the uniqueness of the enzymatic binding sites for the lumazine moieties destined to be donor or acceptor of the 4-carbon fragment. Although this and other riboflavin synthestases exhibit zero- to first-order dependence on lumazine concentration, suggesting widely dissimilar affinity constants with respect to donor and acceptor lumazine binding sites, the enzyme from *E. ashbyii* does reveal a second-order dependence on lumazine concentration.[124]

Recent chemical and enzymatic experiments using hydrogen isotopes have provided insight into the mechanism of this intriguing reaction. As noted in Fig. 14, the 4-carbon fragment transfer is stereospecific, both nonenzymatically[102,103] and enzymatically.[8,110] The observation that protons of the 7-methyl substituent of the lumazine exchange readily with solvent is fundamental; the proposed explanation involves the existence of a highly delocalized anionic species. Given this character, Patterson and Wood[103] have presented a mechanistic hypothesis, the

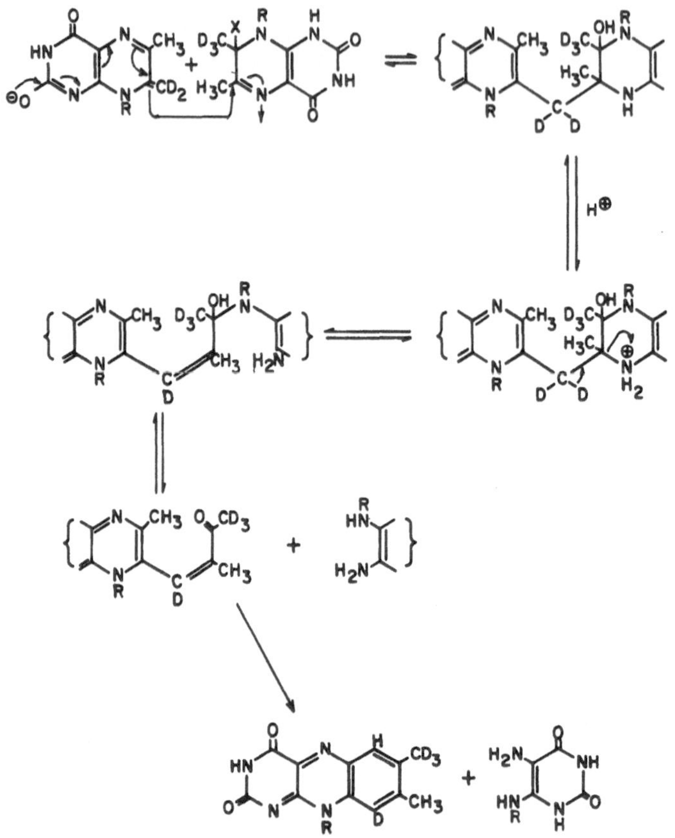

Fig. 15. Proposed mechanism for the conversion of 6,7-dimethyl-8-ribitylluma-zine to riboflavin (from Patterson and Wood[103]). For clarity, deuterium labels are shown only on carbon.

essential aspects of which are given in Fig. 15. In relating chemical conclusions to the enzymatic situation, Patterson and Wood[103] postulate:

> Thus one site might bind the acceptor lumazine molecule in such a way that a proton is readily removed to give the potential carbanion. A nucleophilic group such as OH or SH at the second binding site could readily react with the second lumazine molecule (the donor) converting it into a 7,8-dihydropteridine derivative [e.g., X = O-enzyme or S-enzyme]. Formation of riboflavin might then be expected to take place rapidly and to involve the stereospecific transfer for a 4-carbon atom unit from one lumazine molecule to the other. . . .

A related hypothesis concerning the formation of riboflavin has also been proposed by Beach and Plaut.[8]

5. REFERENCES

1. Albert, A. 1950. Metal binding of pteridines, *Biochem. J.* **47**: xvii–xviii.
2. Aleman, V., and Handler, P. 1967. Dihydroorotate dehydrogenase. I. General properties, *J. Biol. Chem.* **242**:4087–4096.
3. Anfinsen, C. B., and Haber, E. 1961. Reduction and reformation of protein disulfide bonds, *J. Biol. Chem.* **236**:1361–1363.
4. Bacher, A., and Lingens, F. 1968. Accumulation of 2,5-diamino-6-hydroxy-4-ribitylaminopyrimidine in a riboflavin-deficient mutant of *Saccharomyces cerevisiae, Angew. Chem. internat. Edit.,* **7**:219–220.
5. Bacher, A., and Lingens, F. 1969. The structure of the purine precursor in riboflavin biosynthesis, *Angew. Chem. internat. Edit.,* **8**:371–372.
6. Bacher, A., and Lingens, F. 1971. Biosynthesis of riboflavin. Formation of 6-hydroxy-2,4,5-triaminopyrimidine in RIB$_7$ mutants of *Saccharomyces cerevisiae, J. Biol. Chem.* **246**:7018–7022.
7. Baugh, C. M., and Krumdieck, C. L. 1969. Biosynthesis of riboflavin in *Corynebacterium* species: the purine precursor, *J. Bacteriol.* **98**:1114–1119.
8. Beach, R. L., and Plaut, G. W. E. 1970. Stereospecificity of the enzymatic synthesis of the *o*-xylene ring of riboflavin, *J. Am. Chem. Soc.* **92**:2913–2916.
9. Beinert, H. 1960. Flavin coenzymes, *in:* "The Enzymes" (P. D. Boyer, H. Lardy, and K. Myrbäck, eds.), pp. 339–416, Academic Press, New York.
10. Beinert, H., and Hemmerich, P. 1965. Evidence for semiquinone-metal interaction in metal-flavoproteins, *Biochem. Biophys. Res. Commun.* **18**:212–220.
11. Bothe, H., Hemmerich, P., and Sund, H. 1971. Some properties of phytoflavin isolated from the blue-green alga *Anacystis nidulans, in:* "Flavins and Flavoproteins" (H. Kamin, ed.), pp. 211–238, Third International Symposium, University Park Press, Baltimore.
12. Brady, F., Rajagopalan, K. V., and Handler, P. 1971. Preparation and properties of flavin-free metalloflavoproteins, *in:* "Flavins and Flavoproteins" (H. Kamin, ed.), pp. 425–440, Third International Symposium, University Park Press, Baltimore.
13. Brown, G. M., and Reynolds, J. J. 1963. Biogenesis of the water-soluble vitamins, *Ann. Rev. Biochem.* **32**:419–462.
14. Brown, L. E., and Hamilton, G. A. 1970. Some model reactions and a general mechanism for flavoenzyme-catalyzed dehydrogenations, *J. Am. Chem. Soc.* **92**:7225–7227.
15. Brühmüller, M. 1971. Thesis, University of Freiburg.
16. Bruice, T. C., Main, L., Smith, S., and Bruice, P. Y. 1971. Preequilibrium complex formation and nucleophilic addition (and its position) as factors in flavin-catalyzed oxidations, *J. Am. Chem. Soc.* **93**:7327–7328.
17. Brustlein, M., and Hemmerich, P. 1968. Photoreduction of flavocoenzymes by pyruvic acid, *FEBS Lett.* **1**:335–338.
18. Byrom, P., and Turnbull, J. H. 1968. Excited states of flavine coenzymes. IV. Kinetics of the photoreduction of lumiflavine by methionine, *Photochem. Photobiol.* **8**:243–254.
19. Cairns, W. L., and Metzler, D. E. 1971. Photochemical degradation of flavins. VI. A new photoproduct and its use in studying the photolytic mechanism, *J. Am. Chem. Soc.* **93**:2772–2777.
20. Chen, R. F., Vurek, G. G., and Alexander, N. 1967. Fluorescence decay times: proteins, coenzymes and other compounds in water, *Science* **156**:949–951.
21. Coffey, D. S., Neims, A. H., and Hellerman, L. 1965. Studies on crystalline D-amino

acid oxidase. II. Isolation of a reduced ^{14}C-labeled substrate–enzyme intermediate after the action of sodium borohydride, *J. Biol. Chem.* **240**:4058-4064.

22.   De Kok, A., Spencer, R. D., and Weber, G. 1968. Static and dynamic fluorescence quenching in the internal complex of FAD and in lipoamide dehydrogenase, *Fed. Proc.* **27**:298.

23.   De Kok, A., Veeger, C., and Hemmerich, P. 1971. The effect of light on flavins and flavoproteins in presence of α-keto acids, *in:* "Flavins and Flavoproteins" (H. Kamin, ed.), pp. 63-81, Third International Symposium, University Park Press, Baltimore.

24.   Dixon, M. 1971. The acceptor specificity of flavins and flavoproteins. III. Flavoproteins, *Biochim. Biophys. Acta* **226**:269-284.

25.   Dixon, M., and Kleppe, K. 1965. D-Amino acid oxidase. I. Dissociation and recombination of the holoenzyme, *Biochim. Biophys. Acta* **96**:357-367.

26.   Dubourdieu, M., and LeGall, J. 1970. Chemical study of two flavodoxins extracted from sulfate reducing bacteria, *Biochem. Biophys. Res. Commun.* **38**:965-972.

27.   Dudley, K. H., Ehrenberg, A., Hemmerich, P., and Müller, F. 1964. The flavine series. IX. Spectra and structures of the species concerned in the flavine redox system, *Helv. Chim. Acta* **47**:1354-1383.

28.   Dyke, S. F. 1965. "The Chemistry of the Vitamins," Interscience, New York.

29.   Edmondson, D. E., and Tollin, G. 1971. Circular dichroism studies of the flavin chromophore and of the relation between redox properties and flavin environment in oxidases and dehydrogenases, *Biochemistry* **10**:113-123.

30.   Edmondson, D. E., and Tollin, G. 1971. Chemical and physical characterization of the Shethna flavoprotein and apoprotein and kinetics and thermodynamics of flavin analogue binding to the apoprotein, *Biochemistry* **10**:124-132.

31.   Edmondson, D. E., and T llin, G. 1971. Flavin-protein interactions and the redox properties of the Shethna flavoprotein, *Biochemistry* **10**:133-145.

32.   Ehrenberg, A. 1970. Flavin radical metal chelates, *Vitam. Horm.* **28**:489-504.

33.   Ehrenberg, A., Eriksson, L. E. G., and Müller, F. 1966. Electron-spin resonance studies of flavins, *in:* "Flavin and Flavoproteins" (E. C. Slater, ed.), pp. 37-46, First International Symposium, Elsevier, Amsterdam.

33a. Elliott, D. L., and Bruice, T. C. 1973. Evidence for an intermediate adduct in the ethylenediaminetetracetic acid mediated photoreduction of flavins, *J. Am. Chem. Soc.* **95**:7901-7902.

34.   Frisell, W. R., and MacKenzie, C. G. 1970. Sarcosine dehydrogenase and dimethylglycine dehydrogenase (rat liver; monkey kidney). *Methods Enzymol.* **17**:976-981.

35.   Fonda, M. L., and Anderson, B. M. 1968. D-amino acid oxidase. III. Studies of flavin adenine dinucleotide binding, *J. Biol. Chem.* **243**:5635-5643.

36.   Galston, A. W. 1967. Regulatory systems in higher plants, *Am. Sci.* **55**:144-160.

37.   Gascoigne, J. M., and Radda, G. K. 1965. Reaction of dihydrolipoic acid with flavines. Biochemical model system, *Chem. Commun.* 211-212.

38.   Ghisla, S., Hartmann, U., and Hemmerich, P. 1970. The synthesis of succinate-dehydrogenase riboflavin. *Angew. Chem. internat. Edit.*, **9**:642-643.

39.   Ghisla, S., and Hemmerich, P. 1971. Synthesis of the flavocoenzyme of monoamine oxidase, *FEBS Lett.* **16**:229-232.

39a. Ghisla, S., Massey, V., Lhoste, J.-M., and Mayhew, S. G. 1974. Fluorescence and optical characteristics of reduced flavins and flavoproteins, *Biochemistry*, **13**:589-97.

40.   Gibson, Q. H., and Hastings, J. W. 1962. Intermediates in the bioluminescent oxidation of reduced flavin mononucleotide, *Biochem. J.* **83**:346.

41.   Giri, K. V., and Krishnaswamy, P. R. 1954. Studies on the synthesis of riboflavin

by a mutant yeast, *Saccharomyces cerevisiae, J. Bacteriol.* **67**:309-313.

42. Goodwin, T. W. 1963. Riboflavin and related compounds, *in:* "The Biosynthesis of Vitamins and Related Compounds," Academic Press, New York.

43. Gordon-Walker, A., Penzer, G. R., and Radda, G. K. 1970. Excited states of flavins characterised by absorption, prompt and delayed emission spectra, *Eur. J. Biochem.* **13**:313-321.

44. Gupta, N. K., and Vennesland, B. 1964. Glyoxylate carboligase of *Escherichia coli:* a flavoprotein, *J. Biol. Chem.* **239**:3787-3789.

45. Harvey, R. A., and Plaut, G. W. E. 1966. Riboflavin synthetase from yeast. Properties of complexes of the enzyme with lumazine derivatives and riboflavin, *J. Biol. Chem.* **241**:2120-2136.

46. Hellerman, L., Coffey, D. S., and Neims, A. H. 1965. Studies on crystalline D-amino acid oxidase. I. Selective inhibition in the action of sulfhydrylbinding reagents, *J. Biol. Chem.* **240**:290-298.

47. Hemmerich, P. 1960. Synthesis in the lumiflavine series. VIII. Condensation of 8-methylisoalloxazines with aldehydes, *Helv. Chim. Acta* **43**:1942-1946.

48. Hemmerich, P. 1970. Model studies on flavin dependent oxidoreduction, *Vitam. Horm.* **28**:467-487.

49. Hemmerich, P., Bhaduri, A. P., Blankenhorn, G., Brüstlein, M., Haas, W., and Knappe, W.–R. Model studies towards demonstration of covalent $2e^-$-transfer intermediates and their structure in flavin-dependent CH- and O_2-activation, *in:* "The Second International Symposium on Oxidases and Related Oxidation-Reduction Systems," in press, Academic Press, New York.

50. Hemmerich, P., Ghisla, S., Hartmann, U., and Müller, F. 1971. Chemistry and molecular biology of flavin in the fully-reduced state, *in:* "Flavins and Flavoproteins" (H. Kamin, ed.), pp. 83-106, Third International Symposium, University Park Press, Baltimore.

51. Hemmerich, P., Nagelschneider, G., and Veeger, C. 1970. Chemistry and molecular biology, *FEBS. Lett.* **8**:69.

52. Hemmerich, P., and Spence, J. 1966. Interaction of flavin with the MO(V, VI)-and Fe(II, III)-redox systems, *in:* "Flavins and Flavoproteins" (E. C. Slater, ed.), pp. 82-98, First International Symposium, Elsevier, Amsterdam.

53. Hendriks, R., and Cronin, J. R. 1971. The flavin of Chromatium cytochrome *C*-552, *Biochem. Biophys. Res. Commun.* **44**:313-318.

54. Hinkson, J. W. 1968. *Azotobacter* free-radical flavoprotein. Preparation and properties of the apoprotein, *Biochemistry* **7**:2666-2672.

55. Horecker, B. L. 1950. Triphosphopyridine nucleotide-cytochrome c reductase in liver, *J. Biol. Chem.* **183**:593-605.

56. Howells, D. J., and Plaut, G. W. E. 1965. Biosynthesis of riboflavine by a purine-requiring mutant strain of *Escherichia coli, Biochem. J.* **94**:755-759.

57. Kalse, J. F., and Veeger, C. 1968. Relation between conformations and activities of lipoamide dehydrogenase. I. Relation between diaphorase and lipoamide dehydrogenase activities upon binding of FAD by the apoenzyme, *Biochim. Biophys. Acta* **159**:244-256.

58. Kearney, E. B. 1960. Studies of succinic dehydrogenase. XII. Flavin component of the mammalian enzyme, *J. Biol. Chem.* **235**:865-877.

59. Kearney, E. B., Salach, J. I., Walker, W. H., Seng, R. L., Kenney, W., Zeszotek, E., and Singer, T. P. 1971. The covalently bound flavin of hepatic monoamine oxidase, *Eur. J. Biochem.* **24**:321-327.

60. Kearney, E. B., and Singer, T. P. 1955. Prosthetic group of succinic dehydrogenase, *Biochim. Biophys. Acta* **17**:596-597.

61. Kenney, W. C., Walker, W. H., Kearney, E. B., Zeszotek, E., and Singer, T. P. 1970. Amino acid sequence at the active center of succinate dehydrogenase, *Biochem. Biophys. Res. Commun.* **41**:488-491.

62. Kierkegaard, P., Norrestam, R., Werner, P., Csöregh, I., Glehn, M., Karlsson, R., Leijonmarck, M., Rönnquist, O., Stensland, B., Tillberg, O., and Torbjörnsson, L. 1971. X-ray structure investigations of flavin derivatives, *in:* "Flavins and Flavoproteins" (H. Kamin, ed.), pp. 1-22, Third International Symposium, University Park Press, Baltimore.

63. Knappe, W. R., and Hemmerich, P. 1971. 5-(2-Thiolyl)-1,5-dihydroflavin: A model of group transfer in flavin dependent substrate dehydrogenation, *FEBS Lett.* **13**:293-296.

64. Komai, H., and Massey, V. 1971. Alkylation of xanthine oxidase, *in:* "Flavins and Flavoproteins" (H. Kamin, ed.), pp. 399-423, Third International Symposium, University Park Press, Baltimore.

65. Komai, H., Massey, V., and Palmer, G. 1969. The preparation and properties of deflavo xanthine oxidase, *J. Biol. Chem.* **244**:1692-1700.

66. Kotaki, A., Harada, M., and Yagi, K. 1967. Structure and function of D-amino acid oxidase. II. Terminal structure and amino acid composition of hog kidney D-amino acid oxidase, *J. Biochem. (Tokyo)* **61**:598-605.

66a. Kroneck, P., and Spence, J. T. 1973. Model studies for molybdenum enzymes. Reduction of flavins by μ-oxo-bis[oxodihydroxo(L-cysteinato)molybdate (V)], *Biochemistry* **12**:5020-5024.

67. Kurtin, W. E., and Song, P. S. 1968. Photochemistry of the model phototropic system involving flavins and indoles, I, *Photochem. Photobiol.* **7**:263-273.

68. Lingens, F., Oltmanns, O., and Bacher, A. 1967. Intermediates of riboflavine biosynthesis in *Saccharomyces cerevisiae, Z. Naturforsch.* **22b**:755-758.

69. Luckner, M. 1969. Purines, pteridines and alloxazines, *in:* "Biosyn. Alkaloide" (K. Mothes, ed.), pp. 568-592, VEB Deut. Verlag Wiss., Berlin, pp. 568-592.

70. Ludwig, M. L., Andersen, R., Apgar, P. A., and LeQuesne, M. 1971. A preliminary crystallographic study of Clostridial flavodoxin, *in:* "Flavins and Flavoproteins" (H. Kamin, ed.), pp. 171-180, Third International Symposium, University Park Press, Baltimore.

71. Mackler, B. 1961. Studies of DPNH oxidase: Properties of a soluble DPNH dehydrogenase, *Biochim. Biophys. Acta* **50**:141-146.

71a. MacKnight, M. L., Gillard, J. M., and Tollin, G. 1973. Flavin-protein interactions in flavoenzymes: pH dependence of the binding of flavine mononucleotidle and riboflavine to *Azotobacter* flavodoxin, *Biochemistry* **12**:4200-4206.

72. MacLaren, J. A. 1952. The effects of certain purines and pyrimidines upon the production of riboflavin by *Eremothecium ashbyii, J. Bacteriol.* **63**:233-241.

73. Maley, G. F., and Plaut, G. W. E. 1959. Isolation, synthesis, and metabolic properties of 6,7-dimethyl-8-ribityllumazine, *J. Biol. Chem.* **234**:641-647.

74. Massey, V., and Curti, B. 1966. A new method of preparation of D-amino acid oxidase apoprotein and a conformational change after its combination with flavin adenine dinucleotide, *J. Biol. Chem.* **241**:3417-3423.

75. Massey, V., Curti, B., Muller, F., and Mayhew, S. G. 1968. On the reaction of borohydride with D- and L-amino acid oxidases, *J. Biol. Chem.* **243**:1329-1330.

76. Massey, V., Matthews, R. G., Foust, G. P., Howell, L. G., Williams, C. H., Zanetti, G., and Ronchi, S. 1970. A new intermediate in TPNH-linked flavoproteins, *in:* "Pyridine Nucleotide Dependent Dehydrogenases" (H. Sund, ed.), pp. 392-411. Springer-Verlag, New York.

77. Massey, V., Palmer, G., and Ballou, D. 1971. On the reaction of reduced flavins and flavoproteins with molecular oxygen, *in:* "Flavins and Flavoproteins" (H. Kamin, ed.), pp. 349–361, Third International Symposium, University Park Press, Baltimore.

78. Masuda, T. 1957. Chromatography. XXXI. Structure of a green fluorescent substance produced by *Eremothecium ashibyii*, *Pharm. Bull. (Tokyo)* **5**:28–30.

79. Masuda, T. 1957. Chromatography. XXXII. Biosynthesis of riboflavine by *Eremothecium ashbyii*, *Pharm. Bull. (Tokyo)* **5**:136–141.

80. Mayhew, S. G. 1971. Studies on the binding of FMN and other flavin compounds to apoflavodoxin, *in:* "Flavins and Flavoproteins" (H. Kamin, ed.), pp. 185–205, Third International Symposium, University Park Press, Baltimore.

81. Mayhew, S. G. 1971. Studies on flavin binding in flavodoxins, *Biochim. Biophys. Acta* **235**:289–302.

82. McBride, M. M., and Metzler, D. E. 1967. Photochemical degradation of flavines. III. Hydroxyethyl and formylmethyl analogs of riboflavine, *Photochem. Photobiol.* **6**:113–123.

83. McBride, M. M., and Moore, W. M. 1967. The photochemistry of riboflavin. II. Polarographic studies on hydroxyethyl and formylmethyl analogs of riboflavin, *Photochem. Photobiol.* **6**:103–111.

84. McCormick, D. B. 1968. Nature of the intramolecular complex of flavin adenine dinucleotide, *in:* "Molecular Associations in Biology" (B. Pullman, ed.), p. 377, Academic Press, New York.

85. McCormick, D. B. 1970. The tryptophans in flavodoxin and synthetic flavinyl peptides characterized by chemical and photochemical oxidations, *Experimentia* **26**:243–244.

86. McCormick, D. B. 1970. Flavin derivatives via bromination of the 8-methyl substituent, *J. Heterocyclic Chem.* **7**:447–450.

87. McCormick, D. B., Chassy, B. M., and Tsibris, J. C. M. 1964. Coenzyme specificity of D-amino acid oxidase for the adenylate moiety of FAD, *Biochim. Biophys. Acta* **89**:447–452.

88. McNutt, W. S. 1954. The direct contribution of adenine to the biogenesis of riboflavin by *Eremothecium ashibyii*, *J. Biol. Chem.* **210**:511–519.

89. McNutt, W. S. 1956. The incorporation of the pyrimidine ring of adenine into the isoalloxazine ring of riboflavin, *J. Biol. Chem.* **219**:365–373.

90. McNutt, W. S. 1961. The incorporation of the four nitrogen atoms of purine into the pyrimidine and pyrazine rings of riboflavin, *J. Am. Chem. Soc.* **83**:2303–2307.

91. Merkel, P. B., Nilsson, R., and Kearns, D. R. 1972. Deuterium effects on singlet oxygen lifetimes in solutions. A new test of singlet oxygen reactions, *J. Am. Chem. Soc.* **94**:1030–1031.

92. Moore, W. M., and Baylor, C., Jr. 1969. The photochemistry of riboflavin. IV. The photobleaching of some nitrogen-9 substituted isoalloxazines and flavins, *J. Am. Chem. Soc.* **91**:7170–7179.

93. Moore, W. M., Spence, J. T., Raymond, F. A., and Colson, S. D. 1963. The photochemistry of riboflavine. I. The hydrogen transfer process in the anaerobic photobleaching of flavines, *J. Am. Chem. Soc.* **85**:3367–3372.

94. Müller, F., Eriksson, L. E. G., and Ehrenberg, A. 1970. Flavin radical chelates as studied by electron spin resonance and isotopic substitution, *Eur. J. Biochem.* **12**:93–103.

95. Müller, F., Hemmerich, P., and Ehrenberg, A. 1968. Light absorption of flavosemiquinone metal chelates, *Eur. J. Biochem.* **5**:158–164.

96. Müller, F., Hemmerich, P., and Ehrenberg, A. 1971. On the molecular and submolecular structure of flavin free radicals and their properties, *in:* "Flavins

and Flavoproteins'' (H. Kamin, ed.), pp. 107-122, Third International Symposium. University Park Press, Baltimore.

97. Müller, F., Massey, V., Heizmann, C., Hemmerich, P., Lhoste, J.–M., and Gould D. C. 1969. The reduction of flavins by borohydride: 3, 4-dihydroflavin, *Eur. J. Biochem.* **9**:392-401.

98. Nagatsu, T., Nagatsu-Ishibashi, I., and Yagi, K. 1963. Biosynthesis of C[14]-labelled flavin adenine dinucleotide by *Eremothecium ashbyii, J. Biochem. (Tokyo)* **54**:152-155.

99. Negelein, E., and Brömel, H. 1938. Protein der d-aminosäureoxydase, *Biochem. Z.* **300**:225-300.

100. Neims, A. H., DeLuca, D. C., and Hellerman, L. 1966. Studies on crystalline D-amino acid oxidase. III. Substrate specificity and σ-ρ relationship, *Biochemistry* **5**:203-213.

101. Patek, D. R. 1970. Thesis. Purification and characterization of the peptide flavin isolated from sarcosine dehydrogenase of rat liver mitochondria, University of Colorado.

102. Patterson, T., and Wood, H. C. S. 1969. Deuterium exchange of c-methyl protons in 6, 7-dimethyl-8-D-ribityl-lumazine, and studies of the mechanism of riboflavin biosynthesis, *Chem. Commun.* 290-291.

103. Patterson, T., and Wood, H. C. S. 1972. The biosynthesis of pteridines. Part VI. Studies of the mechanism of riboflavin biosynthesis, *J. Chem. Soc., (Perkin I)* 1051-1056.

104. Penzer, G. R. 1970. The chemistry of flavines and flavoproteins: Aerobic photochemistry, *Biochem. J.* **116**:733-743.

105. Penzer, G. R., and Radda, G. K. 1967. The chemistry and biological function of isoalloxazines (flavines), *Quart. Rev. Biol.* **21**:43-65.

106. Penzer, G. R., and Radda, G. K. 1968. The chemistry of flavines and flavoproteins: photoreduction of flavines by admino acids, *Biochem. J.* **109**:259-268.

107. Penzer, G. R., Radda, G. K., Taylor, J. A., and Taylor, M. B. 1970. Chemical properties of flavins in relation to flavoprotein catalysis, *Vitam. Horm.* **28**:441-466.

108. Plaut, G. W. E. 1954. Biosynthesis of riboflavin. I. Incorporation of ^{14}C-labeled compounds into rings B and C, *J. Biol. Chem.* **208**:513-520.

109. Plaut, G. W. E. 1961. Water-soluble vitamins. Part II (folic acid, riboflavin, thiamine, vitamin B$_{12}$), *Ann. Rev. Biochem.* **30**:409-446.

110. Plaut, G. W. E., Beach, R. L., and Aogaichi, T. 1970. Studies on the mechanism of elimination of protons from the methyl groups of 6, 7-dimethyl-8-ribityllumazine by riboflavin synthetase, *Biochemistry* **9**:771-785.

111. Radda, G. K., and Calvin, M. 1964. Chemical and photochemical reductions of flavine nucleotides and analogs, *Biochemistry* **3**:384-393.

112. Rajagopalan, K. V., Brady, F. O., and Kanda, M. 1970. Effect of conformation on the binding of flavins to flavoenzymes, *Vitam. Horm.* **28**:303-314.

112a. Rando, R. R. 1973. 3-Bromoallylamine induced irreversible inhibition of monoamine oxidase, *J. Am. Chem. Soc.* **95**:4438-4439.

113. Risler, J. L. 1971. Fluorescence and phosphorescence of yeast L-lactate dehydrogenase (cytochrome b$_2$). Relative orientations of the prosthetic heme and flavin, *Biochemistry* **10**:2664-2669.

114. Rowan, T., and Wood, H. C. S. 1963. The biosynthesis of riboflavine, *Proc. Chem. Soc.* 21-22.

114a. Ryan, J., and Tollin, G. 1973. Flavine-protein interactions in flavoenzymes. Effect of chemical modification of tryptophan residues upon flavine mononucleotide binding and protein fluoresence in *Azotobacter* flavodotin. *Biochemistry* **12**:4550-4554.

115. Rynd, J. A., and Gibian, M. J. 1970. The oxidation of organic anions by flavins, *Biochem. Biophys. Res. Commun.* **41**:1097-1103.

115a. Shinkai, S., and Bruice, T. C. 1973. The question of covalent intermediate formation in the flavin-catalyzed carbonal to carbinol oxidation-reduction reaction. *J. Am. Chem. Soc.* **95**:7526-7528.

116. Singer, T. P., Salach, J., Walker, W. H., Gutman, M., Hemmerich, P., and Ehrenberg, A. 1971. On the structure of the covalently linked FAD in succinate dehydrogenase, *in:* "Flavins and Flavoproteins" (H. Kamin, ed.), pp. 607-621, Third International Symposium, University Park Press, Baltimore.

117. Song, P. S. 1969. Electronic structures and spectra of flavins: An improved Pariser-Parr-Pople MO and semiempirical unrestricted Hartee-Fock computations, *Ann. N. Y. Acad. Sci.* **158**:410-423.

118. Staal, G. E. J., Helleman, P. W., DeWael, J., and Veeger, C. 1969. Purification and properties of an abnormal glutathione reductase from human erythrocytes, *Biochim. Biophys. Acta* **185**:63-69.

119. Staal, G. E. J., Visser, J., and Veeger, C. 1969. Purification and properties of glutathione reductase of human erythrocytes, *Biochim. Biophys. Acta* **185**:39-48.

120. Steiner, D. F., Cunningham, D., Spigelman, L., and Aten, B. 1967. Insulin biosynthesis: Evidence for a precursor, *Science* **157**:697-700.

121. Strittmatter, P. 1961. The nature of the flavin binding in microsomal cytochrome b_5 reductase, *J. Biol. Chem.* **236**:2329-2335.

122. Strittmatter, P. 1968. Studies on the tertiary structure of cytochrome b_5 reductase, *in:* "Flavins and Flavoproteins," (K. Yagi, ed.), pp. 85-96, Second International Symposium, University Park Press, Baltimore.

123. Suelter, C. H., and Metzler, D. E. 1960. The oxidation of a reduced pyridine nucleotide analogue by flavins, *Biochim. Biophys. Acta* **44**:23-33.

124. Suzuki, Y., and Mitsuda, H. 1971. A second-order kinetic reaction catalyzed by riboflavin synthetase from a high-riboflavinogenic *Eremothecium ashibyii, Biochim. Biophys. Acta* **242**:500-503.

125. Swoboda, B. E. P. 1969. The relationship between molecular conformation and the binding of flavin-adenine dinucleotide in glucose oxidase, *Biochim. Biophys. Acta* **175**:365-379.

126. Swoboda, B. E. P. 1969. The mechanism of binding of flavin-adenine dinucleotide to the apoenzyme of glucose oxidase and evidence for the involvement of multiple bonds, *Biochim. Biophys. Acta* **175**:380-387.

127. Theorell, H., and Nygaard, A. P. 1954. Kinetics and equilibria in flavoprotein systems. I, *Acta Chem. Scand.* **8**:877-888.

128. Theorell, H., and Nygaard, A. P. 1954. Kinetics and equilibria in flavoprotein systems. II, *Acta Chem. Scand.* **8**:1649-1658.

129. Tollin, G., and Edmonson, D. E. 1971. Flavin-protein interactions in the Shethna flavoprotein from *Azobacter, in:* "Flavins and Flavoproteins" (H. Kamin, ed.), pp. 153-166, Third International Symposium, University Park Press, Baltimore.

130. Trus, B. L., Wells, J. L., Johnstone, R. M., Fritche, C. J., and Marsh, R. E. 1971. Crystal structure of the yellow 1:2 molecular complex lumiflavin-bisnaphthalene-2, 3-diol, *Chem. Commun.* 751-752.

131. Vaish, S. P., and Tollin, G. 1970. Flash photolysis of flavins. IV. Some properties of the lumiflavin triplet state, *Bioenergetics* **1**:181-192.

132. Vaish, S. P., and Tollin, G. 1971. Flash photolysis of flavins. V. Oxidation and disproportionation of flavin radicals, *Bioenergetics* **2**:61-72.

133. Varnes, A. W., Dodson, R. B., and Wehry, E. L. 1972. Interactions of transition-metal

ions with photoexcited states of flavins. Fluorescence quenching studies, *J. Am. Chem. Soc.* **94**:946-950.

134. Veeger, C. 1968. Relation between kinetic properties and conformations of flavoproteins, *in:* "Flavins and Flavoproteins" (K. Yagi, ed.), pp. 252-266, Second International Symposium, University Park Press, Baltimore.

135. Veeger, C., Voetberg, H., Visser, J., Staal, G. E. J., and Koster, J. F. 1971. Conformation transitions in flavoproteins, *in:* "Flavins and Flavoproteins" (H. Kamin, ed.), pp. 261-288, Third International Symposium, University Park Press, Baltimore.

136. Visser, J., McCormick, D. B., and Veeger, C. 1968. Relation between conformations and activities of lipoamide dehydrogenase. II. Some aspects of recombination with FAD analogs, *Biochim. Biophys. Acta* **159**:257-264.

137. Visser, J., and Veeger, C. 1968. Relations between conformations and activities of lipoamide dehydrogenase. III. Protein association-dissociation and the influence on catalytic properties, *Biochim. Biophys. Acta* **159**:265-275.

138. Voet, D., and Rich, A. 1971. A hydrogen-bonded complex between riboflavin and an adenosine derivative, and its possible relation to FAD function *in:* "Flavins and Flavoproteins" (H. Kamin, ed.), pp. 23-33, Third International Symposium. University Park Press, Baltimore.

139. Walaas, E. and Walaas, O. 1956. Kinetics and equilibria in flavoprotein systems. V. The effects of pH, anions and partial structural analogues of the coenzyme on the activity of D-amino acid oxidase. *Acta Chem. Scand.* **10**:122-133.

140. Walker, W. H., and Hemmerich, P. 1970. Light-induced alkylation and dealkylation of the flavin nucleus. Stable dihydroflavins: Spectral course and mechanism of formation, *Eur. J. Biochem.* **13**:258-266.

141. Walker, W. H., Kearney, E. B., Seng, R. L., and Singer, T. P. 1971. The covalently bound flavin of hepatic monoamine oxidase, *Eur. J. Biochem.* **24**:328-331.

142. Walker, W. H., Salach, J., Gutman, M., Singer, T. P., Hyde, J. S., and Ehrenberg, A. 1969. ENDOR studies on the covalently bound flavin at the active center of succinate dehydrogenase, *FEBS Lett.* **5**:237-240.

143. Walker, W. H., and Singer, T. P. 1970. Identification of the covalently bound flavin of succinate dehydrogenase as 8 α-(histidyl) flavin adenine dinucleotide, *J. Biol. Chem.* **245**:4224-4225.

144. Walker, W. H., and Singer, T. P. 1971. Structure of the covalently bound flavin active center of succinate dehydrogenase, *Fed. Proc.* **30**:1286 (*Abstr.*).

145. Walsh, C. T., Schonbrunn, A., and Abeles, R. H. 1971. Studies on the mechanism of action of D-amino acid oxidase, *J. Biol. Chem.* **246**:6855-6866.

146. Wang, T. Y., Tsou, C. L., and Wang, Y. L. 1956. Succinic dehydrogenase. I. Isolation, purification and properties, *Scientia Sinica* **5**:73-90.

147. Wang, T. Y., Tsou, C. L., and Wang, Y. L. 1965. Studies on succinic dehydrogenase. V, *Scientia Sinica* **14**:1193-1204.

148. Warburg, O., and Christian, W. 1938. Bemerkung über gelbe Fermente, *Biochem. Z.* **298**:368-377.

149. Weatherby, G. D., and Carr, D. O. 1970. Riboflavin-catalyzed photooxidative decarboxylation of dihydrophthalates, *Biochemistry* **9**:344-350.

150. Weatherby, G. D., and Carr, D. O. 1970. Riboflavin-catalyzed dehydrogenation of dihydrophthalates in the dark, *Biochemistry* **9**:351-354.

151. White, F. H., Jr. 1961. Regeneration of native secondary and tertiary structures by air oxidation of reduced ribonuclease, *J. Biol. Chem.* **236**:1353-1360.

152. Yagi, K., Harada, M., and Kotaki, A. 1966. Trinitrophenylation of D-amino acid oxidase, *Biochim. Biophys. Acta* **122**:182-192.

153. Yagi, K., Yoshitaka, M., Shinpu, K., and Mitsuhiko, T. 1956. Preparation of flavin adenine dinucleotide from *Eremothecium ashbyii, J. Biochem. (Tokyo)* **43**:93-100.

154. Yang, C. S., and McCormick, D. B. 1965. The photochemical degradation of flavins as influenced by the length and extent of hydroxylation of the side chain, *J. Am. Chem. Soc.* **87**:5763-5765.

155. Zelitch, I., and Ochoa, S. 1953. Oxidation and reduction of glycolic and glyoxylic acids in plants. I. Glycolic acid oxidase, *J. Biol. Chem.*, **201**:707-718.

ANALYSIS OF RIBOFLAVIN AND ITS DERIVATIVES IN BIOLOGIC FLUIDS AND TISSUES

Herman Baker and Oscar Frank

1. INTRODUCTION

Flavins are present in all biologic fluids and tissues. Most biologic materials contain many metabolically active compounds incorporating riboflavin derivatives. The most common biologically important flavins are riboflavin and its nucleotides: riboflavin-5'-phosphate (flavin mononucleotide, FMN), and the intramolecular complex of FMN with adenosine-5'-monophosphate (flavin adenine dinucleotide, FAD). The latter two are the principal forms of riboflavin found in nature. FMN and FAD are protein-bound, with the latter usually the most abundant (60-90%) in natural products.[37] Significant amounts of free riboflavin are confined to milk[35] and urine,[37] in which it is, accordingly, dialyzable. In living cells, riboflavin generally occurs as FMN and FAD bound

---

HERMAN BAKER—Professor of Medicine and Preventive Medicine, New Jersey Medical School, College of Medicine and Dentistry of New Jersey. *OSCAR FRANK*—Associate Professor of Medicine, New Jersey Medical School, College of Medicine and Dentistry of New Jersey.

to specific proteins to form oxidative enzymes; these functional forms of flavin are not assayable without proteolytic digestion.[16] In most analytical procedures, it is necessary to treat natural products with acid or enzymes for maximal values, that is, to liberate riboflavin from its protein moiety thus making it more readily extractable for assay. If FMN or FAD content is to be measured, special nonhydrolytic extraction procedures are required.[28]

Three general methods are satisfactory for assaying riboflavin in biologic fluids and tissues: fluorometric, enzymatic, and microbiological. Measurement of growth of riboflavin-deficient animals supplemented with extracts containing riboflavin are not applicable for the riboflavin assay of biologic fluids and tissues. Fluorometric methods have been used to estimate riboflavin and its coenzymes; these methods are considered to be the most sensitive chemical methods available. Such determinations of flavins can be carried out in two ways: measurement of the intensity of the natural fluorescence of flavins or measurement of the fluorescence of lumiflavins derived from flavins.[47] Both methods can be equally applied in similar analytical procedures exploiting certain physicochemical properties of flavins.[28,37,47]

An enzymatic approach to assessing riboflavin status in humans has been recently published.[8,22,44,45] The data presented show that $NADPH_2$-dependent glutathione reductase of red cells reflects riboflavin fluctuations. The occurrence of a $NADPH_2$-dependent glutathione reductase in red cells has long been known; this enzyme has FAD as cofactor.[7,9] Glutathione reductase is sensitive to riboflavin nutritional status; it is lowered in riboflavin deficiency and can be restored in vitro with exogenous FAD or by riboflavin administration.[11,45] Its practical usefulness for nutritional assessment can be judged only after information is available with interaction to other dietary factors and diseases on glutathione reductase activity. This method will be described here.

Aside from many lactic acid bacteria, few free-living bacteria need exogenous riboflavin. The microbiologic assay for riboflavin with Lactobacillus casei is still in use in some laboratories.[30] Leuconostoc mesenteroides (ATCC 10,100) is claimed to be 50 times more sensitive than L. casei for assaying riboflavin and its analogs.[27] More recently, a method based on the ciliate, Tetrahymena pyriformis, for assaying total riboflavin in biologic fluids and tissues of man and animals has been described.[3,5] This protozoan has a sensitive and specific requirement for riboflavin; riboflavin cannot be replaced for growth.[26] Its application to large-scale nutritional surveys has been described.[4] These various microbiological methods will be detailed here.

It is not possible to incorporate all the various modifications of methods being used for assaying riboflavin and its derivatives in biologic fluids and tissues; we can describe only those more commonly used for this purpose.

2. CHEMICAL METHODS

2.1. Fluorometric Assay

Fluorometric assay, a commonly used procedure, is an adaptation of methods described by Burch et al.,[13] Bessey et al.,[10] and Burch.[12] It is based on the following principles: (a) free riboflavin occurs only in minute quantities in most tissues; therefore, total riboflavin in acid extracts is a measure of the riboflavin resulting from hydrolysis of FMN and FAD; (b) differentiation of flavins depends upon the fact that, at neutrality, riboflavin and FMN have the same fluorescence per mole, whereas FAD is only about 14% as fluorescent by this procedure; (c) riboflavin is much more readily extracted by benzyl alcohol from aqueous solution than is FMN or FAD; and (d) FAD is completely hydrolyzed to FMN in 5% trichloroacetic acid in 20 hr at 37°C.

SPECIAL EQUIPMENT. Various fluorometers can be used, but they must be equipped with suitable primary and secondary filters. Farrand Optical Co., Mt. Vernon, N.Y.; American Instrument Co., Silver Spring, Md. (Aminco-Bowman spectrophotometer); and Turner Instrument Co., Palo Alto, Cal., make suitable instruments for this purpose which permit measurements to be made on as little as 10 μl. The Coleman Model 12C photofluorometer cannot be used for the volumes specified in this procedure.

REAGENTS

1. *Trichloroacetic acid, 11%.* Dissolve 11 g trichloroacetic acid in distilled water; bring volume to 100 ml.

2. *K_2HPO_4, 0.2 M.* Dissolve 3.48 g (as K_2HPO_4) (anhydrous) in distilled water; bring volume to 100 ml.

3. *Sodium acetate-acetic acid buffer, 0.05M.* Dissolve 1.7 g sodium acetate in distilled water; add 2.84 ml glacial acetic acid; bring volume to 1 liter with water.

4. *Sodium hydrosulfite solution, 10%.* Dissolve 1 g $Na_2S_2O_4$ in enough 5% $NaHCO_3$ to make 10 ml. *Prepare fresh for each use.*

5. *Benzyl alcohol.* Redistilled, washed, and saturated with redistilled water.

6. *Riboflavin standard. Stock solution:* Dry about 100 mg U.S.P. riboflavin at 105°C for 2 hr and store in dark overnight in a desiccator over P_2O_5 or concentrated H_2SO_4. Weigh 25 mg riboflavin in about 500 ml distilled water and 1.2 ml glacial acetic acid; warm to dissolve. Cool to room temperature and add water to 1 liter in a volumetric flask. Transfer to a dark bottle; add preservative (1 part chlorobenzene, 1 part 1,2-dichloroethane, 2 parts *n*-butyl chloride). This solution contains 25 μg riboflavin per ml. *Working solution.* Dilute 40 ml of stock solution to 100 ml with distilled water just before use; this solution, containing 10 μg per ml of riboflavin, is diluted with 0.01 M HC1 to give riboflavin concentrations of 0.1-0.4 μg/ml (muscle and brain), 1.0-4.0 μg/ml (liver and kidney), and 0.5-2.0 μg/ml for other tissues.

7. *Sodium fluorescein stock solution.* Dissolve 50 mg sodium fluorescein in water to 1 liter. Store in cold. *Working solution:* Dilute 1 ml stock solution to 1 liter with distilled water.

Caution: Do not use corks or rubber stoppers since they may produce interfering fluorescence when they come in contact with the solutions. Glassware should be soaked overnight in concentrated HNO_3 to remove interfering fluorescent substances.

2.1.1. Tissues

TISSUE PREPARATION AND PROCEDURE. A fresh, weighed tissue sample is finely ground in a glass homogenizer at 0-4°C with 10 ml water/g tissue; 0.3 ml cold suspension is mixed with 3 ml of 11% trichloroacetic acid. After 15 min, the sample is centrifuged at 4°C. At the same time, 0.3-ml aliquots of riboflavin standards are carried through the entire procedure. Immediately, 0.2-ml aliquots of the supernatant fluid are placed into calibrated matched fluorometer tubes (3 ml; 10 × 75 mm) containing 1 ml of 0.2 M K_2HPO_4 and are mixed; the final pH should be 6.8. The samples should be kept very cold to prevent hydrolysis of FAD to FMN. Other 0.2-ml aliquots are placed in fluorometer tubes with no K_2HPO_4, tightly sealed with Parafilm,® and incubated in the dark at 37°C overnight or at room temperature for 2 days to permit hydrolysis of FAD to FMN. The hydrolyzed samples with suitable standards are neutralized with 1.0 ml of 0.2 M K_2HPO_4 exactly as for initial samples. After neutralization, care is taken to protect the samples from light; riboflavin and FMN are more sensitive to destruction by light in this concentrated salt solution than in more dilute salt solutions.

MEASUREMENTS. After setting the fluorometer with the fluorescein standard, the fluorescence of the two neutralized extracts is measured (reading "F_1"). Then add 10 µl of 10% sodium hydrosulfite, mix gently, and read again (reading "F_2"). An internal riboflavin standard can be omitted because the high dilution prevents interference from other sources; also the volume change caused by the addition of the reducing agent may be ignored because it is too low to be corrected for volume.

CALCULATIONS. The apparent riboflavin of the initial sample (R_i) and the hydrolyzed sample (R_t) in µg/g tissue is:

$$R_i = 10.94 \times \mu g \text{ riboflavin/ml in standard} \times \frac{(F_1 - F_2)_{sample}}{(F_1 - F_2)_{standard}}$$

$$R_t = 10.94 \times \mu g \text{ riboflavin/ml in standard} \times \frac{(F_1 - F_2)_{sample}}{(F_1 - F_2)_{standard}}$$

Under these conditions, FAD (calculated as riboflavin) has a fluorescence equal to 14% of riboflavin. FMN (calculated as riboflavin) and riboflavin are equal in fluorescence, so that

$$FAD = \frac{R_t - R_i}{0.86}$$

The balance of the flavin consists of FMN and free riboflavin:

$$R_t = FAD + \text{non-FAD riboflavin (FMN + riboflavin)}$$

FREE RIBOFLAVIN AND FMN. Since very little free riboflavin exists in tissues, the measurements described are normally adequate. The following procedure is used. To distinguish between free riboflavin and FMN:

1. Place 2.0 ml cold trichloroacetic acid tissue extract in a glass-stoppered centrifuge tube and neutralize immediately with 0.5 ml of 4 M K_2HPO_4.

2. Shake vigorously with 2.5 ml redistilled benzyl alcohol (saturated with water) and centrifuge to clear the solution.

The low concentrations of free riboflavin in tissues make it desirable to drive the riboflavin into an aqueous solution before measuring fluorescence. To do this:

3. Place 2.0 ml of the benzyl alcohol extract in a glass-stoppered

test tube; shake with 30 ml toluene and 2.0 ml of 0.5 M sodium acetate–acetic acid buffer. This procedure drives the flavins extracted by the benzyl alcohol into the aqueous layer. Standards are carried through the same procedure.

4. Measure the fluorescence as above on a 1.0-ml aliquot. The apparent µg riboflavin/g tissue extracted into benzyl alcohol = R_{BZ}.

CALCULATIONS. The partition coefficients between benzyl alcohol and 10% trichloroacetic acid for riboflavin, FAD, and FMN neutralized as described are 4.1, 0.032, and 0.02, respectively. The apparent riboflavin driven back into the aqueous phase is

$$R_{BZ} = 4.1/5.1 \text{ free riboflavin} + 0.032/1.032 \text{ FMN} + 0.02/1.02$$
$$\times 0.14 \text{ FAD}$$

By letting $R_{non\text{-}FAD}$ = FMN + free riboflavin, then:

Free riboflavin (µg/g tissue) = $1.3\ R_{BZ} - 0.04\ R_{non\text{-}FAD} - 0.003$ FAD

Less sensitive fluorometers require more concentrated extracts of tissues for measurements. An aliquot of the trichloroacetic acid supernatant is neutralized with one-fourth its volume of 4 M K_2HPO_4, instead of five times its volume of 0.2 M K_2HPO_4. Since interfering substances are not diluted out, an internal riboflavin standard should be measured for each sample, followed by reduction with hydrosulfite. Thus, the procedure and the calculation of the apparent riboflavin in each measured sample must be diluted accordingly. Low levels of riboflavin cannot be measured with precision on fluorometers of ordinary sensitivity. A fluorometer of the Farrand type is sensitive enough to measure 0.1 ng riboflavin/ml.

Recovery of riboflavin, FMN, and FAD added to minced tissue averages 95–100%. Values are reproducible within 1% or less.

2.1.2 Serum

The principle and techniques for determination of free riboflavin, FMN, and FAD in serum are the same as those described above for tissues.

Additional equipment besides that described is needed: (a) Serological tubes 6 × 50 mm; (b) Pyrex test tubes, 3-ml and 6-ml capacity; (c) Five 500-µl pipettes; and (d) redistilled chloroform C.P., saturated with water.

PROCEDURE

1. 50 µl of serum is mixed with 1.0 ml of 5% trichloroacetic acid at 0° C in a 3-ml tube. Larger quantities of serum may be used, but

this fact must be taken into account when dilutions and calculations are made.

2. To each of two fluorometric tubes, the first of which contains 0.1 ml of 2.4 M K_2HPO_4, is transferred 0.4 ml of the supernatant. The remaining sample is reserved for the determination of total riboflavin (see below). The apparent riboflavin content A of the tube containing the neutralized extract is measured in the fluorometer within 1-2 hr. *Keep tubes in the dark.* The tube is wiped and three readings are made with the instrument set against fluorescein: an initial reading, R_1; a second reading, R_2, after the addition of the internal riboflavin standard (5 μl, equal to 1 ng riboflavin); and a reduced reading R_3, after the addition of 5 μl of the sodium hydrosulfite solution (see *Reagents* above). Complete blank determinations are also made on reagents, usually in triplicate. A reading on a tube containing redistilled water is made as a measure of the contribution of scattered light and possible fluorescence of the tube itself. To measure the total riboflavin of the filtrate, the fluorometer tube containing the second sample is stoppered with a Parafilm® cork and allowed to hydrolyze in the dark at 37°C overnight. It is then neutralized with 0.1 ml of 2.4 M K_2HPO_4, and its apparent riboflavin content B is measured as described above. Mix all solutions thoroughly and keep tubes free of dust and marks.

CALCULATIONS. Readings R_2 and R_3 are corrected for the dilution resulting from the addition of internal standards and reducing agent and may be designated R_2' and R_3'. The reading for redistilled water is subtracted from the sample readings before correcting for dilution, because the contribution from scattered light would not be affected by dilution:

$$\frac{\text{μg riboflavin added}}{\text{ml serum in aliquot}} \times \frac{R_1 - R_3'}{R_2' - R_1} \times 100 = \text{μg percent riboflavin}$$

Appropriate correction is made in the above figure for blanks that have been treated and calculated in the same manner as the samples.

Because, under the conditions of measurement, FAD before hydrolysis is 14% as fluorescent as riboflavin, then:

$$FAD = \frac{B - A}{0.86}$$

Free riboflavin (+FMN) = $A - 0.14$ FAD = $1.163A - 0.163B$

Ordinarily very little FMN is present in serum.

To determine *total riboflavin*, as little as 25 μl of serum suffices.

The serum is precipitated with 0.5 ml of 5% trichloroacetic acid at room temperature and may be allowed to stand 30 min to 1 hr before centrifuging. A 0.4-ml aliquot is hydrolyzed and measured (as above). Avoid prolonged contact with the trichloroacetic acid as it increases the blank reading.

FREE RIBOFLAVIN, FMN, FAD. To determine *free riboflavin, FMN, and FAD,* a serum filtrate is prepared at 0–5°C, as described above, from 0.2 ml serum and 2.0 ml of 5% trichloroacetic acid in an 8-ml tube. Centrifuge and transfer 1.0 ml of the supernatant to a 3-ml tube containing 0.25 ml of 2.4 M K_2HPO_4 and mix immediately. Free riboflavin + FMN is measured on a 0.5-ml aliquot of this sample *A.* The total riboflavin is measured as above on a 0.4-ml aliquot of the remaining supernatant acid extract *B.* Then 2 ml benzyl alcohol is added to 0.75 ml of the remaining neutral extract. Mix this solution vigorously to extract the free riboflavin, centrifuge 5 min at 3000 rpm, and draw off all the benzyl alcohol. The aqueous extract is then extracted with 1 ml water-saturated chloroform and centrifuged; the chloroform extract removes the last of the benzyl alcohol and clarifies the aqueous phase. A 0.5-ml aliquot of the (upper) aqueous layer is transferred to a fluorometer tube and the apparent riboflavin *C* is measured as above.

CALCULATION. The distribution coefficients for riboflavin, FMN, and FAD between benzyl alcohol and the neutralized trichloroacetic acid extract are 3.8, 0.02, and 0.01, respectively.[13] Thus, when 0.75 ml of the remaining extract is added to 2 ml benzyl alcohol, the free riboflavin = $100 \times (3.8 \times 2)/(0.75 + 3.8 \times 2) = 91\%$, leaving 9% in the aqueous phase. Similarly, it may be calculated that 96% FMN + 98% FAD will be left behind after the benzyl alcohol extraction. The FAD left will show 14% fluorescence as equivalent amount of riboflavin. Thus, if *A, B,* and *C* are equal to the apparent riboflavin in the three samples above: *A* = free riboflavin + FMN + 0.14 FAD; *B* = total riboflavin; and *C* = 0.09 free riboflavin + 0.96 FMN + 0.14 FAD.

It may be calculated that:

$$\text{FAD} = \frac{B - A}{0.86}$$

Free riboflavin = $1.1A - 1.15C + 0.007B$

Since FMN is negligible, then free riboflavin = $1.1(A - C)$

FMN = B − FAD − free riboflavin

2.1.3. Red Cells

Remove plasma, all white cells, and platelets by differential centrifugation. Pack the red cells by centrifuging at 4°C for 1 hr. Remove any supernatant. Remove 20 μl and rinse into 1 ml of 1% NaCl. The suspension may be frozen for analysis. This mixture is then mixed with 3 ml of 13% trichloroacetic acid and allowed to stand 30-60 min, mixed again, and centrifuged for 10 min at 3000 rpm. The clear supernatant is allowed to hydrolyze at 37°C overnight. Aliquots of 0.4 ml are pipetted into fluorometer tubes containing 0.1 ml of 4 M K_2HPO_4. The reducible fluorescence with sodium hydrosulfite is measured as above. These readings must be made promptly because there may be a partial reoxidation of the sample.

2.1.4. Whole Blood

Riboflavin may be determined as for red cells, except that a less dilute extract is prepared. Twenty microliters of blood are delivered into 2 ml of 10% trichloroacetic acid. The mixture is shaken to prevent clumping. The rest of the analyses is carried out as with red cells. Do not permit the acid extract to remain in contact with the protein precipitate for much over 1 hr at room temperature, or 2-3 hr at 4°C.

Recovery of riboflavin and FAD with this fluorometric procedure ranges 98-102%.[13] Riboflavin and FAD content of serum from well-nourished adults in μg percent is: free riboflavin + FMN = 0.3 − 1.3; FAD = 1.8 − 3.0; and total riboflavin = 2.6 − 3.7. The total riboflavin range for *red cells* is 18.0 − 26.2.

2.1.5. Urine

Urine is collected in dark containers with 1 ml glacial acetic acid added as preservative. Urinary riboflavin is extracted into a butanol-pyridine mixture after permanganate oxidation of some interfering substances. The blank is prepared by destruction of the riboflavin internal standard by irradiation with artificial light. The method presented here[34,37] is a modification of other methods.[36,40] The version below was designed to assay riboflavin in urine; it does not differ in specificity and reproducibility from older methods and is less time consuming.

REAGENTS
1. *Acetic acid,* glacial.
2. *Potassium permanganate,* 5%. dissolve 5.0 g $KMnO_4$ in 100 ml water and filter. Prepare fresh weekly.

3. *Hydrogen peroxide, 3%.* Dilute 1 ml of 30% H_2O_2 (Superoxol, Merck) with 9 ml water.

4. *Na_2SO_4* (granular, anhydrous, reagent grade).

5. *Butanol-pyridine mixture.* To 8 ml glass-redistilled pyridine add 92 ml glass-redistilled *n*-butanol. To recover after use, make mixture alkaline with 30% NaOH and filter off the brown precipitate. Distill and collect the 93°-118°C fraction and add enough pyridine to make it 8% by volume.

6. *Fluorescein.* Dissolve 10 mg sodium fluorescein in 1 liter distilled water. For use, dilute 1:200.

7. *Riboflavin standard.* Riboflavin standards should be made as described above. The working standard should contain 1 μg/ml.

EQUIPMENT

Photofluorometer. A Coleman 12C with B_2 and PC-2 filters is suitable.

Wooden irradiation rack. This rack has forty-four 20-mm holes drilled equidistant from a 200-W bulb that is installed in the center. It is approximately 15 cm high and designed to accommodate 19×150 mm cuvettes. It should be open on all sides for ventilation; otherwise, the tubes become too warm. Laboratory test tube racks can suffice if tubes are placed in the racks in single file equidistant from the light source.

SAMPLE.

One milliliter urine can be used directly without extraction.

PROCEDURE.

All operations should be conducted in dim light or with brown "low actinic" glassware.

1. Pipette 0.5 ml glacial acetic acid into glass-stoppered test tubes (16×150 mm). Each sample requires two tubes, *A* and *B*.

2. To *A* and *B* add 1.0 ml urine. Prepare a set of blanks by adding 1.0 ml water instead of urine, *C*. One blank per each series of analyses is needed.

3. Add 0.5 ml distilled water to tube *A* and 0.5 ml riboflavin standard to tube *B*. Treat blank similarly.

4. Add 0.5 ml of 5% $KMnO_4$ to each tube, mix, and let stand for 1 minute.

5. Add 0.5 ml of 3% H_2O_2 to each tube and mix gently.

6. Add 10 ml butanol–pyridine solution.

7. Shake well for 30 sec and let stand in dark for 10 min.

8. Remove, and discard the (bottom) aqueous layer by suction with a long-needle syringe.

9. Add Na_2SO_4 (about 1.5 g) using a small powder funnel.

10. Shake and place in dark for 10-15 min and then decant the clear supernatant into Coleman cuvettes (19 × 150 mm).

11. Set the photofluorometer at 80 with the fluoroscein standard and read each sample.

12. Place the cuvettes into the irradiation rack and irradiate until 80-90% of the riboflavin standard is destroyed. Periodically check the reagent blank containing riboflavin at 15-min intervals to determine the best irradiation time. Usually 1 hr is required if a 200-W bulb is used.

13. Reread all tubes. The average urine containing about 0.5 μg riboflavin per milliliter will read about 20-30 units with a recovery of 15-20 additional units.

CALCULATIONS

1. $A - A'$ (after irradiation) = deflection due to riboflavin destruction in unknown.

2. $B - B'$ (after irradiation) = deflection due to riboflavin destruction in recovery.

3. $C - C'$ (after irradiation) = change in reagent blank fluorescence induced by irradiation.

4.
$$\frac{(A - A') - (C - C')}{[(B - B') - (C - C')] - [(A - A') - (C - C')]} \times 0.5$$

= μg riboflavin in tube.

If 1.0 ml was the original volume of urine used, then this amount of riboflavin was present in 1.0 ml. If dilutions of urine were originally made, the riboflavin content of the sample is calculated by using the dilution factor. For example:

	Unknown cuvette	Recovery cuvette	Blank cuvette
Before irradiation:	30(A)	50(B)	1.0(C)
After irradiation:	8(A')	10(B')	0(C')
Difference	22	40	1.0

Applying the above formula, we then have:

$$\frac{22 - 1.0}{(40 - 1) - (22 - 1)} \times 0.5 = (21/18) \times 0.5 - 0.58 \text{ μg riboflavin per tube}$$

The reagent blank C usually has no change in fluorescene; hence, in most cases, it can be ignored in calculations. The determination for urine can be interrupted for a while after the first readings if immediate irradiation is inconvenient. Tubes can be stoppered with corks. Do not use rubber stoppers because butanol-pyridine disintegrates rubber.

2.2. Enzyme Analysis for Riboflavin Status

In studying inhibition of glutathione reductase by nitrofurantoin, [14,15] the enzymes from rat erythrocytes, liver, and kidney proved to be inactivated by acid treatment, and activity was restored specifically by addition of FAD—the first indication that the glutathione reductase of animal tissues is a flavoenzyme. Further investigation[11] showed that addition of 1 μM FAD increased by two- or threefold the glutathione reductase activity of hemolysates from glutathione reductase-deficient red cells from some subjects without overt nutritional deficiency. [11] Also, administration of 5 mg riboflavin daily for 5 days to a riboflavin-deficient subject doubled glutathione reductase activity with only a slight rise in red cell FAD levels. [9,11,45] Red cell glutathione reductase activity in normal subjects increased only slightly with a modest rise of the FAD levels. Red cell riboflavin levels, as well as glutathione reductase activity per se, were significantly lower in a clinically riboflavin-deficient group as compared to normals; both indices showed significant improvement after treatment. [7] Red cell riboflavin levels did not show much change in normal or, more surprisingly, in deficient subjects. [8] Since enzyme activity depends on the FAD content of red cells and most red cell riboflavin occurs as FAD, a lack of correlation between red cell riboflavin and the enzyme activity is puzzling. Perhaps there are alterations in the conversion of FMN to FAD during a riboflavin deficiency[17] due to an alteration in $NADPH_2$ activity. [43]

At any rate, since red cell glutathione reductase is one of two flavoproteins in the red cell requiring FAD, its measurement has been suggested as a determinant of the nutritional status of riboflavin in man. [21,22,45] The other flavoprotein-containing coenzyme in human red cells is NADH-dependent "diaphorase," but this system has not been applied for analytic work. The method presented here takes into account that $NADPH_2$-dependent glutathione reductase is a flavoprotein having FAD as prosthetic group. In cases of suboptimal supply to red cells, in which the protein part of red cell glutathione reductase has insufficient FAD, its addition to the red cell hemolysate could stimulate the enzyme activity. This result be checked by measuring the diminution of $NADPH_2$ by hemolyzed red cells in the presence of oxidized glutathione in the following overall reaction:

$$GSSG + NADPH_2 \underset{}{\overset{Enzyme FAD}{\rightleftharpoons}} 2\, GSH + NADP$$

Stimulation of enzyme activity *in vitro* depends on the FAD saturation of the protein, which in turn depends on the availability of FAD or riboflavin. Thus the percentage of stimulation of the $NADPH_2$-dependent red cell glutathione reductase in the presence of FAD can be used as an index of riboflavin status.[21,44,45] The method is described below.

REAGENTS

1. 0.1 M *potassium phosphate* buffer, pH 7.4, made in distilled water.

2. *Nicotinamide-adenine dinucleotide phosphate,* reduced $NADPH_2$ (Sigma, St. Louis, Mo.), prepared by dissolving 16.6 mg tetrasodium salt in 10 ml of 1% sodium bicarbonate. Prepare fresh daily and keep in ice.

3. *Oxidized glutathione* (Sigma). Dissolve 46 mg in 10 ml double-distilled water; add 0.1 ml of 1 N NaOH. Prepare fresh daily.

4. *Flavin adenine dinucleotide,* monosodium salt (FAD; Sigma). Dissolve 2.4 mg in 10 ml double-distilled water. Prepared fresh daily and keep in dark.

5. *Dipotassium ethylenediaminetetraacetate* (EDTA-K_2; Sigma). Dissolve 1.5 g in 50 ml double-distilled water.

EQUIPMENT. A Gilford recording spectrophotometer, model 2400, set at 340 nm, 37° C, with a chart speed of 4 mm/inch and a dwell time of 6 sec.[44] If this instrument is not available, one can use an Eppendorf photometer, preferably equipped with devices for changing the cuvettes automatically in a heatable cuvette holder and for recording the periodically measured absorbance of the samples. Set at 340 nm.[22]

2.2.1. Blood

The following assay makes use of only venous blood; results with other tissues have not yet been reported.

Blood is obtained from fasted subjects. Ethylenediaminetetraacetate or "ACD" (7.3 g anhydrous citric acid, 22.0 g sodium citrate dihydrate, 24.5 g D-glucose monohydrate, distilled water to 1 liter) may be used as an anticoagulant. When using ACD, use 3 ml blood for every 0.75 ml ACD solution. Samples must be placed in ice immediately. The blood is washed three times with cold 0.85% soidum chloride solution in about 1:6 ratio. The suspension is centrifuged for 10-15 min—each time about 500 g in glass tubes. The supernatant is discarded; after the third washing, the white cells should be completely removed. The remaining red cell concentrate, which contains about 70-90% red cell, is diluted twentyfold with ice-cold water and hemolyzed by letting it stand in an ice bath for 30 min. The cell debris is removed by centrifugation for 15 min, and the clear supernatant is kept another hr at 0°C. This standing was advantageous since it allowed better reproducibility.[22] The exact dilution of the red cells is not critical as long as identical amounts of hemolysate are used in the procedure.

PROCEDURE. Two cuvettes are necessary for each determination since the red cell glutathione reductase activity is compared with and without FAD addition. Keep all solutions in ice during preparation of the assay. The diluted hemolysate obtained above was assayed for glutathione reductase with the Gilford spectrophotometer set at 340 nm, 37° C (see above, *Equipment*) in the following manner:[44]

1. Two cuvettes were prepared with each containing:

  2.0 ml phosphate buffer   0.1 ml oxidized glutathione
  0.1 ml hemolysate   0.05 ml EDTA-K_2 solution

2. To one cuvette add 0.1 ml FAD solution; add 0.1 ml distilled water to the other cuvette.

3. Allow the cuvettes to equilibrate in the spectrophotometer at 37° C. for 8 min.

4. After equilibration is complete add 0.1 ml $NADPH_2$ solution to each cuvette.

5. Read the change in optical absorption for 10 min.

It is usually helpful to include a reference blood sample routinely in the assays.

CALCULATIONS. The activity coefficient (AC) is defined as the reduction of absorbance (oxidation) of $NADPH_2$ in the presence of FAD (A_2) divided by the reduction of absorbance of $NADPH_2$ without added FAD (A_1) for a given period. In this case, the given period is 10 min, that is:

$$AC = \frac{A_2}{A_1} = \frac{\text{reduction of absorbance } with \text{ FAD for 10 min}}{\text{reduction of absorbance } without \text{ FAD for 10 min}}$$

Classifications of AC based on human studies to date[22, 45] are

  AC = 0.9-1.3. No biochemical evidence of riboflavin deficiency.
  AC = less than 1.0. May be due to inhibition of the reaction by an unknown factor in the FAD.
  AC = 1.3-1.8. Requires attention to and correction of dietary habits as biochemical evidence of riboflavin deficiency is apparent.
  AC = greater than 1.8. Requires medical attention. Riboflavin treatment is rapid in repairing the biochemical lesion, although probable involvement of other B vitamins cannot be discounted.[45]

3. MICROBIAL METHODS FOR ASSAY OF RIBOFLAVIN

3.1. *Tetrahymena pyriformis* Method

This method is based on the protozoan ciliate, *Tetrahymena pyriformis*, syngen 1, mating type II (ATCC No. 30008), which requires riboflavin.[26] The method is extremely useful for measuring total riboflavin in biologic fluids and tissues.[3,5]

TABLE I. *Basal Medium for Riboflavin Assay Using* Tetrahymena pyriformis

Constituents[a]	Amount	Constituents[a]	Amount
Hycase SF[b]	12,000 mg	Pyridoxal HCl[f]	0.3 mg
HEDTA[c]	100 mg	Pyridoxamine 2HCl[f]	0.3 mg
MgSo$_4$·7H$_2$O	400 mg	Pyrodoxine HCl[f]	0.3 mg
KH$_2$PO$_4$	100mg	Ca pantothenate[f]	1 mg
Metals mix[d]	100 mg	DL-Thioctic (lipoic) acid[f]	0.1 mg
Ca^{2+}[e]	50 mg	Glycine	100 mg
Citric acid·H$_2$O	200 mg	Sodium acetate (anhyd.)	600 mg
L-Tryptophan	100 mg	Na$_3$ guanylate·4H$_2$O[g]	120 mg
DL-Methionine	100 mg	Yeast adenylic acid[g]	25 mg
Diacetin	1 ml	Cytidylic acid[g]	30 mg
Nicotinic acid[f]	1 mg	Uracil[g]	10 mg
Nicotinamide[f]	1 mg	Thymidine	10 mg
Thiamin HCl[f]	0.5 mg	Glucose	1500 mg
Folic acid[f]	0.1 mg	Biotin[f]	0.005 mg
Soluble starch[h]	10,000 mg	Distilled water	to 500 ml

[a] Boil to dissolve components. Upon cooling, the pH is readjusted to 6.0 with KOH. The basal medium is then brought to final volume. Store at 4° C with preservative (see page 52) Medium is stable for 3 months.
[b] Acid-hydrolyzed casein; salt free (Sheffield Chemical Co., Union, N.J.).
[c] Hydroxyethylethylenediamine triacetic acid, a nonmetabolizable metal chelator ("Chel DM Acid," Geigy Pharmaceuticals, Ardsley, N.Y.).
[d] Metals mix: a triturate sufficient for 1000 liters is prepared before preparation of the basal medium. ZnSO$_4$·7H$_2$O, 34.8 g; MnSO$_4$·H$_2$O, 20.8 g; Fe(NH$_4$)$_2$(SO$_4$)$_2$·6H$_2$O, 38.5 g; CoSO$_4$·7H$_2$O, 3.55 g; CuSO$_4$·5H$_2$O, 880 mg; (NH$_4$)$_6$Mo$_7$O$_{24}$·4H$_2$O, 610 mg; Na$_3$VO$_4$·Me16H$_2$O, 370 mg; and H$_3$BO$_3$, 910 mg. Grind in a mortar and store in the cold.
[e] CaCo$_3$, 25g, dissolved in minimal concentrated HCl and brought to 100 ml with distilled water yields a solution containing 100 mg Ca^{++}/1 ml solution.
[f] Vitamins are added from stock solutions.
[g] Dissolve while boiling with a few drops of 10% KOH; then add to other constituents.
[h] Soluble starch (Eastman, soluble reagent ACS). Dissolve by autoclaving separately in distilled water for 10 min. Add to cool basal medium.

MAINTENANCE MEDIUM. The maintenance medium is made by autoclaving 9 ml of 1.1% Proteose-peptone (Difco, Detroit, Mich.) solution for 30 min at 15 psi, pH 7.0, in 25 × 150 mm screw-capped borosilicate tubes. After cooling, 1 ml of a 10% separately sterilized glucose solution is added aseptically. Transfers are made every 3-4 days into fresh maintenance medium; one drop of the culture is used for transfer. The organism grows best at temperatures of 29°-32° C. The tubed medium can be stored in the cold indefinitely.

BASAL MEDIUM. The assay medium is given in Table I.

TABLE II. Methods for Assay of Riboflavin in Human and Rat Biologic Fluids and Tissues

---

Blood: Serum[a]
  1. 1 ml blood or serum plus 1 ml buffer.
  2. Autoclave 5 min and cool.
  3. Add 8 ml Clarase (2 mg/ml) dissolved in distilled water. Mince coagulum and add 1 or 2 drops volatile preservative.
  4. Incubate suspension overnight at 37° C.
  5. Autoclave 5 min.
  6. Centrifuge: add 1.0, 1.5, and 2.0 ml supernatant (Table III).
Urine:
  1. 1 ml urine plus 1 ml buffer.
  2. Autoclave 10 min.
  3. Add 8 ml distilled water.
  4. Centrifuge if necessary; assay 0.5, 1.0, and 1.5 ml supernatant (Table III).
Liver:
  1. Suspend 10 mg lyophilized liver in 1 ml distilled water.
  2. Incubate 3 days at 37° C with 1 or 2 drops volatile preservative.
  3. Autoclave 30 min.
  4. Add 9 ml distilled water.
  5. Centrifuge: assay 0.5, 1.0, and 1.5 ml supernatant (Table III).
Muscle: Brain[a]
  1. Suspend 50 mg lyophilized powder in 1 ml buffer.
  2. Autoclave 15 min and cool.
  3. Add 4 ml Clarase (4 mg/ml) dissolved in distilled water. Add 1 or 2 drops volatile preservative.
  4. Incubate 3 days at 37° C.
  5. Autoclave 15 min.
  6. Centrifuge; assay 0.5, 1.0, and 1.5 ml supernatant (Table III).

---

[a] An enzyme control, treated as the specimen, is included to check the riboflavin content of the enzyme; the riboflavin contamination usually is insignificant.

TABLE III. Preparation of Standard Riboflavin and Sample Curves[a]

| Flask number | Riboflavin (ng/ml) | Made from riboflavin standards | | Distilled water additions (ml) |
		Addition (ml)	Standard (μg/ml)	
1	0	0	0	2.5
2	1	0.5	0.01	2.0
3	3	1.5	0.01	1.0
4	10	0.5	0.1	2.0
5	30	1.5	0.1	1.0
6	100	0.5	1.0	2.0
7	300	1.5	1.0	1.0

Flask number	Sample number	Sample additions (ml)	Distilled water additions (ml)
8	1	1.0	1.5
9	1	1.5	1.0
10	1	2.0	0.5

[a]A control flask (No. 1), consisting of 2.5 ml basal medium and 2.5 ml distilled water without riboflavin added, is included in the standard curve to check the riboflavin carryover from the inoculum; the carryover usually is negligible. Samples follow in a consecutive order of three flasks (for example, No. 8, 9, 10; 11, 12, 13; and so forth), additions to the flasks are facilitated by placing them in vertical rows so that common water additions, basal medium addition with an Aupette® (Clay-Adams, New York), and sample volumes can be pipetted without error. An enzyme control is treated like the samples.

SAMPLES AND PROCEDURES. The preparation of biologic fluids and ly-ophilized tissues used for assay is outlined in Table II. To prepare the buffer dissolve 3.3 g sodium citrate·$2H_2O$ and 1.2 g citric acid·H_2O in distilled water, then add water to 1 liter; the pH should be 5.0. The enzyme (Clarase-Diastase, Fisher Scientific Co.) is dissolved in water. In surveying commercially available enzymes (Pronase,® papain, Mylase P,® several phosphatases), we found Clarase best. Clarase is a standardized preparation; enzyme activity did not vary from batch to batch and there was no riboflavin contamination.

3.1.1. Whole Blood and Serum

Whole blood is citrated. Serum is collected by permitting blood to clot at room temperature and centrifuging off the clot. Blood, serum, and urine may be stored frozen before assay. Autoclaving in acid buffer and enzyme treatment (Table II) deproteinizes flavin mononucleotide and flavin adenine dinucleotide into their free forms. Autoclaving after incubation of the blood- or serum-buffer enzyme suspension stops enzymatic action. The supernatant is obtained by centrifuging off the debris. The procedure then follows that outlined in Tables II and III. Final dilutions of the blood or serum are 1:50, 1:33, and 1:25, respectively, when the procedure (Table III) is followed. We prefer blood for assay, since values almost always fall on the linear portion of the curve; serum values sometimes fall on the less sensitive, that is, less steep portion. Values derived from the dilutions used in the assay are reproducible, usually within 5% for each dilution used when values fall on the linear portion of the curve; day-to-day sample reproducibility is within 10%. Recovery of 100 ng/ml of riboflavin added to biologic fluid was 93–101%; recovery of 50 ng/mg of lyophilized tissue was 86–94%.

3.1.2. Urine

An aliquot of a 24-hr urine sample is used for assays since it represents total daily riboflavin excretion. Enzyme treatment is unnecessary— neither riboflavin nor any of its forms is bound to protein in the urine. Urine is autoclaved with buffer to precipitate salts that may be toxic to the assay organism; if proteinuria exists, this procedure will free the riboflavin. The urine (treated as outlined in Table II) is assayed, as for blood and serum, and the results are expressed as total riboflavin in a 24-hr sample; final dilutions of urine are 1:100, 1:50, 1:33 for assay (Tables II and III). If aliquots of a 24-hr sample are used, one may calculate the riboflavin in the total aliquot.

3.1.3. Tissues

Tissues obtained by needle biopsy or autopsy, or from animals are freed from coagulum and adhering tissues, sliced thin, washed five times in saline solution, homogenized in saline in a blender or with a tissue grinder, and then lyophilized. This procedure standardizes determinations since wet weight values fluctuate. The nitrogen content of the tissue should be determined as a measure of tissue protein; this step is necessary when dealing with diseased tissues. Other indices, for example, deoxyribonucleic acid phosphorus, may serve as well.[20]

3.1.4. Liver

Liver is prepared for assay as described in Table II. Enzyme is not used since liver contains all enzymes necessary for liberating riboflavin during the autolytic period. The procedure outlined (Tables II and III) has 0.1, 0.2, and 0.3 mg dried liver/ml of assay medium.

3.1.5. Muscle and Brain

The tissues are prepared for assay as indicated in Tables II and III, and 1, 2, and 3 mg dried tissue/ml of final assay medium are used. We found that enzymatic hydrolysis is necessary to liberate riboflavin from these tissues in contrast to liver.

STANDARD AND SAMPLE CURVES. The standard and sample curves are plotted by making additions to 2.5 ml basal medium per 25-ml flask (micro-Fernbach Kimble) as outlined in Table III. Riboflavin equivalents are used for the standard curve. Because riboflavin does not dissolve easily, Na-riboflavin-5-PO_4 dihydrate was used as a standard; 1.0 mg equals 0.73 mg riboflavin. One hundred milligrams are dissolved in 73 ml hot distilled water. This solution contains 1 mg/ml of riboflavin. Tenfold dilutions of this stock solution are made serially in distilled water to obtain working standards of 0.01, 0.1, and 0.1 μg/ml of riboflavin. Fresh standards are prepared monthly and stored frozen in amber polyethylene bottles.

All results are calculated by plotting the concentration of riboflavin in the standard curve (nanograms per milliliter) on a log scale (abscissa) and optical density as the arithmetic ordinate; calculations must take final dilutions into account.

STERILIZATION, INOCULATION, INCUBATION, AND CALCULATION. When the additions to the individual flasks have been completed (Tables II and III), the flasks are covered with No. 6, autoclavable polypropylene stoppers (Pioneer Plastics, Jacksonville, Fla.), placed into Pyrex utility trays (Corning No. 232), and autoclaved for 30 min. Pressure within the autoclave is released slowly by manual or automatic "slow exhaust" to prevent boiling over. Upon removal from the autoclave, the trays are placed on a table (preferably metal for rapid cooling) away from direct light and drafts. The trays containing the sterile flasks are immediately covered with duplicate inverted trays and permitted to cool to room temperature. Tray covers are removed temporarily for the inoculation of flasks. Two milliliters of a 3- to 4-day-old maintenance culture are suspended in 10 ml sterile distilled water; one drop of the suspension is then added to each assay flask. The cover is replaced, and the edges of the adjoining top and bottom tray are sealed with tape. The tray cover makes a convenient writing surface. Assay flasks are incubated for 3 days at 29–32° C. Growth is expressed in optical density units as measured with a Welch Densichron® equipped with a red-sensitive probe (Sargent-Welch Co., Chicago, Ill.). Optical density of 1.0 equals 0.5–0.55 g dried organism per liter.

For reading growth densities, any sensitive photoelectric instrument with a linear output is suitable. It is convenient to use instruments sensitive enough to measure absorbancies up to 2.0 and to graph for each organism the corrected absorbance plotted against readings; the correct value is derived by extrapolation to infinite dilution. A Klett–Summerson photoelectric colorimeter with a red filter (640–700 nm) reduces error due to the color of the medium; a Coleman Jr. Spectrophotometer at 650 nm may also be used.

Growth densities (ordinate) of the standard vitamin concentrations per milliliter (abscissa) are plotted on semilogarithmic paper (Keuffel and Esser, #46-5490, three-cycle), and values of the unknown are calculated from the standard curve.

Calculations for obtaining total riblflavin content are:

FLUIDS
> a = concentration of vitamin standard (ng/ml) as derived from sample OD
> b = volume of sample when diluted with buffer or water
> c = total volume of sample in growth flasks
> d = ml (volume) sample used for test
> e = ml (volume) diluted sample (sample + diluent) added to the assay flask

$$\frac{a \cdot b \cdot c}{d \cdot e} = \text{ng riboflavin in sample/ml}$$

For urine; multiple by total 24-hr volume and express per 24-hr sample.

TISSUES
> a = concentration of vitamin standard (ng/ml) as derived from sample OD
> c = total volume in growth flasks
> d = ml (volume) of sample used for test
> e = ml (volume) of diluted sample)sample + diluent) added to the assay flask

$$\frac{a \cdot c}{d \cdot e} = \text{ng riboflavin/mg sample}$$

As mentioned, enzyme controls usually have insignificant riboflavin content; if the control does contain some riboflavin activity, it should be subtracted from the sample.

TABLE IV. Riboflavin Values in Biologic Fluids and Tissues from Normal Subjects

Sample	Source and number of samples	Range	Mean
Blood (ng/1 ml)	Human subject, 798	100–500	200 ± 85
	Rat, 210	150–350	260 ± 63
Serum (ng/1 ml)	Human subject, 798	38–240	100 ± 60
	Rat, 210	30–100	60 ± 24
Urine (mg/24 hr)	Human subject, 85	0.3–2.5	1.0 ± 0.5
Liver (ng/1 mg)	Human subject, 29	20–60	40 ± 9
	Rat, 70	100–300	160 ± 50
Muscle (ng/1 mg)	Human subject, 14	14–25	18 ± 3
	Rat, 72	3–10	6 ± 2
Brain (ng/1 mg)	Human Subject, (whole brain), 4	7–17	13 ± 3
	Human subject (gray matter) 4	8–13	11 ± 2
	Rat, (whole brain) 18	15–35	20 ± 5

Table IV gives representative "normal" ranges and mean riboflavin levels in human and rat biologic fluids and tissues. The ranges given represent a survey of nonhospitalized subjects selected at random; all had been in good health. Values 20% below the lowest range figures listed were arbitrarily designated as indicative of riboflavin deficiency. Justification for this designation was derived from the observations that subjects with poor dietary habits usually had levels 20% below the lower limit of normal as listed in Table IV.

Enzyme (Clarase) digestion of fluids and tissues was necessary; autoclaving in buffer did not release all the bound vitamin. Overnight enzyme hydrolysis permitted increased riboflavin release (Table II). Subsequent autoclaving, acid digestion, and longer enzymatic hydrolysis did not increase riboflavin titer.

Tetrahymena pyriformis responds equally well on a molar basis to riboflavin, FMN, and FAD; use of *T. pyriformis* therefore permits estimation of total riboflavin.

3.2. *Lactobacillus casei* Method

Few free-living bacteria require riboflavin; nearly all of those that do require riboflavin are lactic acid bacteria.

Lactobacillus casei also uses FMN and FAD. The growth response is not proportional to the molar concentration of riboflavin in these analogs.[30] Interfering substances, for example, fatty acids in biologic fluids and tissues,[25,37] may detract from the usefulness of *L. casei* as a specific reagent for riboflavin in such materials. Also, *L. casei* responds to many other riboflavin analogs that may or may not have biologic activity.[48]

The classic microbiologic assay for riboflavin with *L. casei*[37] is based upon the many publications of Snell.[41,42] We modified this method to simplify preparation of media and other steps. The method given here eliminated high blanks and some of the drifts seen with the standard methods.[37] It has worked well for us in assaying fat-free, riboflavin-rich materials; however, for biologic fluids and tissues we prefer to use *T. pyriformis* because of its sensitivity and specificity for riboflavin and its congeners.

CULTURE; MAINTENANCE MEDIUM; BASAL MEDIUM. *Lactobacillus casei* (ATCC 7469) is obtainable from the American Type Culture Collection (Rockville, Md.). The culture is maintained in the medium listed in Table V. Follow footnotes for instructions. The medium for riboflavin assay is given in Table VI. It can also be used to assay for serum folate if folic acid is omitted and 0.5 mg riboflavin is included.[3] It may be stored at 4°C for 2 months with added preservative (see page 52).

SAMPLES AND PROCEDURES. Preparation of biologic fluids and tissues used for riboflavin assay with *L. casei* is the same as listed in Tables II and III for the *T. pyriformis* assay method (pages 64–65).

TABLE V. Maintenance Medium for Lactobacillus casei

Constituent[a]	Milligrams
Proteose-peptone 2[b]	750
Yeast extract[b]	750
Glucose	1000
KH_2PO_4	200
Tomato juice-filtrate[c]	10 ml
Tween 80[d]	10
L-Cysteine HCl	100
Distilled water	To 100 ml

[a]The pH is adjusted to 6.8–7.0 with KOH. Ten-ml quantities are distributed into 20 × 125 mm screw-capped test tubes and autoclaved for 30 min. The organism is maintained by transferring one drop into sterile maintenance medium, and incubating overnight at 37°C; storage between weekly transfers is at 4°C. *For inoculum*, one drop is transferred to sterile maintenance medium and incubated for 18–24 hr, or 1 ml of a maintained culture to sterile maintenance medium is incubated for 6–8 hr; cultures are incubated at 37°C in the dark.
[b]Difco, Detroit, Mich.
[c]Filtrate is adjusted to pH 7.0 with KOH before addition to the maintenance medium.
[d]Polyoxyethylene sorbitan monooleate (Atlas Powder Co., Wilmington, Del.). A 10% solution is made in 50% alcohol.

TABLE VI. *Medium for Riboflavin Assay Using Lactobacillus casei*[a]

Constiuents	Concentration in final medium (mg/liter)
Hy-Case[b]	5,000
L-Tryptophan	100
Adenine[c]	10
Guanine HCl[c]	10
Uracil[c]	10
Xanthine[c]	20
L-Asparagine·H$_2$O	300
L-Cysteine HCl	250
Folic acid	0.01
p-Aminobenzoic acid	1.0
Pyridoxine HCL	2.0
Thiamin HCl	0.2
Ca pantothenate	0.4
Nicotinic acid	0.4
Biotin	0.01
Glucose	20,000
Glutathione (reduced)	2.5
Salt mix[d]	5 ml
Na acetate (anhydrous)	20,000
K$_2$HPO$_4$	500
KH$_2$PO$_4$	500
MnSO$_4$H$_2$O[e]	100
Distilled water	To 500 ml

[a]pH 6.6-6.8 (adjusted with H$_2$SO$_4$ or KOH). Boil to dissolve components.
[b]Salt-free hydrochloric acid hydrolysate of casein (Sheffield Chemical Co., Union, N.J.)
[c]Dissolve while boiling with a few drops of 10% KOH; then add to other components.
[d]1.0 ml contains MgSO$_4$·7H$_2$O, 40 mg; NaCl, 2 mg; MnSO$_4$·4H$_2$O, 2 mg; FeSO$_4$·7H$_2$O, 2 mg.
[e]Added slowly after pH adjustment; medium must be cold.

STANDARDS AND SAMPLE CURVES. Preparations are the same as for the *T. pyriformis* assay (pages 64-65) with one exception: The standards and sample curves (Table III) are added to 2.5 ml basal medium/10-ml flasks (microFernbach, Kimble Glass, Toledo, Ohio).

STERILIZATION, INOCULATION, INCUBATION, AND CALCULATIONS. These are the same as for *T. pyriformis*, except: (a) The inoculum is prepared by suspending 1 ml of a 6- to 8-hour culture (see footnote, Table V) in 10 ml sterile distilled water; one drop of this suspension is added to each assay flask (Table III); the riboflavin carryover is negligible. (b) Assay flasks are incubated for 18-24 hours at 37°C. The suspension should be well agitated before turbidity measurements are made.

MEASUREMENT OF ACIDITY. An alternate method for measurement of turbidity after 18-24° C incubation is acidimetry of the lactic acid produced by *L. casei* as a concomitant of growth; the more growth, the more acid. For titration of acid, the flasks must be incubated for at least 60 hr. If necessary, they can be left in the cold (4°C) for up to 2 days before analysis.

REAGENTS. Bromthymol blue solution (0.1%). Dissolve 100 mg bromthymol blue in a few ml of 95% ethyl alcohol, add 1.6 ml 0.1 N NaOH, and dilute to 100 ml with distilled water.

NaOH (0.1 N). Dissolve 4.4 g of NaOH pellets in a little water and dilute to 1 liter. There is no need to standardize this solution, but it is necessary to use the same batch of reagent for titration of any one series of flasks.

PROCEDURE. Transfer the contents of each flask to a 50-ml Erlenmeyer flask, rinse the tube with 5 ml distilled water, and add the rinsing to the flask. Add about 0.2 ml of 0.1% bromthymol blue (medicine dropper) and titrate with 0.1 N NaOH to a green color—about pH 6.8. All flasks should be titrated to the same end point. A convenient end point to use is the yellow-to-green change normally observed on addition of a small amount (0.5-1.0 ml) of 0.1 N NaOH to the blank flask of the standard curve. For extensive assays, use a glass-electrode titration assembly, which has the advantage of eliminating the elusive end point.

A standard curve (ml 0.1/N NaOH *vs.* ng riboflavin/flask) is plotted on linear graph paper. The riboflavin content of each tube is determined by interpolation from the standard curve, and the concentration of riboflavin in the sample is calculated by application of the appropriate dilution factors.

4. COMMENTS AND CLINICAL APPLICATIONS

Life on earth cannot exist in the absence of flavin coenzymes. The particular flavin that satisfies all the requirements of an independent organism, whatever the type, is riboflavin. Riboflavin is essential for growth and tissue repair in all animals from protozoa to man. [3,25]

Many laboratory procedures available are not entirely satisfactory for appraising overall riboflavin nutrition. Urinary excretion of riboflavin is quite variable; thus, caution should be used in interpreting such findings. Because of interfering substances and technical difficulties, chemical and animal methods have not been used widely for biologic fluids and tissues. Such difficulties have restricted riboflavin estimation to the urinary excretion in terms of μg/g of creatinine, with inconsistent results. *Tetrahymena pyriformis* as assay organism for riboflavin in biologic fluids and tissues has proved valuable in assessing riboflavin status in man and animals. [3,5] The riboflavin requirement for *T. pyriformis* is specific, sensitive, rapid, and reproducible enough for assaying large numbers of biologic fluids and tissues. Superaddition of amino acids and vitamins; lecithin; diacetyl tartaric acid ester of tallow glycerides, lauric, palmitic, myristic, and oleic acids; triolein, cholesterol; lanosterol; β-sitosterol; mevalonic acid lactone; farnesol; and squalene at 1.0–10 mg/ml did not relieve galactoflavin inhibition or spare riboflavin for *T. pyriformis*. Lipids and fatty acids result in too high riboflavin values when other assay organisms, for example, *Lactobacillus casei*, [25,37,42] are used—an obvious drawback when dealing with fatty acid- and lipid-rich fluids and tissues. In any assay of tissue and biologic fluids, growth stimulation of the assay organism by unknown factors is often difficult to avoid. In the assay of fluids and tissues for riboflavin by the *L. casei* method, [37,42] we noted growth stimulation and drift in blood and tissues. Tween® 80 (polyoxyethylene sorbitan monooleate) was helpful in stimulating the standard curve, but it spared the riboflavin content of the assay samples. Presumably, traces of other fatty acids and other compounds in the fluids and tissues affect *L. casei* and thus yield false riboflavin values. Obviously, removal of traces of from 1 ml aliquots of biologic fluids would result in great losses of sample material and time, especially if many samples are to be surveyed. Because *T. pyriformis* in riboflavin-limited media was not stimulated by fats or other compounds in blood and tissues, or by ingredients of the medium, use of *T. pyriformis* obviated the drawbacks listed for lactobacilli.

The *T. pyriformis* method has proved adaptable to routine or large-scale surveys, [3,5,18,31,49] because it is sensitive and specific for riboflavin, it is simple, the equipment is inexpensive, and few special precautions are required. In surveys of riboflavin and other B-complex vitamins in over 200 chronic alcoholics with liver disease, [18,31,32] 25% had decreased (<80 ng/ml) circulating riboflavin (subclinical deficiency). The low riboflavin values were attributed to dietary deficiencies—among them inadequate food intake. In 642 New York City school children we also noted evidence of subclinical riboflavin deficiency. [4,49]

In 32 randomly selected subjects, riboflavin disappearance after intravenous administration of 5 mg FMN indicated that the half-time clearance for riboflavin in 27 subjects with riboflavin levels above 100 ng/ml was slower than it was in 5 subjects with levels below 80 ng/ml. [5] Disappearance of administered riboflavin may be useful for rapidly measuring tissue avidity for riboflavin. Because rapidity of the clearance of administered riboflavin from the circulation will be directly related to the tissue pool, a rapid riboflavin disappearance would be indicative of depleted stores. In animals, such studies could be done with ^{14}C-labeled riboflavin. In five patients on a starvation regimen for the treatment of obesity, it took approximately 5 months for laboratory evidence of riboflavin deficiency to appear.[5] Circulating riboflavin levels continued to decline during this time until food and riboflavin were given; the levels then rose. During the first week of food deprivation urinary riboflavin increased despite food deprivation. It declined rapidly thereafter; food and riboflavin administration increased the urinary excretion of the vitamin. These results indicate that riboflavin stores in obese patients are adequate for at least 5 months before hyporiboflavinemia becomes evident.

Well-nourished human subjects have increased urinary excretion of riboflavin during a short period of fasting: The excretion rate is as much as 10–15 times that during the period when food was consumed.[46] Our results[5] with subjects placed on a vitamin and food-deprived regimen confirm these findings. Although urinary riboflavin increases during negative nitrogen balance, the increased riboflavin excretion during fasting remains unexplained. Therefore, caution is needed in interpreting urinary riboflavin values. Increased riboflavin excretion during negative nitrogen balance must always be considered if one is interpreting data collected during nutritional surveys or assessing the nutritional status of subjects with histories of faulty nutrition or inadequate intake due to illness. Circulating riboflavin thus emerges as the earliest and thus the most useful index of riboflavin status for prolonged studies or for nutritional surveys.

The *T. pyriformis* method compared well with fluorometric analysis in normal and riboflavin-deficient rat liver.[5] The results are almost identical for riboflavin-deficient tissues. The fluorometric procedure, however, was slow and poorly suited for large-scale studies because of the involved preliminary preparative procedures. Special precautions must be taken: Tissues have to be finely ground at 0–4°C and, until neutralized, the samples must be kept as cold as possible to prevent hydrolysis of FAD. Other sample aliquots must then be kept at room temperature in the dark for 2 days to complete hydrolysis of FAD to FMN; after incubation and neutralization, care must be taken to protect the samples from light because both riboflavin and FMN are very sensitive to destruction by light in the concentrated salt solution needed for the final fluorometric determination. Caution must be taken to dilute the samples properly to prevent interference from other substances present.

The calculations are laborious. If the lengthy preliminary procedures and the extra precautions necessary for fluorometric analysis, with only a slight gain in sensitivity, e.g., 0.1 ng/ml with the fluorometric analysis vs. 0.5 ng/ml with the *T. pyriformis* assay (values practically meaningless in analysis of biologic fluids and tissues), are considered, the *T. pyriformis* method has fewer pitfalls and permits more assays per unit effort. The fluorometric assay has the advantage of delineating the various flavins, for example, FMN and FAD; it is preferred for such use.

The erythrocyte glutathione reductase activity seems to be a sensitive index of the riboflavin status in humans[7,8,22,45] since it evaluates the metabolic utilization of dietary riboflavin. The sensitive response of the erythrocyte glutathione reductase enzyme to FAD *in vitro*, assumed to be representative of the response of the tissues to riboflavin, enables assessment of the metabolic status of riboflavin in man. Erythrocyte glutathione reductase activity coefficients identify individuals receiving marginal amounts of riboflavin as well as individuals suffering from severe ariboflavinosis. This method can therefore be useful for the evaluation of the riboflavin status of individuals. However, the specificity of the erythrocyte glutathione reductase activity is known to be changed by other diseases, for example, hematologic disease, riboflavin antagonists,[38] and other pharmacologic agents.[9,14] The effects of other vitamin deficiencies for example, B_6, on the enzyme activity remain to be evaluated.[11,45] Special precautions should be taken in interpreting glutathione reductase activity in diabetics. Alternations of glutathione activity appear to be related to lesions in carbohydrate metabolism; thus, it was noted that diabetics may have *increased* erythrocyte glutathione reductase activity, which was supposedly unrelated to riboflavin metabolism.[33]

Our results with galactoflavin[5] point up the similarity of riboflavin metabolism in *T. pyriformis*, man, and animals[29,38]; none utilizes riboflavin in the presence of excess galactoflavin and the riboflavin requirement cannot be spared by other metabolites. Recent reports on development of a riboflavin deficiency anemia, with galactoflavin as the riboflavin antagonist, suggest that riboflavin deficiency may be involved in the development of some anemias.[1,29] Other factors may also contribute to these hemopoietic abnormalities, for example, decreases in liver storage of folic acid and citrovorum factor (N^5-formyl-tetrahydrofolic acid).[24]

It has been shown that tetrahydrofolate (THF) synthesis, hence, DNA synthesis, is indirectly crippled by lack of riboflavin in rats and may explain the erythrocyte dysplasia common in riboflavin deficiency.[39,43] A DNA synthesis crippled by riboflavin deficiency can be expected to be revealed by a decrease in proliferating cells. Folate treatment could not reestablish THF synthesis during riboflavin deficiency, even though this treatment mobilized some residual riboflavin from body stores. Despite the increased circulating riboflavin, tissue riboflavin levels remained depressed—a fact indicating that hepatic avidity for riboflavin may decrease during a riboflavin-deficient state and lead to inability to turn over exogenous folates due to impaired synthesis of flavoprotein enzymes. Results also show that nicotinate deficiency also mimics riboflavin deficiency;[43] it depresses THF synthesis by depressing riboflavin stores. The macrocytic anemia of pellagra[23] could reflect such an indirect depression of tissue riboflavin initiated by a nicotinate deficiency. Thus, THF biosynthesis would be depressed and macrocytosis becomes manifest. The hypochromic anemia also seen in pellagra may reflect depletion of tissue flavoproteins, which would also disrupt normal ferrokinetics.[1,18]

In summary, one vitamin deficiency cripples the functioning of other vitamins and leads to convergence of symptomatology.[43] Hence, riboflavin-deficiency anemia and pellagra do not reflect single vitamin malfunctions but, rather, insufficient catalysts for the smooth functionings of systems dependent on conjoint vitamin function. Methods designed to measure the function of an FAD-dependent enzyme must take this fact into account. Apoenzyme deficiency must be considered because it may disrupt coenzyme function; such is the case with the thiamin-dependent transketolase.[2] Thus, it is not uncommon to find subjects who are apparently healthy but show biochemical changes of deficiency, as well as subjects who show clinical but not biochemical evidence of deficiency because all biochemical systems are not altered at the same rate.[8] One should therefore employ a procedure that measures the intact vitamin riboflavin sensitively and specifically and that permits evaluation of the total riboflavin status, not only that of one of the riboflavin-dependent enzymes. Such enzymes may or may not be important in assessing overall riboflavin nutriture. Our experience[3] has shown that the protozoan method is best suited for determining *total* riboflavin status in man and animals. It has served well in large-scale nutritional surveys,[4,31,49] clinical situations,[32] and experimental approaches.[43] Once the method is established, it can also be adapted for multivitamin analyses. *Tetrahymena pyriformis* can be used to assay riboflavin and at the same time to measure vitamin B_6, nicotinate, and pantothenate by utilizing the same chemicals and equipment.[3] This method can also uncover early "subclinical" deficiencies, that is, instances when no overt clinical signs of deficiency are obvious. Prolonged lowered circulating vitamin levels would be the first signs of impending clinical and biochemical signs.[3-6]

Circulating vitamin levels are the earliest indicators of impending bio-chemical and clinical signs; depressed vitamin levels occur before any of the biochemical or clinical lesions appear. Tissue vitamin storage still permits enzymes to function; however, depressed circulating levels indicate that tissues sources of enzymatic function will soon become depleted as well.

We have attempted here to detail some of the many methods designed to assay for riboflavin in biologic fluids and tissues. Many other methods are designed for other purposes as well;[28] the reader must choose the one that is most suitable for his needs and equipment. We have tried to make less grueling the search for an adequate method.

5. REFERENCES

1. Alfrey, C. P., and Lane, M. 1970. The effect of riboflavin deficiency on erythropoiesis, *Seminars in Hematol.* 7:49-54.
2. Baker, H. 1967. Thiamine discussion, *Amer. J. Clin. Nutr.* 20:543-546.
3. Baker, H., and Frank, O. 1968. Riboflavin, in: "Clinical Vitaminology; Methods & Interpretation," pp. 45-53, Interscience Pubs., New York.
4. Baker, H., Frank, O., Feingold, S., Christakis, G., and Ziffer, H. 1967. Vitamins, total cholesterol, and triglycerides in 642 New York City School Children, *Amer. J. Clin. Nutr.* 20:850-857.
5. Baker, H., Frank, P., Feingold., S., Gellene, R. A., Leevy, C. M., and Hutner, S. H. 1966. A riboflavin assay suitable for clinical use and nutritional surveys, *Amer. J. Clin. Nutr.* 19:17-26.
6. Baker, H., Frank, O., and Hutner, S. H. 1969. Subclinical malnutrition, *Science* 172:313.
7. Bamji, M. B. 1969. Glutathione reductase activity in red blood cells and riboflavin nutritional status in humans, *Clin. Chim Acta* 26:263-269.
8. Bamji, M. B. 1971. Assessment of riboflavin deficiency in humans, *J. Sci. & Ind. Research*, 29:S44-S46.
9. Bamji, M. B., and Sharada, D. 1971. Physiological implications of reduced glutathione reductase activity of red blood cells in human ariboflavinosis, *Clin. Chim. Act* 31:409-12.
10. Bessey, O. A., Lowry, O. H., and Love, R. H. 1949. Fluoremetric measure of the nucleotides of riboflavin and their concentration in tissues, *J. Biol. Chem.* 180:755-769.
11. Beutler, E. 1969. The correction of glutathione reductase deficiency by riboflavin administration, *J. Clin. Invest.* 48:1957.
12. Burch, H. B. 1957. Fluorometric assay of FAD, FMN and riboflavin, in: "Methods in Enzymology," (S. P. Colowick and N. O. Kaplan, eds.), Vol. 3, pp. 960-962, Academic Press, New York.
13. Burch, H. B., Bessey, O. A., and Lowry, O. H. 1948. Fluorometric measurements of riboflavin and its natural derivatives in small quantities of blood serum and cells, *J. Biol. Chem.* 175:457-470.
14. Buzard, J. A., and Kopko, F. 1963. The flavin requirement of some inhibition characteristics of rat tissue glutathione reductase, *J. Biol. Chem.* 238:464-468.

15. Buzard, J. A., Kopko, F., and Paul, M. F. 1960. Inhibition of glutathione reductase by Nitrofurantoin, *J. Lab. Clin. Med.* **56**:884-890.

16. Cerletti, P., Strom, R., and Giordano, M. G. 1963. Flavin peptides in tissues: The prosthetic group of succinic dehydrogenase, *Arch Biochem. Biophys.* **101**:423-428.

17. Fass, S., and Rivlin, R. S. 1969. Regulation of riboflavin-metabolizing enzymes in riboflavin deficiency, *Amer. J. Physiol.* **217**:988-991.

18. Fennelly, J., Frank, O., Baker, H., and Leevy, C. M. 1964. Peripheral neuropathy of the alcoholic. I. aetiological role of aneurin and other B-complex vitamins, *Brit Med. J.* **2**:1290-1292.

19. Foy, H., Kandi, A., Harris, E. B., and Preston, J. K. 1968. Isotopic and cytological estimation of marrow erythroid activity in normal and riboflavin deficient baboons, *Acta Haematol.* **39**:118-127.

20. Frank, O., Luisada-Opper, A., Sorrell, M. F., Thomson, A. D., and Baker, H. 1971. Vitamin deficits in severe alcoholic fatty liver of man calculated from multiple reference units, *Exptl. & Molecular Pathol.* **15**:191-197.

21. Glatzle, D., Weber, F., and Wiss, O. 1968. Enzymatic test for the detection of a riboflavin deficiency. NADPH dependent glutathione reductase of red cells and its activation by FAD *in vitro. Experientia* **24**:1122-1123.

22. Glatzle, D., Körner, W. F., Christeller, S., and Wiss, O. 1970. Method for the detection of a biochemical riboflavin deficiency, *Intern. J. Vit. Res.* **40**:166-183.

23. Goldsmith, G. A. 1964. The B-vitamins: Thiamine, Riboflavin, Niacin, *in:*"Nutrition" (G. H. Beaton and E. W. McHenry, eds.), Vol. 2, Academic Press, New York.

24. Halevy, S., and Guggenheim, K. 1958. Metabolism of pteroylglutamic acid and liver nucleic acids levels in certain vitamin deficiencies, *J. Nutr.* **65**:77-88.

25. Horwitt, M. K. 1960. Thiamine, riboflavin, and niacin, *in:* "Modern Nutrition in Health and Disease" (M. G. Wohl, and A. S. Goodhart, eds.), 2d ed., pp. 334-337, Lea & Febiger, Philadelphia.

26. Kidder, G. W., and Dewey, V. 1951. The biochemistry of ciliates in pure culture, *in:* "Biochemistry and Physiology of Protozoa," (A. Lwoff, ed.), Vol. 1, pp. 323-400, Academic Press, New York.

27. Kornberg, H. A., Langdon, R. S., and Cheldelin, V. H. 1948. Microbiological assay for riboflavin, *Anal. Chem.* **20**:81-83.

28. Koziol, J. 1971. Fluorometric analyses of riboflavin and its coenzymes, *in:* "Methods in Enzymology" (D. B. McCormick, and L. D. Wright, eds.), Vol. 18, Part B, pp. 253-290, Academic Press, New York.

29. Lane, M., Alfrey, C. P., Mengel, C. E., Doherty, M. A., and Doherty, J. 1964. The rapid induction of human riboflavin deficiency with galactoflavin, *J. Clin. Invest.* **43**:357-373.

30. Langer, B. W., Jr., and Charoensiri, S. 1966. Growth response of *Lactobacillus casei* (ATCC 7469) to riboflavin, FMN and FAD, *Proc. Soc. Exptl. Biol. & Med.* **122**:151-152.

31. Leevy, C. M., Baker, H., tenHove, W., Frank, O., and Cherrick, G. R. 1965a. B-complex vitamins in liver disease of the alcoholic, *Amer. J. Clin. Nutr.* **16**:339-346.

32. Leevy, C. M., Cardi, L., Frank, O., Gellene, R. A., and Baker, H. 1965b. Incidence and significance of hypovitaminemia in a randomly selected municipal hospital population, *Amer. J. Clin. Nutr.* **17**:259-271.

33. Long, W. K., and Carson, P. E. 1961. Increased erythrocyte glutathione reductase activity in diabetes mellitus. *Biochem. & Biophys. Research Comm.* **5**:394-399.

34. Manual for Nutrition Surveys. 1963. Urinary Riboflavin by a Modification of the Method of Slater and Morell, 2d ed., pp. 140-142. Interdepartmental Committee on Nutrition for National Defense, U.S. Government Printing Office, Washington, D.C.

35. Modi, V. V., and Owen, E. C. 1957. Flavin adenine dinucleotide metabolism and lactation, *Biochim. Biophys. Acta* 24:423-425.
36. Morell, D. B., and Slater E. C. 1946. Modification of fluorometric method of detecting riboflavin in biological materials, *Biochem. J.* 40:644-652.
37. Pearson, W. N. 1967. Riboflavin, *in:* "The Vitamins" (P. György, and W. N. Pearson, eds.), Vol. 7, pp. 99-136, Academic Press, New York.
38. Prosky, L., Burch, H. B., Bejrablaya, D., Lowry, O. H. and Combs, A. M. 1964. The effects of galactoflavin on riboflavin enzymes and coenzymes, *J. Biol. Chem.* 239:2691-2695.
39. Rivlin, R. S. 1970. Riboflavin metabolism, *New Eng. J. Med.* 283:463-472.
40. Slater, E. C., and Morell, D. B. 1946. Fluorometric determination of riboflavin in urine, *Biochem. J.* 40:652-657.
41. Snell, E. E. 1950, "Vitamin Methods" (P. György, ed.), Vol. 1, pp. 340-505, Academic Press, New York.
42. Snell, E. E. 1954. Microbiological methods, *in:* "The Vitamins" (W. H. Sebrell, Jr., and R. S. Harris, eds.), Vol. 3, pp. 372-373, Academic Press, New York.
43. Tamburro, C., Frank O., Thomson, A. D., Sorrell, M. F., and Baker, H. 1971. Interactions of folate, nicotinate, and riboflavin deficiencies in rats. *Nutr. Reports Intern.* 4:185-189.
44. Tillotson, J. A., and Sauberlich, H. E. 1971. Effect of riboflavin depletion and repletion on erythrocyte glutathione reductase in the rat, *J. Nutr.* 101:1459-1466.
45. Tillotson, J. A., and Baker, E. M. 1972. An enzymatic measurement of the riboflavin status in man, *Amer. J. Clin. Nutr.* 25:425-431.
46. Windmueller, H. G., Anderson, A. A., and Mickelson, O. 1964. Elevated riboflavin levels in urine of fasting subjects, *Amer. J. Clin. Nutr.* 15:73-83.
47. Yagi, K. 1971. Simultaneous microdetermination of riboflavin, FMN and FAD in animal tissues, *in:* "Methods in Enzymology" (D. B. McCormick, and L. D. Wright, eds.), Vol. 18, Part B, pp. 290-305, Academic Press, New York.
48. Yang, C. S., Charalampos, A., and McCormick, D. B. 1964. Microbiological and enzymatic assays of riboflavin analogues, *J. Nutr.* 84:167-172.
49. Ziffer, H., Frank, O., Christakis, G., Talkington, L., and Baker, H. 1967. Data analysis strategy for nutritional survey of 642 New York City school children, *Amer. J. Clin. Nutr.* 20:858-865.

CHROMATOGRAPHIC AND RADIOISOTOPIC METHODS FOR THE ANALYSIS OF RIBOFLAVIN AND THE FLAVIN COENZYMES

Arpad G. Fazekas

1. INTRODUCTION

This chapter will describe chromatographic and radioisotopic methods for the analysis of riboflavin (RF) and the flavin coenzymes in animal tissues. Chromatographic separations of the three major tissue flavins—flavin adenine dinucleotide (FAD), flavin mononucleotide (FMN), and RF—have been in wide use since the early 1950s and are summarized in excellent review articles[21] and textbooks.[16,14] The first part of this chapter, therefore, deals only with the most important and practical chromatographic methods, including those that have been successfully used in the author's laboratory.

In spite of earlier extensive studies,[1,25] a great deal remains to

ARPAD G. FAZEKAS—Department of Medicine, University of Montreal and Laboratory of Endocrinology, Notre-Dame Hospital, Montreal, Quebec, Canada.

be learned about the distribution and utilization of riboflavin in the body. Very little is known about the dynamics of flavin coenzyme synthesis by various tissues and about the factors influencing those processes. The availability and introduction of radioisotopically labeled riboflavin for such studies open up new horizons and territories in flavin biochemistry. In order to derive the full benefits of this powerful tool, however, new analytical methods had to be devised, utilizing the principles of radiochemistry and introducing the latest analytical methods into the field of flavin biochemistry.

The second and longer part of this chapter describes these new methods that are currently being used in the author's laboratory for the determination of radioactive flavins in animal tissues. These methods have been successfully used for both *in vivo* and *in vitro* studies of flavin coenzyme synthesis by various tissues including rat liver, kidney, adrenals, brain, heart, or human erythrocytes.

2. THE CHROMATOGRAPHIC SEPARATION OF FLAVINS

2.1. Column Chromatographic Procedures

A large variety of column chromatographic procedures have been utilized for the separation of riboflavin and the flavin coenzymes.[4] Cellulose powder was introduced by Whitby[19] for the purification of FMN and FAD from baker's yeast extracts. Cellulose column chromatography—with water, saturated with *i*-amyl alcohol as solvent—was used for the isolation and purification of FAD from rat liver by Kokai *et al.*[11] and Fazekas and Kokai.[5] Separation of RF, FMN, and FAD has been achieved on DEAE–cellulose columns by Rao *et al.*[17] These three flavins can be separated in .the above elution order on Dowex-1 ion exchange resin columns.[24]

The quick separation of FAD + FMN from RF can be achieved by chromatography on a carboxymethyl cellulose (Whatman CM-70) ion-exchange column.[5] The resorcinolformaldehyde resin R-15 has been found to be useful for the adsorption and separation of flavin nucleotides from free RF.[13] Molecular filtration on Sephadex gel columns can be used with advantage for the purification of crude extracts of biological material.[5] The complete separation of FAD, FMN, and RF can be achieved on a 35-cm-long Sephadex G-15 column.[6,7] The columns are prepared as follows: The Sephadex powder (G-15) is suspended in an

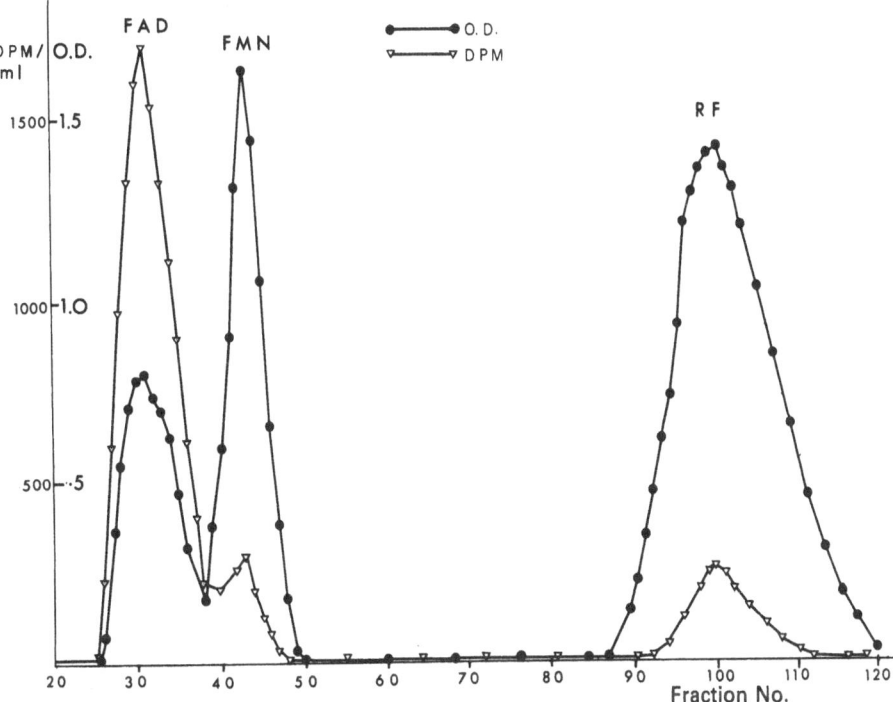

Fig. 1. Distribution of radioactivity in adrenal tissue flavins. Flavins were separated on a 350 × 25 mm Sephadex G-15 column and 1 ml fractions collected. The quantity of nonradioactive carrier was 100 μg each of FAD, FMN, and RF.

appropriate volume of distilled water and then permitted to swell for 24 hr. The swollen gel is then poured into a glass column of 10 mm internal diameter and allowed to settle to a height of 35 cm. After the gel is settled, a 1-ml tissue extract is layered on the top (with a Pasteur pipette). Distilled water is then used as the eluant. The three flavins separate as distinct bands: FAD is eluted first, followed closely by FMN, while RF is retained much longer. The flavins are collected in separate tubes manually. The elution pattern is shown in Fig. 1. It should be emphasized here that FAD and FMN isolated from biological material are not spectrophotometrically pure following chromatography on Sephadex G-15. For their complete purification, subsequent thin-layer chromatography (TLC) is necessary.[5] This method has been used successfully in conjunction with carrier flavins for the determination of radioactive flavins in animal tissues.[6,7] The outline of the method is shown in Fig. 2.

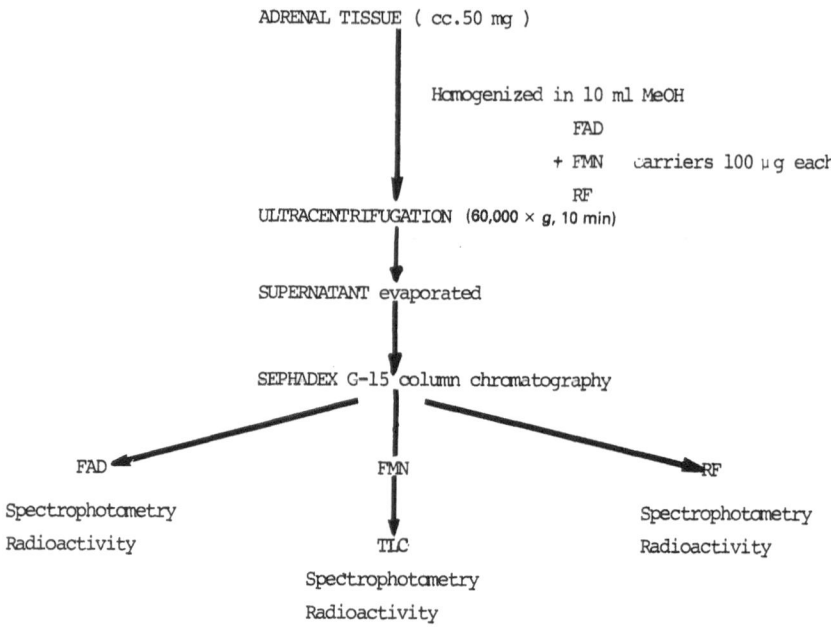

ADRENAL TISSUE (cc.50 mg)

Homogenized in 10 ml MeOH

FAD

+ FMN   carriers 100 μg each

RF

ULTRACENTRIFUGATION (60,000 × g, 10 min)

SUPERNATANT evaporated

SEPHADEX G-15 column chromatography

FAD   FMN   RF

Spectrophotometry   Spectrophotometry
Radioactivity   TLC   Radioactivity
                        Spectrophotometry
                        Radioactivity

Fig. 2. Flow sheet for the determination of radioactive flavins in adrenal tissue.

2.2. Paper Chromatography of Flavins

This analytical tool has been most frequently utilized for the analytical separation of various flavins. The separations are achieved in most cases by ascending[3,20] or circular[8] paper chromatography. Descending preparative paper chromatography was used by Kovacs and Fazekas[12] for the purification of FAD from baker's yeast. The best separations are obtained with the following two solvent systems: (a) the upper layer of n-butanol:acetic acid:water (4:1:5, v/v/v), and (b) 5% aqueous solution of Na_2HPO_4.[9] This latter solvent also separates riboflavin from its degradation products—lumiflavin and lumichrome. Individual flavins can be localized on the paper by examination under ultraviolet light. They can be eluted with 10% acetic acid or by the warm water extraction method of Yagi.[22] For other solvent systems the reader is referred to Kilgour et al.[10]

2.3. Thin Layer Chromatographic Separation and Purification of Flavins

Thin layer chromatographic purification and separation of three major tissue flavins (RF, FMN, FAD) was introduced first by Kokai,

Fazekas, and Domjan.[11] These authors used silica gel-G (Merck) layers of 250 μm thickness. Of the variety of solvent systems tested, the 5% aqueous solution of $Na_2HPO_4 \cdot H_2O$ proved to be the most efficient. Details of this method can also be found in Fazekas and Kokai.[5] Precoated silica gel TLC sheets (250 μm) manufactured by Merck (without fluorescence indicator) can also be conveniently used.[6] Prior to use, the sheets are washed (by running) in 50% aqueous methanol, dried at room temperature, and stored in a cabinet. For the complete separation of the flavins (RF, FMN, FAD) a 15-cm-long run is satisfactory. Alternatively, a 2% solution of anhydrous Na_2HPO_4 can also be used as the solvent. After the plates have been dried, the flavins are visualized under u.v. light and the spots scraped into 50-ml beakers containing 5 ml of 50% aqueous methanol. Extraction of flavins is complete after 10 min, during which time the beakers are occasionally shaken. The silica gel is then sedimented by centrifugation at 1500 rpm for 3 min. The clear supernatant solution is used for the quantitative assay of the flavins. Recoveries from the TLC plates range between 75% and 80% by this method. More recently, Yagi and Oishi[23] have described the thin layer chromatographic separation of some fat-soluble riboflavin derivatives.

3. RADIOISOTOPIC METHODS FOR THE STUDY OF 2-^{14}C-RIBOFLAVIN CONVERSION TO FLAVIN COENZYMES BY ANIMAL TISSUES *IN VIVO* OR *IN VITRO*

3.1. Extraction, Separation, and Determination of Radioactive Flavins in Animal Tissues.

3.1.1. Principle

The radioactive flavins in animal tissues are determined by the nonradioactive carrier method, utilizing the principle of reverse isotope dilution. The radioactive flavins are extracted from the tissue sample in the presence of known amounts of the three flavins (RF, FMN, FAD). The flavins are separated by column chromatography on DEAE-Sephadex A-25, followed by the determination of their specific activity (disintegrations/min/μg flavin). The specific activity obtained multiplied by the added mass of nonradioactive carrier yields the total radioactivity incorporated into each flavin.

3.1.2. Special Equipment

Potter-Elvehjem-type glass-Teflon homogenizer; preparative ultra-centrifuge; spectrophotometer (visible range); rotary evaporator (Buchi); glass chromatography columns, 30 × 1 cm with Teflon stopcock (Fisher); liquid scintillation spectrometer.

3.1.3. Reagents

Crystalline riboflavin, FMN, and FAD (Sigma). Sephadex A-25 anion exchanger (Pharmacia, Uppsala) 1% ammonium sulfate $[(NH_4)_2SO_4]$ solution; Aquasol (New England Nuclear Corp.) scintillation liquid; methanol (analytical grade) 2-^{14}C-riboflavin (Amersham & Searle Corp.).

3.1.4. Preparation of Nonradioactive Carrier Flavin Solutions

To prepare the carrier solutions, 5 mg of each flavin are dissolved in 50 ml distilled water to yield solutions containing 100 μg/ml. Riboflavin (Sigma) and FAD (Sigma) are usually of satisfactory purity. FMN, however, requires careful checking since it generally has some degree of riboflavin contamination, usually between 3% and 10%. We can choose between two alternatives: (a) either to purify the FMN on a Sephadex G-15 column prior to use and to prepare the standard solutions from purified FMN, or (b) to subtract the quantity of RF contamination in the FMN carrier when calculating the results.

Practical experience shows that the carrier flavin solutions have to be prepared fresh every day. For example, about 20% of the FMN is degraded into RF in 24 hr even at the slightly acidic pH of distilled water used in most laboratories. FAD is also unstable in solution while RF is more stable in solution then either FMN or FAD and can be stored in the dark at acidic pH for several days. In our laboratory, riboflavin solutions more than 2 days old are no longer used.

3.1.5. Extraction of Flavins

The tissue sample to be analyzed is placed in a Potter-Elvehjem-type glass homogenizer equipped with a Teflon pestle. The usual quantity of liver, kidney, or heart tissue used in our laboratory is 50 mg. After the addition of 7 ml methanol and 1.0 ml each of nonradioactive FAD, FMN, and RF (100 μg/ml), the tissue is homogenized for 3 min. After homogenization the mixture is centrifuged in an ultracentrifuge (preparative) at 60,000 × g for 10 min. During this step, care has to be taken

TABLE 1. Efficiency of Methanol Extraction of Total Radioactive Flavins from Rat Liver Homogenates[a]

Experiment number	Homogenate (dpm/ml)	Methanol extract (dpm/ml)	Recovery (%)
1	616	605	98
2	731	715	97
3	622	621	100
4	840	822	97
5	610	584	96

[a]Rats (female, Wistar, 200 g) were injected with 2.5 µCi 2-^{14}C-RF *in vivo* subcutaneously 1 hr prior to sacrifice. Livers (50 mg) were extracted as described in the text. Samples of the homogenates and the methanol extracts after centrifugation at 60,000 × g for 10 min were taken for measurement of radioactivity.

not to use cellulose–acetate centrifuge tubes, since these are dissolved by methanol. Tubes of polyallomer (Beckman) are suggested. The high-speed centrifugation is necessary to sediment all the fine particles in order to obtain a clear extract. Filtration through analytical filter paper is not satisfactory.

The entire procedure gives a 98% yield of total radioactivity present in rat liver (Table I) 1 hr following the *in vivo* injection of 2-^{14}C-RF, which verifies the efficiency of the extraction. The role of methanol is dual: precipitation of proteins, thereby liberating flavins attached to protein molecules; and inactivation of the flavin-destroying phosphatases. These enzymes can also be inactivated by heating the tissue at 80° C for 5 min prior to extraction, as suggested and used by Yagi.[22] This procedure, however, was found to destroy approximately 15% of the endogenous radioactive FAD and is therefore not recommended (Table II). Furthermore, heating decreases the efficiency of the methanol extraction by approximately 8% (Table II). The use of 50% methanol gives equally good extraction of all flavins. However, under these

TABLE II. Effect of Heating of Rat Liver Tissue on the Recovery of Radioactive Flavins by Aqueous Methanol Extraction[a]

Treatment	Experiment number	RF	FMN	FAD	Total dpm
No heating	1	2040	2586	5606	10,232
	2	2117	2636	5827	10,580
Heating	1	2590	2310	4590	9,490
	2	2550	2520	4900	9,970

[a]Samples of rat liver were heated at 80° C for 5 min before the addition of nonradioactive carriers and extraction with aqueous methanol. Tests were carried out with 50-mg liver samples taken from each of two animals. Results are expressed as dpm/100 mg tissue.

conditions, some phosphatase activity still persists. This might result in the partial destruction of the FMN carrier, especially if the extracts are not processed immediately after their initial centrifugation. The nonradioactive flavins facilitate by their mass action the extraction of radioactive flavins by displacing them from their binding sites.

After centrifugation the supernatant solutions are decanted into 50-ml round-bottom flasks (with 20/40 ground joints) and evaporated to dryness *in vacuo* at 50° C in a flask evaporator (Rotavapor R Buchi, Switzerland).

3.1.6. Separation of Flavins on DEAE-Sephadex A-25 Anion Exchange Columns

The Sephadex columns are prepared as follows: The DEAE-Sephadex A-25 powder is suspended in an appropriate volume of distilled water and then permitted to swell for 3 hr at room temperature. The Sephadex suspension is best used when it is freshly prepared or has been stored no longer than 24 hr. Gels stored in the swollen state for longer periods of time may still be used to achieve separation of the flavins, but the bands obtained are somewhat broader than optimal.

The swollen gel is then poured into a glass chromatographic column (10 mm internal diameter) equipped with a Teflon stopcock and left to settle to a height of 15 cm. The end of the column is blocked with a small piece of cotton wool. After the column is settled the gel is washed with 10 ml distilled water.

The dried tissue extract in the round-bottom flask is then dissolved in 1 ml of distilled water and transferred to the column by means of a long Pasteur pipette with a fine tip. The solution is carefully layered

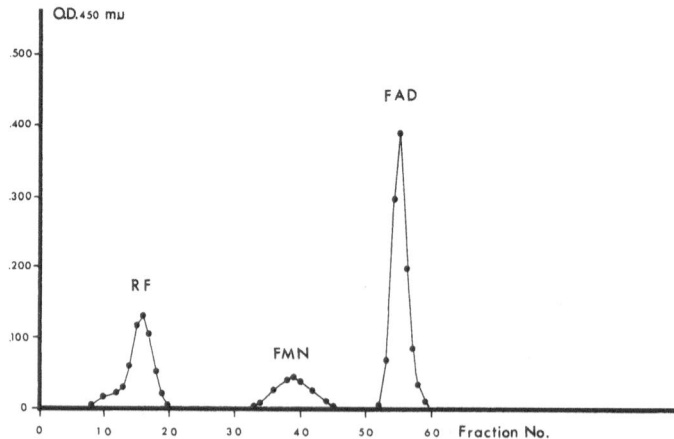

Fig. 3. Separation of FAD, FMN, and RF on a DEAE-Sephadex A-25 column.

onto the top of the column to avoid stirring the gel. The flask is then rinsed with 0.5 ml distilled water, which is also transferred to the column. After the extract has entered the gel, elution is started with 2 ml distilled water. When the water has entered the column, elution is continued with 1% ammonium sulfate solution. Since RF has no charge, it passes through the gel and can be eluted with distilled water alone. By contrast, FMN and FAD, because of their anionic charges, are bound to the gel and eluted by the displacing action of ammonium sulfate. RF is eluted first, followed by FMN and FAD. The band of FMN is broader than that of FAD. The elution pattern is shown in Fig. 3.

The flavins are collected manually in separate graduated volumetric tubes. The flavin bands are easily distinguishable by their color. In this manner an experienced technician can run four or five columns at the same time.

3.1.7. Quantitative Determination of Radioactivity of the Flavin Fractions

After the column chromatography has been completed, the three flavin-containing tubes (RF, FMN, FAD) are mixed in the vortex stirrer and their volumes are noted (to calculate the recovery of cold carrier). A 1-ml aliquot of each tube is transferred with a volumetric pipette into the liquid scintillation vials. After the addition of 14 ml Aquasol scintillation liquid, the samples are capped, shaken vigorously, and counted in a liquid scintillation spectrometer. (It is convenient to use the blue channel of a Packard, Tri-Carb, Model 3375, with the following settings: amplification: 7; channel selection: ^{32}P (^{14}C); discriminator settings: E 40, F 1040; background: to be determined.) The use of Aquasol (a water-miscible, organic solvent-based solution) yields an efficiency of about 80–90% for ^{14}C on the blue channel. Another useful scintillation fluid for flavins is 4% BBOT [2,5-bis(2-(5-tert-butylbenzoxazolyl))-thiophene] in toluene:methanol (1:1), which gives about 60% efficiency at the above channel settings. The efficiency for each unknown sample is read from a calibration curve prepared using a standard ^{14}C-series with varying degrees of quenching by the automatic external standard-ization method, which has been found to work very well at this water:Aquasol ratio.

3.1.8. Quantitative Estimation of the Mass of Flavins by Spectrophotometry

Following their chromatographic separation, the individual flavins are quantitated by spectrophotometry at 450 nm. Readings are taken against 1% ammonium sulfate solution, and flavin concentrations are expressed as $\mu g/ml$ for each flavin fraction, based on calibration curves prepared from the original standard stock solutions which have been used as carriers. The calibration curves should range from 0 to 50 $\mu g/ml$. The specific activity of each flavin is then calculated by dividing the number of dpm by the number of μg flavin in 1 ml flavin fraction.

3.1.9. Calculation of Results

The total radioactivity incorporated (tdpm) into the three different flavin fractions is calculated by multiplying the specific activity with the mass of nonradioactive carrier added for each flavin:

$$tdpm = \text{specific activity} \times \mu g \text{ carrier flavin}$$

where

tdpm = total disintegrations per minute (incorporated)
Specific activity = $dpm/\mu g$ flavin (calculated as above)
μg carrier flavin = 100 μg

When the values are referred to 100 mg wet tissue weight (since 50 mg tissue was extracted in this assay), then

$$tdpm/100 \text{ mg tissue} = dpm/\mu g \times 200$$

Examples of the experimental protocol and calculations are given in Table III.

TABLE III. Typical Results of Assay of FMN and FAD Synthesis in Normal Rat Liver (Experimental Protocol Sample)[a]

Liver sample	Flavin	Fraction volume (ml)	Optical density[b]	Flavin ($\mu g/ml$ solution) (c.e.)[c]	Recovery of carrier (%)	Solution (dpm/ml)	Specific activity (dpm/μg)	Dpm/ 100 mg tissue
	FAD	6.2	0.162	12.4	76.8	730.0	58.90	11,780
1	FMN	10.5	0.143	6.3	66.1	58.7	9.32	1,860
	RF	7.1	0.405	12.1	85.9	71.3	5.90	1,181
	FAD	6.5	0.142	11.0	71.5	592.0	53.8	10,763
2	FMN	11.2	0.118	5.2	58.2	30.4	5.67	1,134
	RF	6.0	0.496	14.8	88.8	102.6	6.91	1,380

[a]Tissue sample: 50 mg; carriers: 100 μg each.
[b]Determined at 450 nm.
[c]c.e. = column eluate.

3.2. General Remarks about the Method

Because of the sensitivity of flavins toward light, the experiments should be carried out in a laboratory illuminated with dimmed or red light. This procedure is especially important in the context of the present method because the photolytic destruction follows the sequence: $FAD \rightarrow FMN \rightarrow RF$. Since the major tissue flavin is FAD, most of the radioactivity is present in this compound and its destruction will result in the migration of radioactivity into FMN and ultimately RF. Consequently, the results obtained will be falsely high for FMN and RF since their specific activity will become higher. The other source of danger is the phosphatase activity of the tissue itself. The use of 70% methanol for the extraction procedure apparently destroys enzymatic activity in the tissue during homogenization and gives good recovery values for the flavin carriers. Under these conditions there is no appreciable breakdown of FAD carrier, and FMN breakdown to RF is negligible (between 1 and 2%). The percentage of recoveries for the three nonradioactive carriers range between 90 and 95% for RF; 55 and 75% for FMN; and 80 and 85% for FAD (Table III). Differences of recoveries among the three flavin fractions are probably caused by losses encountered during extraction, transfer, and column chromatography. The relatively lower recovery of FMN is probably due to its partial absorption by the tissue sample during extraction.

Although flavins in animal tissues are stable enough to allow the storage of tissue samples in the frozen state for their later analysis, prolonged freezing is not recommended. A considerable proportion of FAD was found to be destroyed after 60 days of storage at $-20°$ C. As a consequence, riboflavin radioactivity is increased after 60 days and that of FMN is variable, and it is therefore not advisable to store tissue samples for longer than 2 weeks. Analyses should ideally be carried

TABLE IV. *Simultaneous Determinations of Flavin Content of the Same Liver Sample*[a]

	dpm/100 mg tissue		
Flavin	Assay 1	Assay 2	Assay 3
FAD	4269	4140	4120
FMN	762	790	778
RF	2538	2592	2516

[a] Assays were performed on the same sample of liver (stored at $-20°$ C for 60 days).

out on the same day and tissue extracts should never be stored longer than overnight at $-20°$ C. Under these conditions, reproducibility of results is obtained (Table IV).

3.3 Application of the Method for *in Vivo* or *in Vitro* Studies of Flavin Coenzyme Synthesis

The present method may be used equally well for the study of flavin coenzyme biosynthesis both *in vivo* and *in vitro*. When radioactive riboflavin is injected into the living animal either subcutaneously[6,7] or intraperitoneally,[25] the animals are killed at the desired time interval following the injection. The organs to be analyzed are then immediately cooled and the assays performed. The incorporation of radioactivity proceeds actively into the liver and kidney flavin fractions and peak levels are reached 90 min following the injection.[7a] The quantity of radioactivity incorporated into tissue flavin is strongly influenced by the dose of 2-^{14}C-RF injected (Table V). These results clearly show that the 2.5 and 5.0 μCi/200 g body weight doses can be considered as tracer doses. By contrast, 20 μCi/200 g body weight results in relatively increased accumulation of RF and FMN in relation to FAD, suggesting that tracer kinetics no longer prevail. Normal values (mean $\pm$ SEM) 1 hr after the s.c. injection of 2.5 μCi 2-^{14}C-RF into female 200-g Wistar rats (10 animals) were as follows: liver—FAD: 9550 $\pm$ 470, FMN: 1203 $\pm$ 118, RF: 1435 $\pm$ 240; kidney—FAD: 14,932 $\pm$ 592, FMN: 4074 $\pm$ 467, RF: 9083 $\pm$ 1159.

TABLE V. *Effect of the Size of Injected Dose on the Incorporation of ^{14}C-RF Into Rat Liver Flavins in Vivo*[a]

Dose injected (μCi/200 g body weight)	Animal	dpm/100 mg liver		
		FAD	FMN	RF
2.5	1	9,630	1,150	1,330
	2	8,830	870	1,400
5.0	1	18,300	2,500	980
	2	19,900	2,800	1,200
20.0	1	45,800	11,900	10,000
	2	65,200	19,700	12,670

[a]Normal animals (3 $\times$ 2) were injected subcutaneously with varying doses of ^{14}C-RF dissolved in 1.0 ml saline and killed 60 min following the injection.

TABLE VI. The Biosynthesis of Flavin Coenzymes from 2-^{14}C-RF by Human Erythrocyte Homogenates in Vitro[a]

Experiment number	dpm/flask	
	FAD	FMN
1	3600	20,100
2	3340	19,200
3	3340	19,208
4	2920	13,650
5	2180	11,210

[a]Blood was drawn into heparinized tubes. Red blood cells were freed of white cells by centrifugation, then washed twice with an equal volume of isotonic saline, and homogenized in Krebs-Ringer phosphate solution. 1.5 ml red blood cell homogenate (equivalent to 0.75 ml RBC) was incubated in each flask with 2-^{14}C-RF (570,000 dpm) and 5 μM ATP in a total volume of 1.9-ml Krebs-Ringer phosphate solution for 2 hr at 45° C. Following incubation, nonradioactive flavin carriers and 6 ml methanol were added to each flask and the radioactive flavins determined as described in the text.

The method described above can be adapted for other organs (brain, heart) as well, but the rate of incorporation of radioactivity will be much less (brain: one-tenth of liver FAD rate; heart: one-third of liver FAD rate). Working with such tissues, 100 mg can be used for the analysis as starting material. When larger quantities of tissue are used, a considerable amount of lipid may interfere with the column chromatography. The elimination of lipids from the extract can be achieved by partitioning it with an equal volume of diethyl-ether.

Following *in vitro* incubation, the tissue slices are thoroughly rinsed with iced isotonic saline, then transferred to the homogenizer and homogenized with the flavin carriers and methanol as described above.

Kinetic studies performed with quartered rat adrenal tissue have shown that flavin synthesis *in vitro* can be reliably measured by a method essentially identical with the one described by Fazekas and Sandor.[6] Furthermore, the flavin synthesizing capacity of human erythrocytes *in vitro* can be determined by this method (Table VI), as can the radioactive flavin content of the blood of rats following injection of 2-^{14}C-RF.[7a] The residual heme, which contaminates the extract, is readily separated from the flavins on the Sephadex A-25 column and is eluted before RF. Thus it does not interfere with the spectrophotometric assay of the nonradioactive carriers. This method is useful for the investigation of flavin coenzyme synthesis by surviving rat liver slices *in vitro* from 2-^{14}C-RF (Fig. 4). As this time-study shows, both RF uptake and flavin coenzyme synthesis increase during 90 min of incubation.[7a]

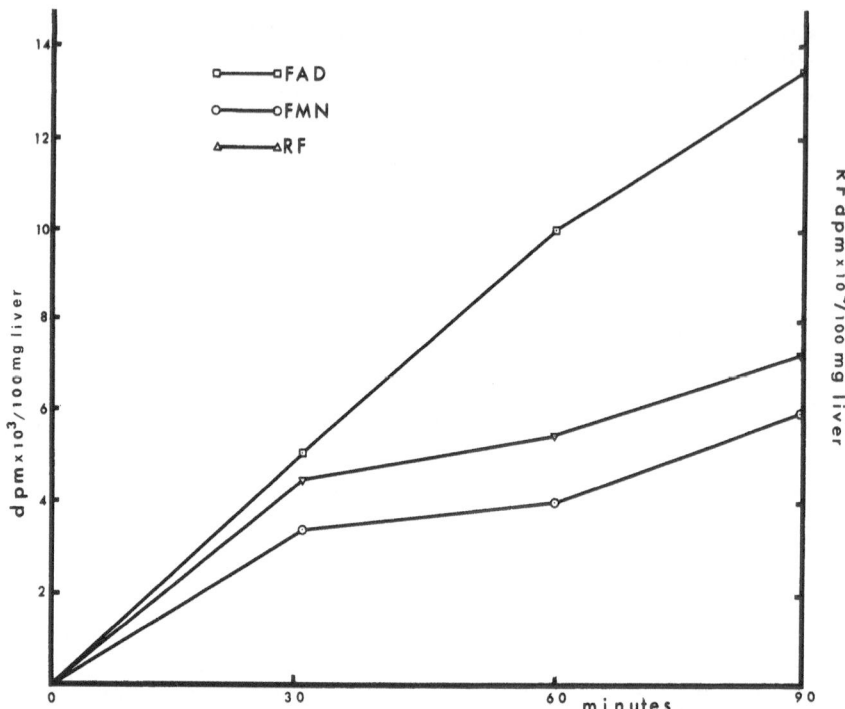

Fig. 4. The *in vitro* biosynthesis of flavin nucleotides (FAD, FMN) from 2-^{14}C-RF by surviving rat liver slices. In each flask, 100 mg of liver slices were incubated with 0.25 μCi of 2-^{14}C-RF in 2 ml Krebs–Ringer phosphate solution, containing 200 mg/100 ml glucose, at 40° C.

4. COMPETITIVE PROTEIN BINDING ASSAY OF RIBOFLAVIN

The application of competitive protein binding for the assay of various hormones in biological fluids has gained considerable ground recently.[26] This type of saturation analysis is based on a reversible association between a binding protein with high affinity and high specificity and a relatively small molecule, the ligand. The interaction between the binding protein and the ligand is reflected by the equation:

$$L + P \underset{k_2}{\overset{k_1}{\rightleftharpoons}} LP$$

At equilibrium

$$k_1(L)(P) = k_2(LP)$$

and if

$$K = k_1/k_2$$

then

$$K = \frac{(LP)}{(L)\cdot(P)}$$

where K is the association constant of the binding protein with the ligand and (P), (L), and (LP) are the molar concentrations, respectively, of the free protein P, free ligand L, and the protein bound ligand LP.

When the concentration of the binding protein is kept constant, the fraction of bound ligand decreases with increasing ligand concentration, and a plot of bound ligand against total ligand concentration will give an S-shaped curve. Thus, at equilibrium the fraction of bound ligand is a function of the total amount of ligand present, and measurement of the bound fraction permits the calculation of the unknown total ligand concentration. This can be easily and simply achieved by using a radioactively labeled tracer ligand as an indicator. The tracer behaves as the nonradioactive ligand. Hence, for this type of assay one needs a specific binding protein and a radioactive ligand in tracer amounts.

The existence of riboflavin-binding proteins in the egg white and yolk has been known for some time.[18,15] More recently, Clagett and his co-workers[2] have shown the presence of a highly specific riboflavin binding protein in chicken plasma (see Chapter 4).

In our preliminary studies presented here we used the egg white as a source of riboflavin binding protein. The egg white was separated, then homogenized in a Potter–Elvehjem-type glass-Teflon homogenizer, followed by dilution in distilled water to a 1% concentration. This solution was then filtered through wool in order to eliminate the precipitated particles. To 100 ml of the protein solution 2-^{14}C-RF tracer was added (final concentration: 5000–6000 dpm/ml). The mixture was then stored in the refrigerator at 3° C for 2 hr. During this period the tracer reached equilibrium.

The assay was carried out as follows: For the preparation of the standard curve, various amounts (50–500 ng) of nonradioactive RF are measured (from a stock solution containing 10 μg/ml) into disposable culture tubes (13 × 100 mm, Becton, Dickinson Co.,) in duplicate and made up to an equal volume (0.1 ml) with distilled water. To each tube, 1 ml of the tracer-protein solution is then added and the tubes shaken vigorously. The tubes are then placed in a refrigerator (+3° C) for 1 hr to equilibrate. The separation of bound riboflavin from free

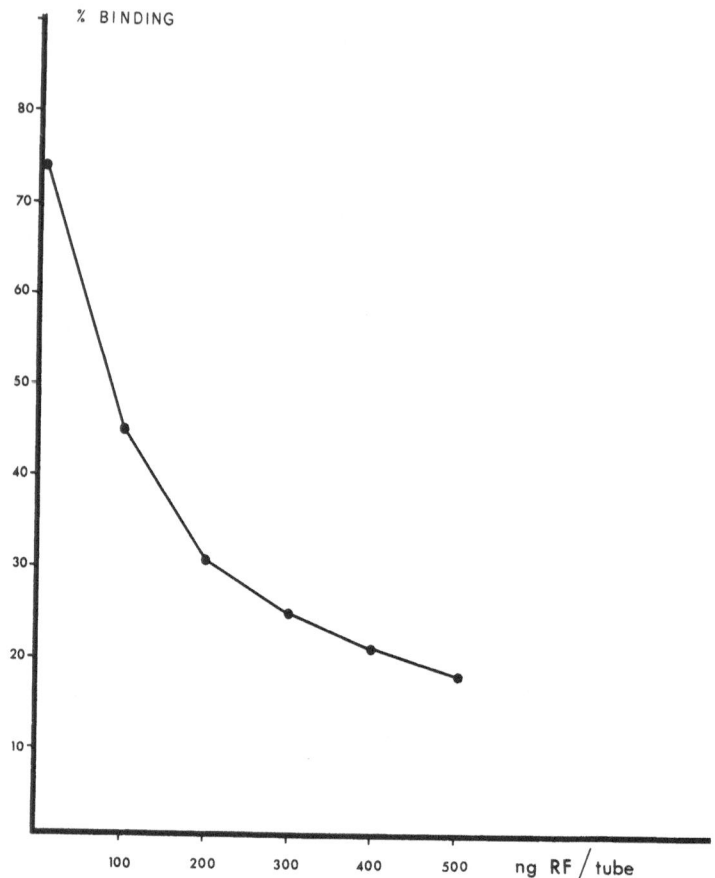

Fig. 5. Competitive protein binding assay for riboflavin. Standard curve. Tracer solution: 1% egg white in distilled water containing 6000 dpm/ml 2-^{14}C-RF.

riboflavin is achieved by the adsorption of the free fraction to Florisil (60–100 mesh, Fisher). To each tube, 80 mg of washed Florisil is added. The tubes are shaken for 2 min, then left to stand for 2 min, during which time the Florisil settles to the bottom. Since free riboflavin is bound by Florisil, only the protein bound riboflavin (radioactivity) will remain in the supernatant fraction. Exactly 0.5 ml of the supernatant solution (volumetric pipette) is then pipetted into scintillation vials, 10 ml of scintillation liquid is added (Aquasol), and the samples are counted for radioactivity.

A typical binding curve is shown in Fig. 5. Binding of 2-^{14}C-RF in the tracer solution is usually around 75%, and the useful range of the standard curve is from 25 to 500 *ng* RF per tube.

Results suggest that this method is suitable for the determination of free riboflavin in biological samples—for instance, human urine[27] or blood.

5. REFERENCES

1. Bessey, O. A., Lowry, O. H., Davis, E. B., and Dorn, J. L., 1958. The riboflavin economy of the rat, *J. Nutr.* **64**:185-202.
2. Clagett, C. O. 1971. Genetic control of the riboflavin carrier protein, *Fed. Proc.* **30**:127-129.
3. Crammer, F. L. 1948. Paper chromatography of flavine nucleotides, *Nature* **161**:349-350.
4. Diamant, E., Sanadi, D. R., and Huennekens, I. M. 1952. The isolation of flavin nucleotides, *J. Am. Chem. Soc.* **74**:5440-5444.
5. Fazekas, A. G., and Kokai, K. 1971. Extraction, purification and separation of tissue flavins for spectrophotometric determination, *in:* "Vitamins and Coenzymes, Methods in Enzymology" (D. B. McCormick and L. D. Wright, eds.), Vol. XVIII, Part B, pp. 385-398, Academic Press, New York.
6. Fazekas, A. G., and Sandor, T. 1971. Flavin nucleotide coenzyme biosynthesis and its relation to corticosteroidogenesis in the rat adrenal, *Endocrinology* **89**:397-407.
7. Fazekas, A. G., and Sandor, T. 1971. The *in vivo* effect of adrenocorticotrophin on the biosynthesis of flavin nucleotides in rat liver and kidney, *Can. J. Biochem.* **49**:987-989.
7a. Fazekas, A. G., and Sandor, T. 1973. Studies on the biosynthesis of flavin nucleotides from 2-^{14}C-riboflavin by rat liver and kidney, *Can. J. Biochem.* **51**:772-782.
8. Giri, K. V., and Krishnaswamy, P. R. 1956. Circular paper chromatography, part X. Separation, identification and quantitative estimation of riboflavin and flavin compounds, *Indian Inst. Sci.* **38**:232-244.
9. Huennekens, F. M., Sanadi, D. R., Diamant, E., and Schepartz, A. I. 1953. The occurrence of a new flavin dinucleotide (FAD-X), *J. Am. Chem. Soc.* **75**:3611-3612.
10. Kilgour, G. L., Felton, S. P., and Huennekens, F. M. 1957. Paper chromatography of flavins and flavin nucleotides, *J. Am. Chem. Soc.* **79**:2254-2256.
11. Kokai, K., Fazekas, A. G., and Domjan, G. 1967. The determination of tissue flavins by spectrophotometry, *Kisérl. Orvostud.* **19**:241-248.
12. Kovacs, E., and Fazekas, A. G. 1962. Ein einfaches Verfahren zur Herstellung von Flavin-Adenin-Dinucleotid (FAD), *Naturwiss.* **15**:349-350.
13. Koziol, F. 1971. Fluorometric analyses of riboflavin and its coenzymes, *in:* "Vitamins and Coenzymes, Methods in Enzymology" (D. B. McCormick and L. D. Wright, eds.), Vol. XVIII, Part B. pp. 253-285, Academic Press, New York.
14. McCormick, D. B., and Wright, L. D., eds. 1971. Vitamins and coenzymes, *in:* "Methods in Enzymology," Vol. XVIII, Part B, Sec. VIII, Academic Press, New York.
15. Ostrowski, W., and Krawczyk, A. 1963. The riboflavin flavoprotein from egg yolk, *Acta Chem. Scand.* **17**:5241-5245.
16. Pearson, W. N. 1967. Riboflavin, *in:* "The Vitamins. Chemistry, Physiology, Pathology, Methods" (G. Gyorgy and W. N. Pearson, eds.), Vol. VII, pp. 99-136, Academic Press, New York.

17. Rao, N. A., Felton, S. P., Huennekens, F. M., and Mackler, B. 1963. Flavin mononucleotide: The coenzyme of reduced diphosphopyridine nucleotide dehydrogenase, *J. Biol. Chem.* **238**:449-455.

18. Rhodes, M. B., Bennett, N., and Feeney, R. E. 1959. The flavoprotein-apoprotein system of egg white, *J. Biol. Chem.* **234**:2054-2060.

19. Whitby, L. G. 1953. A new method for preparing flavin-adenine dinucleotide, *Biochem. J.* **54**:437-442.

20. Whitby, L. G. 1950. Enzymic formation of a new riboflavin derivative, *Nature* **166**:479-480.

21. Yagi, K. 1962. Chemical determination of flavins, *Methods Biochem. Anal.* **10**:319-356.

22. Yagi, K. 1956. Simplified lumiflavin method for the microdetermination of flavin compounds in animal tissues, *J. Biochem.* **43**:635-644.

23. Yagi, K., and Oishi, N. 1971. Separating determination of flavins using thin layer chromatography, *J. Vitaminol.* **17**:49-51.

24. Yagi, K., Okuda, J., and Matsuoka, Y. 1955. Separation of flavins by ion-exchange resins, *Nature* **175**:555-556.

25. Yagi, K., Nagatsu, T., Nagatsu-Ishibashi, I., and Ohashi, A. 1966. Migration of injected C^{14}-labelled riboflavin into rat tissues, *J. Biochem.* **59**:313-315.

26. Murphy, B. E. P. 1970. Methodological problems in competitive protein binding techniques, *in:* "Karolinska Symposia on Research Methods in Reproductive Endocrinology" (E. Diczfalusy, ed.), Second Symposium, Steroid Assay by Protein Binding, pp. 37-60, Karolinska Institutet, Stockholm.

27. Frazekas, A. G., Menendez, C. E., and Rivlin, R. S. 1974. A competitive protein binding assay for urinary riboflavin, *Biochem. Med.* **9**:167-176.

ABSORPTION, PROTEIN BINDING, AND ELIMINATION OF RIBOFLAVIN

William J. Jusko and Gerhard Levy

The absorption, distribution, metabolism, and excretion of riboflavin have been studied most extensively in man and in the rat. These studies have revealed considerable species differences in the intestinal absorption, protein binding, biliary excretion, and renal excretion of the vitamin. Fortunately, the pharmacologic innocuousness and the availability of good methods for the quantitative analysis of riboflavin in biological fluids and tissues have permitted detailed investigation of the pharmacokinetic characteristics of the vitamin in man. Most of these studies have been carried out with relatively large doses of riboflavin (>0.1 mg/kg), considerably in excess of the amounts that satisfy nutritional requirements. Such studies are therefore useful more for elucidating mechanisms of absorption and elimination of the vitamin, rather than for illustrating the quantitative aspects of these processes when riboflavin is derived entirely from normal dietary sources.

WILLIAM J. JUSKO AND GERHARD LEVY—Department of Pharmaceutics, School of Pharmacy, State University of New York at Buffalo, Buffalo, New York.

This report was written while WJJ was Assistant Professor of Pharmacology, Boston University School of Medicine and Veterans Administration Hospital, Boston, Massachusetts.

1. ABSORPTION

1.1. Normal Patterns of Riboflavin Absorption

Considerable differences in absorption and disposition of riboflavin among species have led to confusion concerning the degree and mechanism of intestinal absorption of riboflavin. In man, riboflavin is absorbed to an appreciable degree by a specialized transport process that appears to be localized in the proximal small intestine. Evidence for this, to be described in greater detail in subsequent paragraphs, takes the following nature:

1. Site specificity of intestinal absorption is shown by the absorption of as much as 60% of an oral dose of riboflavin, while similar doses administered rectally yield only about 10% absorption.
2. Studies of the absorption of riboflavin administered in various pharmaceutical dosage forms have shown that the vitamin must be released promptly (i.e., in the proximal region of the intestinal tract) from the product, or absorption will be diminished.
3. Saturability of intestinal absorption of riboflavin has been demonstrated by the administration of 5- to 300-mg doses of the vitamin of which decreasing fractions are recovered in the urine as the dose is increased.
4. Specialized transport is also indicated by the fact that riboflavin absorption from oral doses can occur at an extremely rapid rate, while the physicochemical properties of the vitamin suggest that passive diffusion across the intestine should be slow.

1.1.1. Intestinal Absorption in Man

The absorption of riboflavin and FMN has usually been studied in man by following the urinary excretion of the vitamin. This method of elucidating the absorption characteristics of the vitamin in man is valid as long as: (a) large doses (>5 mg) are used, (b) comparison is made of data obtained after oral and parenteral doses, (c) the time course of excretion is followed until no further elimination of the dose occurs (8-24 hr), and (d) concentration-dependent effects on the renal clearance of riboflavin are recognized as a confounding factor. (These precautions apply as well to the examination of plasma concentration data.) The application of pharmacokinetic principles is helpful because they sort out the simultaneously acting variables and because plasma

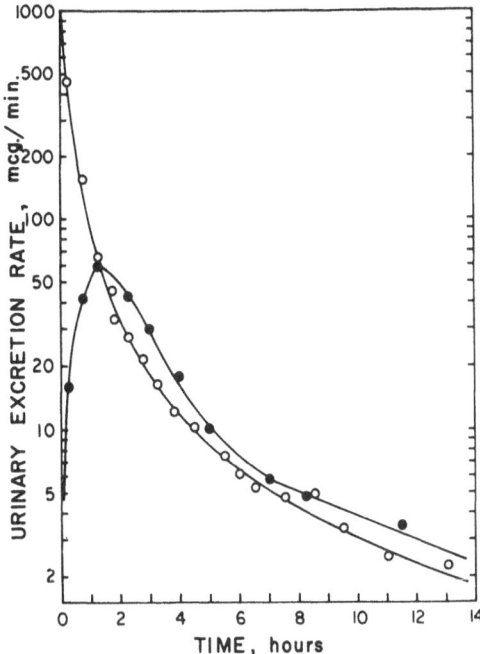

Fig. 1. Urinary excretion rate of riboflavin in a normal adult as a function of time oral (●) and intravenous (o) administration of 30 mg riboflavin as FMN. Adapted from Jusko and Levy. [50,53]

and urine drug levels will differ appreciably, depending on whether the degree and time course of drug absorption is governed by first-order or Michaelis–Menten kinetics.

Figure 1 shows the time course of urinary excretion of riboflavin after oral and intravenous administration of 30 mg riboflavin as FMN (riboflavin-5'-phosphate) to a normal adult male subject. [50,53] Ninety percent of the i.v. dose was excreted into the urine, while only 44% of the oral dose was recovered. The ratio of urinary recoveries indicates that about 50% of the oral dose was absorbed. The curvilinear decline in the logarithm of excretion rates is caused by the relatively slow tissue distribution of the vitamin and the concentration dependence in its renal clearance. Upon completion of the absorption process, urinary excretion rates decline in parallel for both the oral and parenteral dosage forms. The rapid absorption of riboflavin is reflected by the early appearance of peak excretion rates and the subsequent parallel decline of the oral and i.v. curves when the vitamin is given orally in solution. These types of data are one indication that riboflavin absorption is probably limited

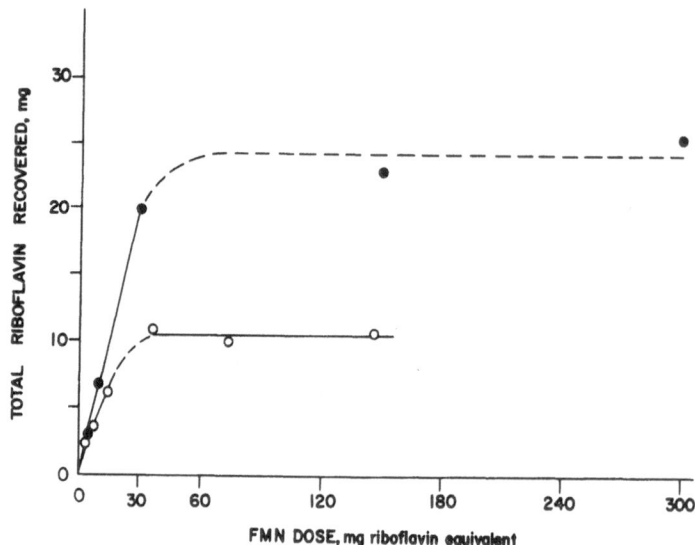

Fig. 2. Urinary recovery of riboflavin in normal adults after oral administration of various doses of FMN following a standard breakfast. The limited absorption capacity is evident in the high dose range. Upper data were obtained by Jusko and Levy[50] and lower data by Stripp.[124] From Jusko and Levy.[50] (Reproduced with permission of the copyright owner.)

to the proximal small intestine because continued absorption would have decreased the slope of the curve after the excretion peak. A similar absorption pattern is usually observed when the vitamin is administered in various pharmaceutical dosage forms in that the absorption phase is limited to 2–3 hr even though only a fraction of the dose is absorbed.

When large oral doses of the vitamin are administered in solution to adults, the upper limit in intestinal absorption of riboflavin appears to be about 25 mg under ordinary conditions.[50] Figure 2 shows urinary recoveries of riboflavin after oral doses of 5–300 mg riboflavin were given as FMN to normal adult subjects. The vitamin was ingested in the form of sodium FMN since the solubility is limited and it was desired to maintain the vitamin in solution. The upper data, from Jusko and Levy,[50] reflect the optimal absorption of the vitamin since it was administered with food that causes maximal riboflavin absorption. The lower data, from Stripp,[124] involved no control of dietary conditions, and absorption was less efficient. Both sets of data show relatively constant fractional absorption of the dose of vitamin over the range of about 5–30 mg. If food is ingested prior to the riboflavin dose, maximum absorption is achieved when the doses of the vitamin exceed about

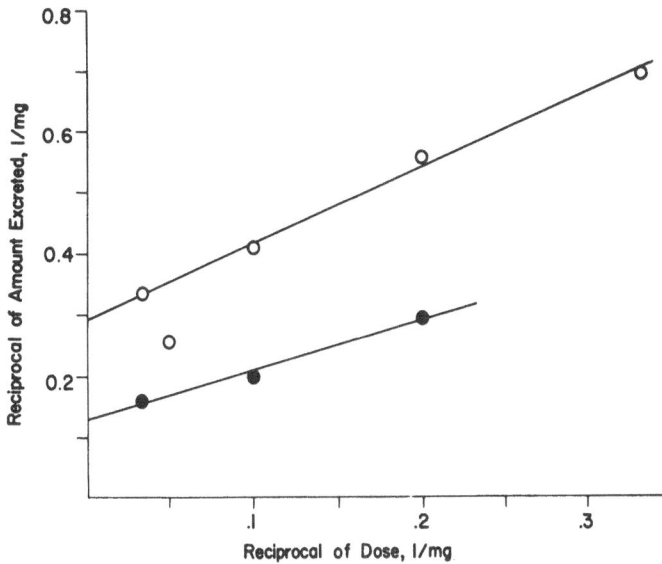

Fig. 3. Lineweaver–Burk-type plot of the reciprocal of the amount of riboflavin recovered in the urine versus the reciprocal of the oral dose given on an empty stomach to two normal adults. From Levy and Jusko. [70] (Reproduced with permission of the copyright owner.)

50 mg. This condition occurs at even smaller doses when the vitamin is given to fasting subjects. About 45% of a 5-mg dose, 30% of a 10-mg dose, and 16% of a 30-mg dose are recovered in the urine of fasting adult subjects. [70] Such data, indicative of a capacity-limited transport process, can be quantitated in terms of Michaelis–Menten kinetics, as shown in Fig. 3. The Lineweaver–Burke type of graph reflects the dose-dependent absorption of riboflavin by two fasting adult males. The linearity of the data is consistent with a specialized absorption process having a maximum capacity and a half-saturation constant. The subject represented by the lower line absorbed relatively more of the vitamin; the difference in absorption was attributed to either a longer duration of absorption (slower gastrointestinal transit) or a greater gastrointestinal surface area in the first subject.

Two of the major characteristics of a specialized intestinal transport process are saturability and site specificity. The latter is markedly evident in man when riboflavin absorption from the small intestine and colon are compared. Table I shows urinary recoveries of riboflavin after administration of about 5 mg of the vitamin by various routes to a male adult. Although absorption from the small intestine is incomplete,

TABLE I. *Effect of Route of Administration on Urinary Recovery of a 5-mg Dose of Riboflavin in a Normal Human Subject*[a]

Route of administration	Urinary recovery, %
Oral, empty stomach	35.8
Oral, after breakfast	49.8
Intravenous	72.0
Rectal	6.2

[a]Data from Levy and Jusko.[70]

colonic absorption is about one-eighth of that from the small intestine. Other studies have also demonstrated the poor absorption of riboflavin from the colon in man. Campbell and Morrison[13] recovered 3% of a rectal dose of 5 mg riboflavin in the urine compared to 66% recovery of an oral dose. Sorrell and co-workers[121] measured blood levels of riboflavin after direct installation of 20 mg riboflavin into the large intestine of surgical patients. When their data are compared to blood-level data obtained after intravenous injection of riboflavin,[53] the extent of absorption of the vitamin from the large intestine can be estimated as less than 15%.

1.1.2. Intestinal Absorption in Animals

The gastrointestinal absorption of riboflavin differs considerably in man and animals. Prior to the elucidation of the specialized transport process for riboflavin in man, studies in animals yielded little indication of the complexity of riboflavin absorption from the gastrointestinal tract. Several studies of riboflavin transport were made in various *ex vivo* animal intestinal preparations. Spencer et al.[122] used everted intestinal sacs from rats and hamsters and the *in vivo* ligated loop technique in rats to investigate riboflavin transport. They did not find accumulation against a concentration gradient and, in fact, noted that the intestinal sac was relatively impermeable to the vitamin. Similar results were later obtained by Turner and Hughes.[135] Both studies involved the use of relatively high concentrations (1×10^{-4} M) of riboflavin, which may have saturated the transport process. However, subsequent studies by Spencer and Bow[123] with physiological concentrations (7×10^{-6} M) of radiolabeled riboflavin showed uptake of riboflavin into the intestinal wall, but serosal-to-mucosal concentration ratios greater than unity, indicative of uphill transport across the intestine, could not be demonstrated. It was thus concluded that riboflavin absorption in isolated and *in vivo* rat intestinal preparations occurred only by passive diffusion. Additional studies of the passive transport of riboflavin across the everted rat intestine have been made by Mayersohn and Gibaldi.[85] Riboflavin transfer was decreased by materials that cause tissue fluid uptake (glucose and xylose), while carbohydrates that cause no tissue fluid uptake (mannitol) do not affect transfer of riboflavin and other compounds. Hayton *et al.*[44] found that riboflavin absorption from the *in situ* rat intestine was comparable to such poorly absorbed compounds as phenol red and tetracycline. The poor absorption of the vitamin from the rat intestine has led to the use of riboflavin phosphate as a "nonabsorbed" complexing agent in studies of the inhibiting effect of complex formation on absorption of various well-absorbed drugs.[125]

Middleton and Grice[88] studied ^{14}C-riboflavin absorption in the intact rat. About 27% of an orally administered dose of 10 μg riboflavin was recovered in the urine; 10% of the dose was found in the feces. Surgical removal of most of the small intestine had only a slight effect on these recovery values, and absorption from the large intestine was found to be slightly less than from the small intestine. It was concluded that riboflavin was absorbed throughout the intestine of the rat with maximal absorption occurring in the ileum. Absorption of riboflavin from the colon of the rat, as in man, appears to be limited. Kasper[62] gave colonic doses of FMN as large as 6 mg/kg to rats that were maintained on a riboflavin-free diet and observed very poor growth in comparison with the growth of animals given tenfold smaller oral doses.

Christensen[17] administered oral doses of 0.2–4.0 mg riboflavin as FMN to normal rats and found a relatively constant 5% of the dose in the urine and 12% in the feces after 72 hr. Metabolism was suggested as the fate of most of the remainder of the vitamin.[18] Comprehensive studies of riboflavin absorption and disposition in the rat were recently carried out by Axelson and Gibaldi.[5] A summary of the data obtained after oral and intraperitoneal administration of 0.2- and 1.0-mg doses of riboflavin as FMN to various combinations of normal, riboflavin-deficient, fasted, fed, and bile-duct–ligated animals is shown in Table II. Normal, fasted rats (*G* and *J*) excreted 51–63% of i.p. doses of the vitamin in the urine, while the recovery of a 1.0-mg oral dose (*F*) was only 10%. It was estimated that about 20% of a 1-mg oral dose of riboflavin is absorbed in the rat. However, these data show that the study of riboflavin absorption and disposition in the rat is complicated by factors such as disproportionate increases in biliary excretion with increasing body levels of the vitamin (Section 3.2), decreased tissue binding with higher body levels, and increased retention in the tissues of riboflavin-deficient rats. These factors, as well as the poor intestinal

TABLE II. Urinary Recovery of Riboflavin after FMN Administration to Rats under Various Experimental Conditions[a]

Group	Dose, μg	Number of animals	Route of administration	Nutrition status	Dietary state	Bile duct	Amount excreted in urine, μg[b]		Total urinary recovery, %[b]
							in 24 hr	in 72 hr	
A	1000	10	Oral	Deficient	Fasted	Intact	15 ± 9	44 ± 21	4 ± 2
B	1000	5	Oral	Deficient	Fed	Intact	8 ± 6	44 ± 33	4 ± 3
C	1000	5	I.p.	Deficient	Fasted	Intact	404 ± 38	413 ± 36	41 ± 4
D	1000	11	Oral	Deficient	Fasted	Ligated	18 ± 7	58 ± 26	6 ± 3
E	1000	8	I.p.	Deficient	Fasted	Ligated	657 ± 68	721 ± 74	72 ± 7
F	1000	6	Oral	Normal	Fasted	Intact	65 ± 31	98 ± 40	10 ± 4
G	1000	7	I.p.	Normal	Fasted	Intact	490 ± 35	509 ± 49	51 ± 5
H	200	5	I.p.	Deficient	Fasted	Intact	...	59 ± 5	29 ± 3
I	200	5	I.p.	Deficient	Fasted	Ligated	...	57 ± 9	29 ± 5
J	200	10	I.p.	Normal	Fasted	Intact	...	125 ± 28	63 ± 14

[a]Data from Axelson and Gibaldi.[5]
[b]Mean ±1 standard deviation.

absorption of riboflavin in the rat, make this animal unsuitable as a model for extrapolation of riboflavin pharmacokinetics to man.

1.1.3. Mechanism of Intestinal Absorption

The absorption and excretion characteristics of the vitamin are essentially identical whether riboflavin or FMN is administered orally[50] This fact is probably due to the rapid and complete dephosphorylation of FMN to riboflavin in the small intestine. Okuda[101-103] found that FMN is rapidly decomposed enzymatically to free riboflavin in pancreatic juice and in homogenates of the small intestinal mucosa, and when it is injected into the lumen of the small intestine of rats. Similar results were obtained by Turner and Hughes,[135] who used isolated rat intestinal preparations. Phosphomonoesterase activity appears most pronounced in the jejunum and is somewhat less active in the duodenum and ileum of the rat. Riboflavin, formed from FMN or given directly, is eventually converted or reconverted to FMN in the intestinal mucosa. Yagi and Okuda[145] and Chen and Yamauchi[16] have reported that riboflavin is phosphorylated enzymatically in the mucosa during absorption in the rat. Tedeschi and Canali[128] found predominantly FMN in the mesenteric blood of rabbits after introduction of FMN or riboflavin into the intestinal tract; thus, the vitamin appears to be transferred into the mesenteric circulation as FMN. It seems that the FMN is dephosphorylated in the intestinal lumen, is rephosphorylated in the intestinal mucosa, and appears initially in the blood as FMN. Thereafter, dephosphorylation of FMN to riboflavin occurs rapidly in the blood; Stripp[124] found only free riboflavin in the venous blood of man after oral administration of FMN. Rapid dephosphorylation of FMN in whole blood occurs in man[54] and in the rat.[99]

Most of the evidence that suggests that the intestinal absorption of riboflavin involves a phosphorylation-dephosphorylation process has been obtained in the rat, in which, in contrast, only little of the vitamin is absorbed. Since considerable species difference exists in almost all aspects of riboflavin transport, it is not certain whether the mechanism of riboflavin absorption in man also involves a similar transport mechanism. However, there is no evidence of competitive inhibition in the intestinal absorption of riboflavin and thiamine in man.[72] Since phosphorylation is involved in[113] thiamine transport it probably is not the primary mechanism for the specialized intestinal transport of riboflavin in man.

1.1.4. Developmental Aspects

The effect of age on the gastrointestinal absorption of riboflavin has been studied primarily in man. Jusko *et al.*[55] administered oral saturation doses of FMN (150 mg riboflavin per square meter) with a standard meal to 23 subjects between the ages of 3 months and 40 years. Various urinary excretion parameters indicative of the absorption and elimination of riboflavin were related to the age of the subjects. The percent urinary recovery, which is proportional to the absorption capacity of the subjects and the duration of the absorption process, showed the greatest age dependence. The total urinary recovery of the vitamin increased gradually from about 6% at 0.25 years to about 12% at 40 years of age, a statistically significant increase (see Fig. 4). The percent urinary recovery was only a small fraction of the dose because the administered amount was greatly in excess of that which can be absorbed (see Fig. 2). This fact permitted the assumption that absorption occurred at maximum capacity. Since the half-life for elimination of most of the dose and the ratio of the peak excretion rate to dose (indicative of the absorption capacity) did not change with age, it was concluded that the intestinal transit rate, which controls riboflavin retention at absorption sites in the proximal small intestine, is primarily responsible

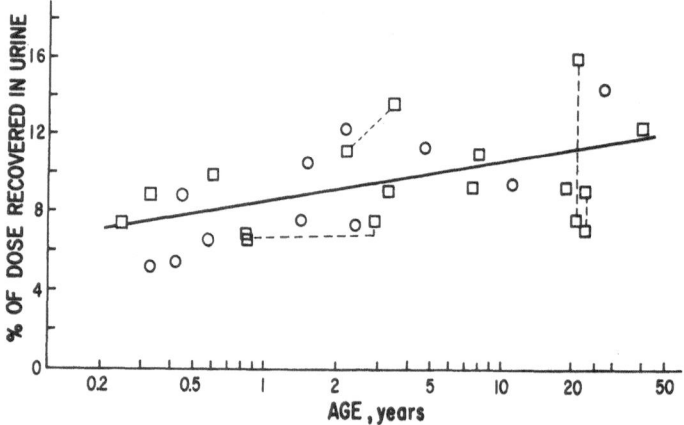

Fig. 4. Relationship between the percent urinary recovery of riboflavin and age of normal human subjects after oral administration of 150 mg/sq m riboflavin as FMN. Squares and circles represent male and female subjects, respectively. Dashed lines connect repeated tests in the same subject and solid line shows the least-squares regression fit of the data (intercept = 8.34% at 1 yr, slope = 2.22, r = 0.57, p < 0.01). From Jusko *et al.*[55] (Reproduced with permission of the copyright owner.)

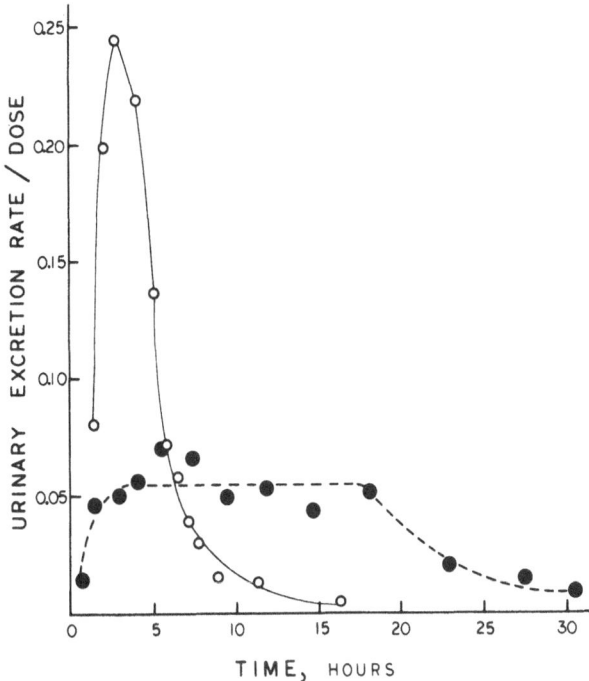

Fig. 5. Urinary excretion rate/dose (μg/min/mg) of riboflavin as a function of time after oral administration of 150 mg/sq m riboflavin as FMN to a 10-month-old infant (o); and a 5-day-old infant (●). From Jusko *et al.*[56]

for the age-dependent change in riboflavin absorption at ages greater than 3 months.

Similar studies were carried out in 5- to 6-day-old infants to whom oral and intramuscular doses of FMN had been given.[56] Figure 5 shows the striking difference in the time course of urinary excretion of riboflavin after oral administration of saturation doses to a 5-day-old infant and a 10-month-old infant. The maximum urinary excretion rate in the 10-month-old is several times higher than that of the neonate, but the latter shows a much longer duration of absorption (14–16 hr). As a consequence, the total amount of riboflavin excreted in the urine is similar at both ages, namely, 6–8% of the administered dose. A limited renal capacity was not responsible for the low excretion rate in the neonate, although the renal clearance of the vitamin was somewhat lower in the neonate than in older subjects. Although detailed studies were carried out in only two newborn infants, the slow and prolonged excretion of riboflavin in the newborn appears to be due to slow, but sustained, intestinal absorption. In spite of an apparently immature intestinal transport mechanism, the human neonate seems to be capable of absorbing an adequate amount of riboflavin for nutritional purposes.

Developmental aspects of riboflavin absorption from the gastrointestinal tract have not been investigated systematically in other species. Cordona and Payne, [28] using an *ex vivo* everted sac preparation, observed that riboflavin transfer was 45% greater in the mature chicken compared to immature female chickens.

1.1.5. Absorption from Other Body Sites

The most common route of administration of riboflavin is that via the gastrointestinal tract. No direct evidence seems to indicate absorption of riboflavin from the stomach. Chen and Liao[15] administered riboflavin orally to rats and, 1 hr later, observed no vitamin in the mucous membrane of the stomach.

Absorption of riboflavin from intramuscular injection sites in man is rapid and leads to essentially complete recovery of the vitamin in the urine. After i.m. injection of about 17 mg/m^2 of FMN in solution, the maximum urinary excretion rate occurs within 30 min and urinary recoveries averaged 79% in four normal adults[51] and 93% in two newborn infants. [56]

Riboflavin is absorbed percutaneously in the rat. Schaefer and co-workers[119] used the growth of rats as an index of absorption of topical biweekly doses of 250 and 500 μg riboflavin. The animals were restrained from licking the site of application. Comparison of body weights after 2 and 5 weeks of dosing showed that some degree of riboflavin absorption through the skin occurred. However, topical application was less efficient than oral administration of the vitamin.

1.1.6. Physicochemical Properties in Relation to Absorption

The physicochemical properties of riboflavin and FMN are not compatible with rapid or appreciable absorption by passive diffusion. The partition coefficient for riboflavin between chloroform and either pH 1 or pH 7 aqueous solution is less than 0.001, and the molecular weight of riboflavin is 376. These properties preclude rapid diffusion through biological membranes, such as the intestine, which behave as lipoid-sieve barriers and have a molecular weight cutoff of about 200–400 for passage of non-lipoid-soluble compounds. [141] The larger molecular weight (514), negative charge, and even poorer lipid solubility of FMN suggest that it too will diffuse only very slowly across intestinal membranes. Because of these characteristics, the intestinal absorption of

TABLE III. *Physical Properties of Riboflavin Crystal Types*[a]

Type	Microscopic appearance	Solubility, mg/ml at 25° C
A	Long hairlike fibers	0.05-0.1
B	Short thin needles	0.15-0.25
C	Short wide needles	0.50-1.40

[a]From Brumfield and Gross.[10]

the vitamin would be extremely slow unless transport occurs by a specialized process.

Other physicochemical properties that may, at times, affect the absorption or disposition of riboflavin and FMN include the crystal form of the vitamin, its solubility in aqueous solution, and the ease with which riboflavin forms complexes or chelates with other substances. As shown in Table III, riboflavin has three crystal forms, each with different water solubilities. Type B (Regular Type, Roche) is the material most often encountered in pharmaceutical preparations.[115] Riboflavin-5'-phosphate, as the sodium salt, is the preferred form of the vitamin for many pharmaceutical purposes because of its appreciable solubility of 112 mg/ml at pH 6.9. A slight disadvantage to FMN may be its greater susceptibility (compared to riboflavin) to formation of chelates with divalent metals.

A large number of substances are capable of forming complexes

TABLE IV. *Substances Found to Complex or Chelate with Riboflavin or FMN*

Divalent metals[a]	
Cu^{++}	p-aminobenzoate[c]
Zn^{++}	Benzoate salts[c]
Co^{++}	Salicyate salts[c]
Fe^{++}	Sodium saccharin[c]
Mn^{++}	Vanillin[c]
Cd^{++}	Tyrosine amide[c]
Caffeine[b]	Tryptophan[c]
Theophylline[b]	Urea[c]
Dimethyluracil[b]	Sodium deoxycholate[c]
Benzyl alcohol[c]	Napthol sulfonates[c]
Gentisic acid salts[c]	Ascorbic acid[d]
Boric acid salts[c]	Anthraquinone derivatives[e]
Nicotinamide[c]	Cinnamate derivatives[e]
2,4-Dihydroxybenzoic acid[c]	Anisate[e]

[a]Foye.[33] [b]Guttman and Athalye.[41] [c]Brumfield and Gross.[10] [d]Huttenrauch.[46] [e]Harbury and Foley.[42]

or chelates with riboflavin or FMN. For example, nicotinamide, which is included in 5% concentration in a commercial intravenous solution of riboflavin (Eli Lilly and Co.), increases riboflavin solubility from about 0.1 to 10 mg/ml.[10] Table IV summarizes the variety of other drugs and chemicals which are known to complex or to chelate with riboflavin or FMN. Since complexation of the vitamin with the other substance can alter the pharmacologic properties of either or both compounds, results of experimental studies that involve the use of drugs or chemicals together with riboflavin or FMN should be interpreted cautiously. For example, boric acid can produce riboflavin deficiency in many species,[116] presumably by a mechanism of complex formation with riboflavin,[41] which decreases tissue uptake and protein binding and thus enhances the renal excretion of the vitamin.

1.2. Factors Affecting Riboflavin Absorption

1.2.1. Effects of Natural Substances

1.2.1A. FOOD. The gastrointestinal absorption of riboflavin is increased appreciably in the presence of food, particularly at doses greater than 10 mg.[50] Figure 6 shows the urinary excretion rates of riboflavin as a function of time after administration of 30 mg riboflavin with and without previous ingestion of a standard meal consisting of 60 g of cornflakes and 500 ml of milk. About 60% of the vitamin is absorbed when taken with food, but only 15% of the dose is absorbed when the vitamin is taken on an empty stomach. The inset of Fig. 6 shows the linear relationship obtained between dose and urinary recovery of riboflavin when the vitamin is given with food. Also shown is the nonlinear absorption of riboflavin in the absence of food. Similar urinary recoveries in the presence of food were obtained by Morrison and Campbell[93] with riboflavin doses of 1–20 mg. The physical bulk of the meal partly accounts for the increased absorption of riboflavin since the urinary recovery of the vitamin increases from 15 to 22% if it is given with 600 ml of water instead of 200 ml of water. The major effect of food probably involves a decreased rate of intestinal transit, which increases the degree and duration of vitamin exposure to absorption sites in the small intestine. If very large doses of FMN are given (150–300 mg), ingestion of a second meal 3–4 hr after the first appears to cause additional absorption of the as yet unabsorbed vitamin still present in the upper gastrointestinal tract. This procedure causes secondary peaks in the

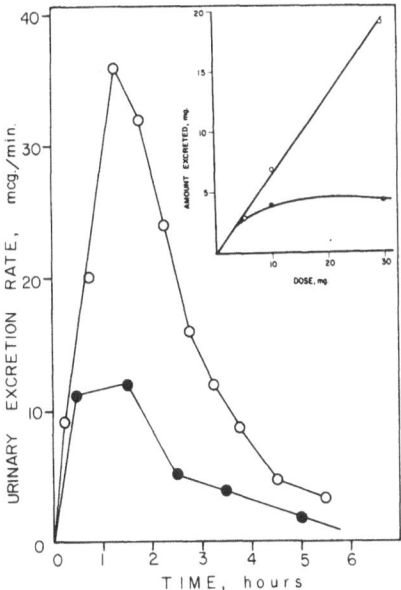

Fig. 6. Mean urinary excretion rate of riboflavin as a function of time after oral administration of 10 mg riboflavin to four normal adults on an empty stomach (●); and after a standard breakfast (o). Inset shows urinary recoveries of riboflavin after oral administration of 5- to 30-mg doses of FMN under the same conditions. Adapted from Jusko and Levy.[50]

urinary excretion rate *vs.* time profile which were originally thought to be the result of enterohepatic cycling of the vitamin.[50]

1.2.1B. BILE SALTS. The stimulation of bile flow by food, coupled with the possible role of bile salts in riboflavin absorption, may be involved in the enhancement of riboflavin absorption by food. Mayersohn *et al.*[84] determined the effect of sodium deoxycholate on the intestinal absorption of riboflavin and FMN in normal human subjects (Table V). There was a significant increase in urinary recovery of riboflavin after administration of the vitamin with the bile salt. This increase was probably not an effect of the bile salt on metabolism or urinary excretion or riboflavin: Murata *et al.*[97] showed that ursodeoxycholate actually decreased the urinary excretion of the vitamin after subcutaneous administration of 10 mg riboflavin to tuberculosis patients. Earlier studies by Onishi[104] and by Arakawa *et al.*[3] demonstrated that ursodeoxycholate, when incubated with riboflavin in the intestinal lumen of dogs and guinea pigs, increases the concentration of phosphorylated riboflavin

TABLE V. *Effect of Sodium Deoxycholate[a] on Gastrointestinal Absorption of 30-mg Doses of Riboflavin and FMN in Man[b]*

Flavin	Number of subjects	Urinary recovery of riboflavin, %		Statistical difference
		Control	With bile salt	
FR	4	18.0	29.5	$p < 0.001$
FMN	5	18.5	23.4	$p < 0.025$

[a] Doses of 600 mg bile salt were given orally 0.5 hr before the vitamin.
[b] From Mayersohn et al. [84]

in the intestinal wall. Mayersohn et al.[84] also showed that 10 mM sodium taurodeoxycholate increases the rate of passive transfer of riboflavin across the everted intestine of the rat. The role of bile salts in the intestinal absorption of riboflavin may include either alteration of intestinal transit or a direct effect on or involvement in the specialized transport process.

1.2.1c. GLUCOSE. Conflicting reports have appeared concerning the possible effects of glucose on riboflavin absorption. Glucose-1-phosphate and ATP have been considered as possible phosphate donors in the synthesis of FMN from riboflavin in the mucosa of the small intestine.[63] This fact could account for the enhanced uptake of riboflavin in the presence of glucose in the small intestine of the chicken that was observed by Cordona.[27] In contrast, Fukuhara[36,37] found that glucose decreased the intestinal absorption of riboflavin in the ligated small intestine of the rabbit; Mayersohn and Gibaldi[85] found that glucose decreased the passive transfer of riboflavin by altering water uptake in the everted rat intestine. Studies of the effect of glucose on riboflavin absorption in man are warranted.

1.2.1d. THIAMIN. It originally appeared that the intestinal absorption of both riboflavin and thiamine involves phosphorylation during transfer across the intestinal mucosa.[16,113] Thus it was of interest to determine whether therapeutic doses of the two vitamins mutually inhibit their absorption by competition for the same transport process. Levy and Hewitt[72] evaluated the urinary excretion of riboflavin and thiamine after oral administration of 41 mg FMN and/or 26.9 mg thiamin (both molar equivalents of 30 mg riboflavin) to normal subjects. Neither vitamin appeared to affect the absorption of the other. This fact suggests that the two vitamins do not share a common specialized absorption pathway in man.

1.2.1E. FOLIC ACID. The possible biochemical interrelationship of riboflavin and folate is of recent interest[108,114] Berlin *et al.*[7] measured the urinary excretion of riboflavin after oral administration of this vitamin to 19 human subjects with and without co-ingestion of folic acid. No effect of folic acid was observed.

1.2.1F. ASCORBIC ACID-CALCIUM. Libby *et al.*[77] administered 10 mg riboflavin to six human subjects with and without separate tablets containing vitamins C and D and an unidentified form of calcium. The urinary recovery of riboflavin decreased to 56% of control values when the mineral-vitamin preparation was coadministered. Although it is not known which material caused the decrease in riboflavin absorption, both ascorbic acid[46] and most divalent metals[33] are capable of forming complexes or chelates with riboflavin and FMN.

1.2.1G. THYROXINE. The metabolism of riboflavin is affected by thyroid hormone as described in Chapter 12. Administration of thyroxine to rats[110] and man[107] appears to decrease the intestinal absorption of riboflavin, but this result requires further substantiation.

1.2.1H. STEROID HORMONES. Cordona and Payne[28] used an everted gut technique to determine the effect of earlier estradiol injections on riboflavin absorption in chickens. The hormone decreased riboflavin transfer into the gut in mature male chickens but had no effect on immature females. Brummer *et al.*[11] gave oral doses of 6 mg riboflavin before and during the administration of triamcinolone and dexamethasone to 11 human subjects. These corticosteroids did not affect the urinary recoveries of riboflavin and several other B vitamins. Verzar[139] showed that adrenalectomized rats will die unless FMN is administered; he claimed that adrenal cortical hormones restore the FMN synthetic process of the intestinal mucosa of rats after inhibition of this process by monoiodoacetic acid. These studies are of interest because Fazekas and Sandor[31] recently found that adrenal steroids affect the synthesis of FMN and FAD from riboflavin in adrenal tissue; a similar relationship in the small intestine may therefore exist. This subject is treated more fully in Chapter 13.

1.2.2. Effects of Drugs

1.2.2A. ANTIBIOTICS. The role of antibiotics in riboflavin nutrition has been studied in rats by Lih and Baumann[78] and reviewed by

Goldsmith.[39] Antibiotics such as tetracyclines, penicillin, and strep-tomycin have a sparing effect on marginal riboflavin diets by apparently influencing synthetic and degradative microorganisms in the gastrointes-tinal tract. Most of such studies were performed in animals, and studies of the effects of antibiotics on riboflavin absorption in man have not been pursued. Doiphode and Bamji[30] recently showed that treatment of human subjects with 0.5 g aureomycin daily for 7 days causes an increase in urinary excretion and a decrease in fecal excretion of endogenous levels of riboflavin. These results might be explained by the well-known[65] antianabolic effects of tetracyclines which could mobilize riboflavin from the labile flavoprotein pool of the liver.

1.2.2B. PROBENECID. Jusko and Levy[51] measured the effects of oral doses of probenecid on the urinary excretion of riboflavin after oral and intramuscular administration of the vitamin to human subjects. Not only does probenecid inhibit the active tubular secretion of riboflavin in man,[54] but the data also suggest that probenecid inhibits the intestinal absorption of riboflavin.

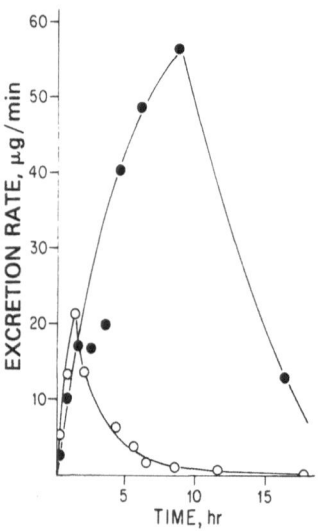

Fig. 7. Effect of an anticholinergic drug on riboflavin absorption. Urinary excretion rate of riboflavin as a function of time after oral administration of 150 mg/m² riboflavin as FMN on an empty stomach. Control (o); after propantheline bromide, 30 mg in the evening before and 30 mg in the morning of the study (●). Data from Levy *et al.*[74]

1.2.2c. ANTICHOLINERGICS. Anticholinergic agents inhibit gastric emptying and decrease intestinal transit rate. These effects result in a longer residence time of materials in the proximal small intestine and thereby prolong contact of riboflavin with its specialized absorption sites. Oral administration of the anticholinergic agent propantheline bromide to fasting healthy adult males 30-60 min before a large oral dose of FMN (150 mg riboflavin equivalent per square meter of body surface area) delayed the absorption of the vitamin (because of slower gastric emptying) but increased considerably the total amount absorbed.[74] Administration of FMN alone resulted in an average 24-hr recovery of 3.6% of the dose in the urine; pretreatment with propantheline bromide increased the average recovery of the vitamin to 8.0% of the dose. Figure 7 shows the pronounced prolongation of the riboflavin absorption phase if the vitamin was taken after administration of the anticholinergic agent. These results are similar to those of food (see Section 1.2.1) and affect mainly the absorption of relatively large, and therefore incompletely absorbed, doses of riboflavin.

1.2.3. Effect of Disease

Most published studies on riboflavin in disease have been designed so that no distinction can be made between possible effects of the disease on absorption and on metabolic retention or biotransformation of the vitamin. The most definitive information is obtained by administering riboflavin orally and parenterally, at different times, to healthy subjects and to patients with various diseases. Since the relative metabolic retention and biotransformation of large doses (>5 mg in human adults) of riboflavin is small, some information on the effect of disease on riboflavin absorption may be obtained even if the vitamin is administered orally only, provided that large doses are employed. This procedure has the obvious disadvantage of limited relevance to nutritional problems. The significance of the studies to be reviewed here should be assessed with this limitation in mind.

1.2.3A. BILIARY ATRESIA. Jusko *et al.*[59] studied the effect of biliary obstruction (mainly due to congenital biliary atresia) on riboflavin absorption in infants and children. A saturation dose of FMN (150 mg riboflavin equivalent per square meter of body surface area) was administered orally, in aqueous solution, immediately after a standard breakfast. There was no apparent difference in the half-life for elimination of the vitamin in the sick children and in normal control subjects in the same age range. The absorption of riboflavin, as judged by the fraction of

TABLE VI. Comparison of Riboflavin Absorption in Normal Children and Patients with Biliary Obstruction[a]

Parameter[b]	Normal subjects	Patients with biliary obstruction	Statistical differences
Number of tests	15	9	—
Urinary recovery, percent of dose	8.90 (2.41)	5.34 (2.74)	$p < 0.01$
Maximum excretion rate per dose, μg/min/mg	0.257 (0.078)	0.127 (0.055)	$p < 0.01$
Age, yr	1.86(1.32)	1.36 (1.14)	N.S.
Weight, kg	10.9 (3.7)	7.73 (2.37)	$p < 0.025$

[a]Data from Jusko et al. [59]
[b]Mean values are shown with standard deviation in parentheses.

the dose recovered in the urine during 24 hr, was significantly impaired in children with biliary obstruction (Table VI). This impairment may be the result of the absence of bile in the intestinal tract. The gastrointestinal transit of a large mixed meal is more rapid in bile-fistula dogs,[1] and bile salts decrease the rate of gastric emptying and the transit rate through the proximal small intestine in rats.[32] Biliary atresia may, therefore, reduce the absorption of large doses of riboflavin by causing more rapid gastrointestinal transit and thereby decreasing the residence time of the vitamin at absorption sites in the small intestine.[59]

1.2.3B. THYROID DISEASE. Intestinal propulsive activity is increased in most thyrotoxic patients while hypomotility of the gastrointestinal tract is a common manifestation of hypothyroidism.[64] The latter condition should increase the residence time of ingested riboflavin at intestinal absorption sites and produce more extensive absorption of the vitamin in hypothyroidism. Conversely, hyperthyroidism may be expected to decrease riboflavin absorption. Ponz[110] found that treatment with thyroxine appreciably decreases the absorption of orally administered riboflavin in rats while the urinary excretion of parenterally administered riboflavin was actually increased. Extensive studies in animals have shown that thyroid hormones also affect the metabolism of riboflavin[114] (see Chapter 12). Levy et al.[75] studied riboflavin absorption in infants and children with thyroid disorders. The kinetics of elimination and the urinary recovery of riboflavin after intramuscular injection of FMN were normal in both hypothyroid and hyperthyroid children (Fig. 8). On the other hand, oral administration of a large dose of FMN resulted in much more than normal absorption by hypothyroid subjects and in below normal absorption by hyperthyroid children. The absorption of

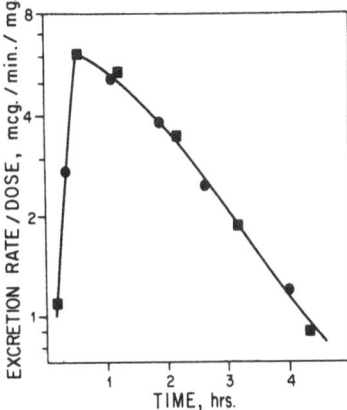

Fig. 8. Urinary excretion rate per dose (μg/min/mg) of riboflavin as a function of time after intramuscular administration of 15 mg/m² riboflavin as FMN to a hypothyroid (●) and hyperthyroid (■) child. Data from Levy et al. [75]

FMN became normal in both groups after successful treatment of the thyroid disorder (Fig. 9). The duration of absorption was considerably prolonged in the hypothyroid children and shorter than normal in hyperthyroidism—results that are consistent with the view that the differences in the extent of absorption are due to differences in intestinal transit rates.

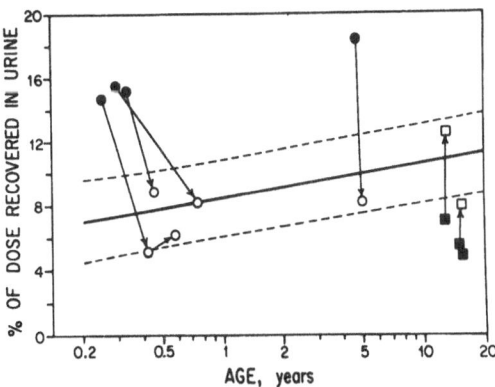

Fig. 9. Percent urinary recovery of riboflavin after oral administration of 150 mg/m² riboflavin as FMN to children who are hypothyroid (●); hyperthyroid (■); and euthyroid after treatment (o,□). Continuous and dashed lines show mean ±1 standard deviation of data obtained in normal subjects (see Fig. 4). Data from Levy et al. [75]

1.2.3C. LIVER DISEASE. Miyao *et al.*[90] investigated the effect of liver damage induced by carbon tetrachloride on the intestinal absorption of riboflavin in rabbits and rats. They also measured blood concentrations and urinary excretion of riboflavin in normal and liver-damaged children after oral administration of 0.5 mg riboflavin kg body weight. Riboflavin absorption appeared to be enhanced somewhat during acute liver damage (acute hepatitis in children; 48 hr after carbon tetrachloride injection in animals) and was diminished during chronic liver disease (liver cirrhosis in children; 6 wk after twice weekly carbon tetrachloride injections in animals).

Clarke[24] gave oral test doses (amount unspecified) of riboflavin to patients with various diseases. The mean urinary excretion of the vitamin was $33.3 \pm 10.2\%$ in 13 normal subjects (collection for 8 hr or more). Two patients with infectious hepatitis excreted less than 1% of the dose, whereas those with chronic liver disease tended to excrete 5–18% of the dose. As expected, the presence of kidney disease also diminished riboflavin excretion.

1.2.3D. OTHER DISEASES. Kagaya[61] measured the concentrations of riboflavin in the portal blood of normal and malnourished (low protein and low riboflavin diet) dogs after intragastric administration of riboflavin. The increase in riboflavin concentration, expecially in esterified form, was markedly smaller in the malnourished dogs than in the normal animals.

Markkanen[81] studied the effect of achlorhydria and partial gastrectomy on riboflavin absorption in human subjects. The average urinary recovery of a 6-mg oral dose was 31.4% in normal subjects, 27.3% in partially gastrectomized patients with acid gastric secretion, 26.5% in partially gastrectomized patients without acid gastric secretion, and only 20% in patients with achlorhydria. However, intersubject variation was large, and none of the differences is statistically significant.

1.2.4. Pharmaceutical Formulation Factors

Since the intestinal absorption of riboflavin is both saturable and limited largely to the upper region of the intestinal tract, the extent of its absorption in man can be affected by the site and rate of release of the vitamin from a pharmaceutical dosage form. Relatively large doses of riboflavin (>5 mg in adults) are almost completely recoverable in the urine of human subjects after intravenous or intramuscular administration[51,54,124]; thus, urinary recovery can serve as an index of the extent of absorption (often called physiological availability or bioavailability) of orally administered riboflavin. A measure of *relative* bioavailability may be obtained by comparing the urinary recovery of riboflavin from a pharmaceutical dosage form to that from an equal dose of riboflavin administered in aqueous solution. This "human bioassay technique" was first employed by Melnick *et al.*[87] to evaluate the absorption characteristics of vitamin tablets in man. They and others[70,94] demonstrated a linear relationship between the oral dose of riboflavin in rapidly released form (aqueous solution or rapidly dissolving tablets) and the total amount of the vitamin recovered in the urine, provided that the dose is in the 5-20 mg range and is taken after a meal. Melnick *et al.* recovered 46% of the dose on the average; Morrison and Campbell[94] recovered 61%; Levy and Jusko[70] obtained an average recovery of 62% of the dose. The difference between the results of Melnick *et al.* and those of the other two groups may result because the former gave the vitamin after dinner, while the latter administered it after breakfast. The area under a plasma concentration *vs.* time curve is not suitable for determining precisely the bioavailability of riboflavin due to the nonlinear nature of its elimination kinetics.

Chapman *et al.*[14] found that sugar-coated tablets of riboflavin that did not disintegrate within 60 min, as measured by a modified U.S.P. XIV tablet disintegration test, were usually not as well absorbed as a control dose given in the form of uncoated, rapidly disintegrating tablets. Enteric-coated tablets of riboflavin with an *in vitro* disintegration time of 120 min yielded a 24-hr urinary recovery of only 41% of the control, while enteric-coated tablets of sodium salicylate with an *in vitro* disintegration time of up to 213 min were fully absorbed.[94] A good correlation appears to exist between the disintegration time of coated riboflavin tablets and the dissolution time of riboflavin,[89] so that the disintegration time reflects the rate of release of riboflavin from the tablets used in the study. Riboflavin must be released rapidly to be available for absorption at specialized absorption sites in the proximal region of the intestinal tract; drugs such as sodium salicylate, which are absorbed from all regions of the intestine, can be released in a more distal region and yet be fully absorbed.

Coating of riboflavin particles, or combination of riboflavin with an ion exchange resin to overcome the objectionable taste of the vitamin in chewable tablets, may reduce its absorption.[95] Similarly, oral administration of riboflavin in prolonged- or sustained-release preparations has been found to decrease its absorption.[40,96] The excretion rate *vs.* time curves show that riboflavin absorption occurs only during the first few hours after administration of a sustained release preparation, i.e., while at least part of the dosage form is presumably in the stomach or in the upper region of the intestinal tract or both. Oral administration of riboflavin in prolonged-release mode (1-2 mg in solution every 2 hr) did not reduce absorption relative to the control since the vitamin, when given in this form, is readily accessible to the intestinal absorption sites. [96]

Studies in rats have shown that the intestinal transit rate of a drug solution is decreased when the viscosity of the solution is increased by addition of methylcellulose. [69] A similar retardation of intestinal transit rate in man should increase the extent of riboflavin absorption due to longer persistence of the vitamin at intestinal absorption sites. Contrary to expectations, no such increase was observed when 30 mg riboflavin as FMN was administered orally in a viscous methylcellulose solution to human volunteers. [45] In a subsequent study, administration of the vitamin in sodium alginate solution produced a 50% increase in absorption. [73] The sodium alginate solution is considerably more viscous than the methylcellulose solution at low shear rates, and it tends to gel when exposed to acidic environments such as gastric fluids. For these reasons, it may be expected to pass much more slowly through the proximal region of the small intestine.

Prolonged absorption of parenterally administered riboflavin can be achieved by appropriate pharmaceutical formulation or by chemical modification (esterification) of the vitamin. Brzezinski and co-workers [12] prepared riboflavin in a 2% aqueous suspension of aluminum monostearate for intramuscular injection and observed significant excretion of the vitamin for 6 weeks after injection. A similar prolonged release was obtained when riboflavin was incorporated in cholesterol pellets that were implanted in the thigh of human subjects. [8]

Some absorption of riboflavin has been observed upon rectal administration to dogs of a large dose (200 mg) in suppositories. [118] Suppositories containing a surface-active agent caused more rapid absorption than suppositories made from only cocoa butter, as judged by the serum concentrations of riboflavin. No indication of the extent of absorption of the vitamin was provided in the cited study.

1.2.5. Riboflavin Derivatives

A large number of fat-soluble fatty acid esters of riboflavin have been synthesized by Yagi and co-workers. [146,148,150] These are intended to function nutritionally through the liberation of riboflavin by the action of pancreatic lipase in the small intestine [146,147] or of nonspecific esterases elsewhere in the body. The limited absorption and rapid excretion properties of riboflavin make development of such compounds potentially beneficial for treatment of vitamin deficiency in situations in which sustained or regular treatment is difficult or malabsorption occurs. Compounds such as riboflavin tetrabutyrate[150] and riboflavin tetranicotinate[66] appear to have the desired properties of sustaining body levels of free riboflavin and preventing the development of ariboflavinosis in rats otherwise deprived of riboflavin. Other compounds such as riboflavin tetrapalmitate do not hydrolyze adequately in body fluids. Since it is partially absorbed unchanged—a characteristic that overcomes the problem of limited gastrointestinal absorption of riboflavin—and subsequently hydrolyzes to riboflavin,[100] riboflavin tetranicotinate appears to be one of the most promising nutritional derivatives of riboflavin.

2. PLASMA PROTEIN BINDING

The degree of plasma protein binding of a compound can influence its transport through, distribution in, and elimination from the body. This influence is exemplified by the genetic absence of a highly specific riboflavin carrier protein in a strain of Leghorn chickens that causes subsequent embryonic death due to riboflavin deficiency. [22]

2.1. Human Plasma Protein Binding

Detailed studies of flavin binding to human plasma proteins have been limited to riboflavin and FMN. Both flavins are capable of interaction with the major serum proteins of man as shown in Table VII.[52] At physiological concentrations of the individual protein fractions, albumin accounts for most of the binding of riboflavin and FMN. The similarity of the data obtained with whole plasma, albumin, and reconstituted plasma indicates that albumin is primarily responsible for binding of the flavins in plasma. This was confirmed by dialyzing riboflavin and FMN in whole plasma against a solution with equal albumin concentration; essentially equal flavin concentrations were found on each side of the membrane at equilibrium. From the data in Table VII, it must be realized that competitive binding processes can decrease the relative contribution of each protein fraction when it is combined as in plasma.

At low concentrations, riboflavin is bound to human plasma to less than half the degree of FMN (Table VII). The interaction of various concentrations of either flavin with albumin is shown in greater detail in Fig. 10. The Scatchard plot of FMN–albumin interaction indicates

TABLE VII. Binding of Riboflavin and FMN to Human Plasma Proteins[a,b]

Protein	Protein concentration, g/100 ml	Fraction bound[c]	
		FR	FMN
Whole plasma[d]	6.5	0.42 ± 0.02	0.81 ± 0.02
Albumin	4.04	0.41 ± 0.01	0.86 ± 0.01
α-Globulin	0.79	0.13 ± 0.06	0.32 ± 0.06
β-Globulin[e]	0.81	0.27 ± 0.02	0.12 ± 0.02
γ-Globulin	0.74	0.07 ± 0.05	0.09 ± 0.02
Fibrinogen	0.34	0.04 ± 0.01	0.14 ± 0.04
Reconstituted plasma	6.72	0.45 ± 0.04	0.84 ± 0.02

[a] From Jusko and Levy.[52]
[b] Flavin concentrations = 0.5 μg/ml
[c] Mean ±1 standard deviation.
[d] Containing 3.9 g-percent albumin.
[e] Present largely in suspension.

that FMN occupies one site ($n = 1$) on the albumin molecule. The poor aqueous solubility and weak binding prevented collection of adequate data to construct a Scatchard plot for riboflavin. The riboflavin–albumin association constant (k) is 1.3×10^3 liters/mol at 30° C and pH 7.4, while that of FMN is more than one order of magnitude greater at 3.2×10^4 liters/mol. These constants were used to predict accurately the actual degree of overall binding of riboflavin and FMN mixtures in human serum after administration of FMN.[52,54] Since riboflavin binding is not very extensive and does not change over the concentration range encountered with usual therapeutic doses, no evidence has been found to indicate that plasma protein binding plays an important role in distribution and elimination of the vitamin in man. The situation is entirely different when consideration is made of riboflavin binding to flavoproteins; these tissue proteins, with binding constants of the order of 10^8 liters/mol,[130] account for the retention of nutritionally important amounts of vitamin in the body.

Very little is known about the role of diseases, drugs, hormones, and physiologic factors on the binding of riboflavin to plasma proteins. For example, it has been found that boric acid decreases riboflavin binding to various animal plasma proteins[116] and that probenecid has no effect on flavin binding in man,[54] but few other studies of this nature have been carried out.

2.1.1. Interaction Mechanism

The mechanism of interaction of riboflavin with plasma proteins is thought to involve hydrogen bonding between the 3-imino group

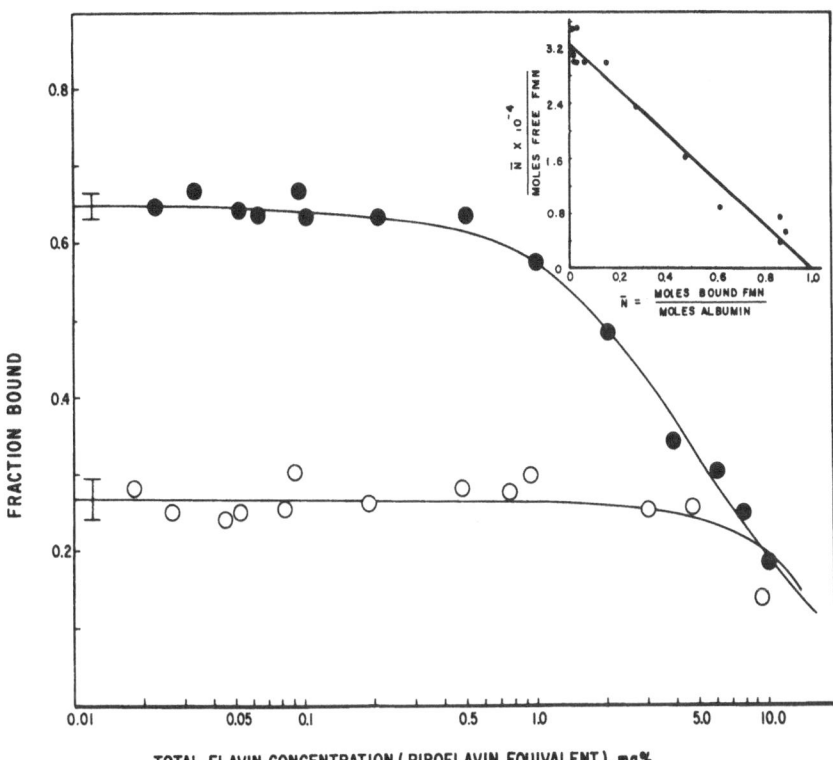

Fig. 10. Binding of riboflavin to 2% human albumin (o), and FMN to 0.4% human albumin (●) as a function of flavin concentration at 30° C. Inset is a Scatchard plot of FMN–albumin binding showing an association constant of 3.2×10^4 liters/mol as the intercept on the ordinate and one binding site as the abscissa intercept. Adapted from Jusko and Levy.[52]

of the isoalloxazine ring of riboflavin and tyrosine hydroxyl groups of the protein. The association constant for FMN binding to human albumin is 20 times larger than that for riboflavin. This difference could be caused by the additional interaction stability incurred by the association of the phosphate anion of FMN with cationic groups of the protein.[52,68,130] This finding is consistent with the physical properties of each flavin because riboflavin is an amphoteric compound (pKa = 10.2, pKb = 1.7) and exists in neutral form at pH 7.4, while FMN is anionic because of the ribose phosphate group (pKa's of 4.5 and 8.5). Support for such mechanism of interaction was obtained from estimates of free energy change (ΔG) and enthalpy (ΔH), which indicate that the driving force of the riboflavin–albumin and FMN–albumin interaction is primarily enthalpic with a magnitude consistent with hydrogen bonding. Other

TABLE VIII. Riboflavin Content[a] of Serum Protein Fractions from Various Species[b]

Species	Riboflavin concentrations, ng/mg nitrogen				
	α-Globulin	β-Globulin	γ-Globulin	Albumin	β-Lipoprotein
Man	2.6 ± 0.3	2.7 ± 0.5	2.0 ± 0.2	1.0 ± 0.1	1.8 ± 0.3
Dog	9.8 ± 1.8	28.4 ± 6.3	9.6 ± 1.8	c	28.0 ± 2.0
Cow	9.6 ± 0.4	11.0 ± 2.2	25.1 ± 2.2	26.0 ± 2.5	29.2 ± 3.5
Horse	17.3 ± 2.3	23.6 ± 1.4	16.9 ± 2.8	c	c
Rabbit	45.0 ± 5.0	6.4 ± 0.3	29.6 ± 6.0	21.4 ± 0.6	6.7 ± 1.8
Sheep	17.1 ± 1.5	18.3 ± 1.5	17.5 ± 3.3	c	c
Pig	c	21.3 ± 1.0	19.7 ± 5.0	c	20.6 ± 3.3

[a] Mean ±1 standard deviation.
[b] From Frank et al.[34]
[c] Value not measured.

flavin derivatives need to be studied to confirm this mechanism for human plasma protein binding of the vitamin.

2.2. Species Differences

The binding of flavins to serum proteins varies considerably among species. Riboflavin is 42 ± 2% bound in human plasma,[52] 19 ± 4% bound in dog plasma,[57] and 21 ± 3% bound in rat plasma[21] at concentrations less than 10 µg/ml. The association constants of FMN and albumin are also appreciably different: 3.2×10^4 liters/mol for man and 1.6×10^3 liters/mol for the cow.[68]

Frank and co-workers[34] measured the vitamin content in Cohn fractions of serum proteins from a variety of species (Table VIII). Large differences in flavin concentrations in each fraction as well as among species were found. These values cannot be compared with usual measurements of fractional binding (Table VII) because the use of a conventional protein-binding technique would be required to determine whether the observations of vitamin content reflect differences in the number of protein-binding sites and their association constants.

2.2.1. Avian Riboflavin Carrier Protein

The level of riboflavin in chicken eggs is regulated by the quantity of a genetically controlled riboflavin-binding protein found in the blood and egg. This is a glycoprotein of 32,000 daltons containing 16 half-cystine residues with no free sulfhydryl groups.[22] Absence of the protein in rdrd (autosomal recessive) genotype hens leads to riboflavinuria due to increased glomerular filtration of the vitamin. This condition produces riboflavin-deficient eggs and results in embryonic death between the tenth and fourteenth day of incubation. Relative degrees of riboflavin binding in serum and egg albumin from normal (RdRd), heterozygous (Rdrd), and recessive hens are shown in Table IX.[143] Administration of at least 5 mg/kg of estradiol to recessive genotype chicks will induce riboflavin-binding protein in the blood.[23] These recent studies explain the early work of Common *et al.*,[25] who showed that estradiol doses of 1–4 mg/per day for 6 days increased serum riboflavin levels in pullets from about 0.03 μg/ml to as much as 5.3 μg/ml without affecting hepatic flavin concentrations. Since laying hens have markedly higher serum riboflavin levels than do cocks and nonlaying hens, it is likely that endogenous gonadal hormone activity controls the plasma levels of riboflavin carrier protein in relation to the reproductive cycle of the hen.

Ostrowski and Krawczyk[105] and Rhodes *et al.*[112] investigated the physicochemical aspects of riboflavin binding to proteins in egg yolk and egg white. This is apparently the avian carrier protein subsequently described by Clagett *et al.*[23] Riboflavin exhibited much stronger binding than did either FMN and FAD; the association constant of the 1:1 complex was found to be about 3.8×10^8 liters/mol at pH 7 and 23.5° C. Comparative studies with riboflavin analogs such as 3-methylriboflavin, lyxoflavin, galactoflavin, and lumiflavin revealed much weaker binding and indicated that both the 3- and the 9-position on the isoalloxazine ring are involved in the highly specific protein binding process.

TABLE IX. *Genetic Determination of Relative Binding Capacities of Riboflavin to Avian Serum and Egg Albumin*[a]

Material	Avian genotype	Relative binding capacity[b]
Serum	RdRd	1.32 μg/ml
	rdrd	0.08 μg/ml
Egg albumin	RdRd	94 ± 15 protein, μg/g
	Rdrd	47 ± 6 protein, μg/g
	rdrd	2.3 ± 0.7 protein, μg/g

[a] Mean Winter *et al.*[143]
[b] Mean ±1 standard deviation.

3. ELIMINATION

Elimination of riboflavin from the body is the result of renal excretion, biliary excretion, minor losses with various body secretions, and metabolic interconversions to other flavins, coenzymes, and flavoproteins. The metabolism and retention of riboflavin are important factors if nutritional levels of the vitamin are considered, or if large doses of the vitamin are used in malnourished patients and animals. Investigations with relatively large doses reveal mainly the mechanisms of excretory pathways, but they do not reflect the quantitative contribution of metabolism and flavoprotein formation to the disposition of physiologic amounts of the vitamin. For example, i.v. doses on the order of 30 mg or more can be quantitatively recovered in the 24-hr urine of normal subjects, [53,124] whereas only about 39% of a 1-mg intravenous dose is found in urine. [98] In subjects with ariboflavinosis, the urinary recovery of 1-mg doses of riboflavin decreases to 15%.

3.1. Renal Excretion

3.1.1. Kinetics and Mechanisms in Man and Animals

Renal excretion of riboflavin in man involves glomerular filtration, tubular secretion, and tubular reabsorption. The contribution of each process to the observed renal clearance depends on the amount of the vitamin in the body. There are considerable species differences in the degree of renal excretion of large parenteral doses of riboflavin, as shown in Table X. The rat and dog behave similarly in that about one-half

TABLE X. *Dose and Species Differences in Degree of Renal Excretion of Riboflavin*

Species	Riboflavin, dose and route	Urinary excretion, %[a]	Reference
Man	0.015 mg/kg i.v.	26–68	Najjar and Holt[98]
Man	0.3 mg/kg i.m.	59–100	Jusko and Levy[51]
Man (infant)	1.1 mg/kg i.m.	92	Jusko et al.[56]
Man	1 mg/kg i.v.	97	Stripp[124]
Dog	3–5 mg/kg i.v.	49–56	Jusko et al.[57]
Rat	1–3 mg/kg i.v.	41–54	Christensen[19]
Rat	1–5 mg/kg i.p.	51–63	Axelson and Gibaldi[5]

[a]Urine collected until no further excretion of the vitamin occurred.

of the administered dose of vitamin is recovered in the urine. Man, on the other hand, excretes nearly all of a large dose of riboflavin in the urine.[4]

The occurrence of renal tubular secretion of riboflavin was first noted by Rennick,[111] using the Sperber technique in unanesthetized chickens. Infusion of probenecid reduced both PAH and riboflavin transport, but tolazoline infusion (1.9 µmol/min) decreased riboflavin excretion by 50% while PAH excretion was either unaffected or slightly increased. These data suggest that riboflavin shares the organic acid and possibly the organic base transport systems of the kidney. Subsequently, Levy and Jusko,[71] in analyzing the data of Stripp,[124] found renal clearances of riboflavin in man to range from 220 to 310 ml/min, indicative of active tubular secretion. This led to further investigation of the renal excretion of riboflavin in man and dogs.[53,57] The renal clearances of riboflavin and creatinine were measured after i.v. injection of the vitamin into a normal adult subject. These clearances are shown as a function of the serum flavin concentration in Fig. 11. At flavin plasma levels of about 1 µg/ml, the renal clearances approach an apparent maximum of 420 ml/min. As flavin levels fall to about 0.02 µg/ml,

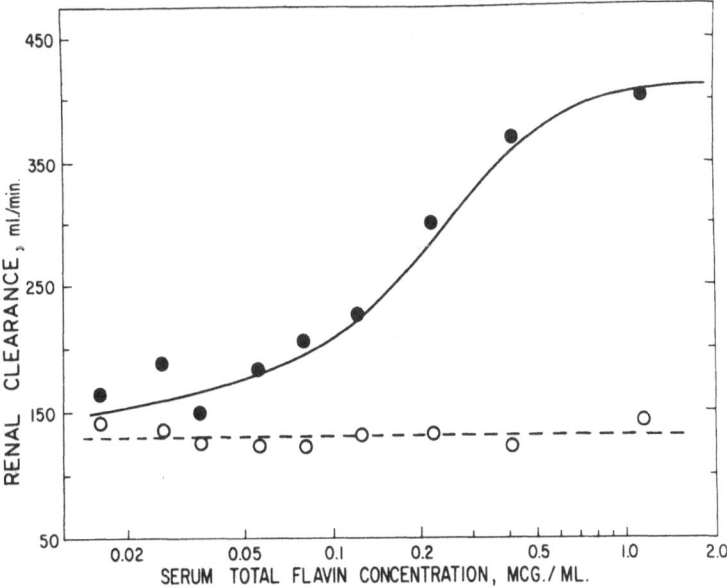

Fig. 11. Renal clearances of riboflavin (●) in an adult human subject as a function of serum total riboflavin concentration. Open symbols are simultaneously obtained creatinine clearances. From Jusko and Levy.[53] (Reproduced with permission of the copyright owner.)

the renal clearances gradually decrease to 140 ml/min, similar to the creatinine clearance. Similar data were obtained in the dog[53]; an apparent maximum clearance of 232 ml/min was observed in a 16-kg dog. These renal clearance data are indicative of renal excretion by a tubular secretion process of high capacity and a tubular reabsorption process that is easily saturated. Further evidence of tubular reabsorption was found in the dog when it was shown that the renal clearance, at low plasma flavin levels, was directly affected by the urine flow rate. When probenecid (1 g) was given to the same human subject for whom data are shown in Fig. 11, the minimum renal clearance value obtained was about 100 ml/min. This value, when corrected for the 40% plasma protein binding of riboflavin, is about the same as the glomerular filtration rate (creatinine clearance of 140 ml/min). This suggests that probenecid may inhibit the tubular reabsorption process as well as the secretory mechanism.

Probenecid appears to inhibit the tubular secretion of riboflavin and PAH to the same degree. Rennick[111] found that infusion of 1.5 mg/min probenecid into chickens reduced both PAH and riboflavin transport by 40%. Jusko and co-workers[57] obtained the log concentration–effect relationship shown in Fig. 12 for the effect of probenecid on riboflavin and PAH excretion in the dog. Parallel slopes for the inhibition of renal excretion of both compounds were found and the maximum inhibitory effect of probenecid was reached at a plasma concentration of about 7 mg/100 ml. A similar serum level (8 mg/100

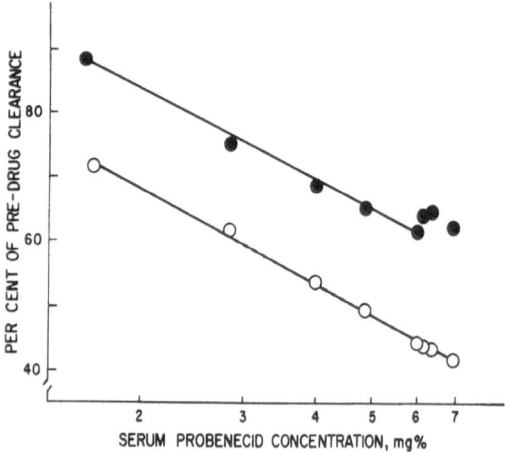

Fig. 12. Log concentration-effect relationship between inhibition of renal clearances of riboflavin (●), and PAH (o), and serum concentration of probenecid in a dog. From Jusko *et al.*[57]

ml) resulted in maximum inhibition of the renal clearance of riboflavin in human subjects. [54]

Christensen [21] investigated the renal excretion of riboflavin in the rat. At plasma concentrations of riboflavin ranging from 0.5 to 20 μg/ml, the riboflavin–inulin clearance ratio varied from 1.2 to 3.2, indicative of active tubular secretion of the vitamin. Doses of 10–75 mg/kg of probenecid depressed the clearance ratio to the range of 0.8–1.0. Renal tubular reabsorption of riboflavin has not been demonstrated in the rat. At plasma riboflavin concentrations of 20 μg/ml, the tubular secretion of riboflavin does not appear even to approach saturation. Precipitation of riboflavin in the kidneys at higher plasma levels prevented the demonstration of a possible maximum (T_m) for the tubular secretion process.

Stop-flow studies were carried out in the dog to elucidate the site of tubular secretion of riboflavin. [57] The pattern obtained, in comparison with that of PAH, suggested that secretion occurred at or slightly distal to the proximal tubular site of PAH secretion. In the same study, renal papilla-to-cortex tissue gradient studies of riboflavin, PAH, and inulin revealed that the riboflavin gradient differs appreciably from those of compounds excreted by glomerular filtration (inulin), filtration and distal tubular reabsorption (urea), filtration and proximal tubular secretion by the organic acid transport system (PAH), and filtration and dual acid–base transport (creatinine). Although these results are by no means conclusive, they suggest that the transport mechanism of riboflavin is somewhat unusual for this compound. The possibility of a phosphorylation-dephosphorylation mechanism of transport was suggested on the basis of an increase of only FMN in the renal tissue after administration of riboflavin. This mechanism could involve the flavokinase system, which converts riboflavin to FMN [86] and phosphatases, which dephos-phorylate FMN. [109] The most reasonable alternative mechanism of riboflavin transport across the renal tubule appears to be that involving a dual sharing of the organic acid–base mechanism. This would be consistent with the amphoteric nature of the riboflavin molecule and would explain the inhibitory effects of both tolazoline and probenecid at low concentrations of these compounds. Clearly, further studies are required to elucidate fully the mechanism of renal transport of riboflavin.

The time course of excretion of riboflavin into the urine after oral and intravenous doses in man is shown in Fig. 1. The elimination of large doses of the vitamin usually shows three phases with half-lives of about 0.2, 1, and 5–12 hr. The most rapid phase reflects distribution of the vitamin from the plasma into tissues. The phase with a half-life of about 1 hr reflects elimination of a major portion of the dose, and its transition into the very slow phase is caused by the concentration-dependent change in renal clearance. A pharmacokinetic analysis of riboflavin elimination in man and dog has been carried out. [53] The relationship of clearance and distribution factors to the appearance of riboflavin in the urine is of importance in considering the effects of age and diseases on the elimination of riboflavin (to be discussed in Sections 3.1.3 and 3.1.4).

3.1.2. Urinary Excretion Products

Administration of either riboflavin or FMN to man results in the urinary excretion mainly of riboflavin. [29,124] Although FMN is capable of undergoing rapid dephosphorylation in the kidney [109] and in whole blood, [54] a small fraction of a dose of FMN can be detected in the urine of man. Estimation of the apparent renal clearance of unchanged FMN suggests that riboflavin and FMN are excreted equally well. [53] Ureter-cannulated patients with kidney disease have been reported to excrete about 20% of intravenous doses of both riboflavin and FMN in the form of the phosphate. [137] This fact would suggest that, upon excretion of FMN, further dephosphorylation takes place in the bladder in those studies where urine samples are not collected frequently and/or in the kidney of normal subjects.

Normal doses of riboflavin or FMN do not appear to produce significant amounts of any other urinary excretion products in man. This fact is demonstrated by the near quantitative recovery of large intravenous doses of the vitamin, [53,124] as measured by fluorometric analysis and by the use of fluorometric and microbiological (L. casei) methods of assay, which yield identical urinary recovery data after administration of 10-mg doses of riboflavin to human subjects. [29]

Degradation products of riboflavin have been detected in the urine of goats after small doses and in man when doses of nearly 1 g riboflavin are given orally. [140] The experiment with 1 g riboflavin in man is somewhat unusual in that part of the unabsorbed vitamin is degraded by bacteria in the gastrointestinal tract to hydroxyethylflavine and to a second compound, both of which are then absorbed and appear in the urine 24 or more hours after the oral dose.

3.1.3. Effect of Age

Riboflavin excretion by human subjects of various ages was studied by Jusko et al. [55,56] Figure 13 shows a comparison of the time course of urinary excretion of riboflavin in a 6-day-old infant and in an adult

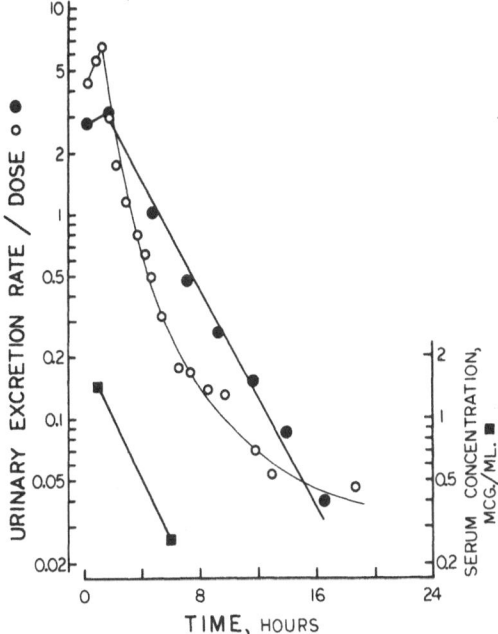

Fig. 13. Urinary excretion rate/dose (μg/min/mg) of riboflavin as a function of time after intramuscular injection of about 17 mg/m^2 riboflavin as FMN to a 6-day-old infant (●), and to an adult subject (o). Serum concentration data are also shown for the infant (■). From Jusko et al.[56]

after i.m. doses of 17 mg/m^2 riboflavin as FMN. Elimination in the adult showed the characteristic curvilinear decline, whereas only mono-exponential elimination was found in the neonate. This difference was attributed to the immature renal function of the infant, since the renal clearances were only 60–78 ml/min/1.73 m^2 in two newborn infants. The rapid initial elimination phase with a 0.2-hr half-life apparent in adult subjects is not observed when the vitamin is given by routes other than intravenous; the time course of absorption obscures this phase.

Oral doses of the vitamin were administered to subjects in the age range of 3 months to 40 years.[55] The rapid and slow half-lives of elimination were obtained from data such as shown in Fig. 14. The logarithm of the amount remaining unexcreted was plotted as a function of time, and the postabsorptive data were used to calculate the appropriate half-life values. It can be noted that absorption takes place only during the first 4 hr and that elimination of most of the dose occurred during the rapid elimination phase, which had an average half-life of 1.4 hr.

The relationship of the rapid and slow half-life of elimination to

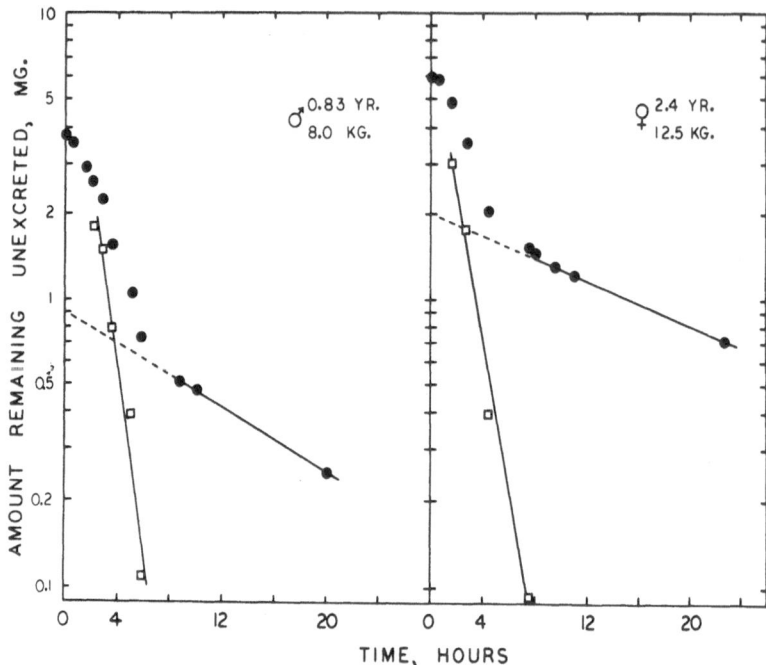

Fig. 14. Amount of riboflavin remaining unexcreted (●), as a function of time after oral doses of 150 mg/m² in a male and a female child. The rapid half-life of elimination was determined (□) from the postabsorptive data using the method of residuals by extrapolating (dashed line) the linear slow phase of elimination to the ordinate. Adapted from Jusko *el al.*[55]

the age (logarithmic scale) of the subjects is shown in Fig. 15. No significant change in the rapid half-life (mean of 1.2 hr) occurred with age. The slow half-life values were variable but showed a barely significant tendency to increase with age. Because these data reflect elimination of only a minor portion of the dose, it could not be ascertained whether this change was due to an effect of age on renal function or to metabolic utilization of the vitamin.

3.1.4. Effects of Diseases and Physiological Factors

The influence of various nutritional and physiological factors on the urinary excretion of riboflavin has been reviewed by Bro-Rasmussen.[9] The amount of riboflavin excreted into urine has often been used to estimate riboflavin intake and as an index of the nutritional status of the subject with respect to this vitamin. However, numerous factors affect the urinary excretion of riboflavin, and caution is necessary in the interpretation of urinary excretion data alone. A complex, dynamic situation is involved in the absorption, distribution, retention, and excretion of riboflavin. Factors such as conversion to coenzyme forms and subsequent attachment to proteins, as well as renal tubular reabsorption, contribute to the retention of small amounts of the vitamin in the body. Intake of food and vitamin preparations and the liberation of riboflavin from tissues and flavoproteins contribute to the appearance of the vitamin in the urine. These factors are complicated further by the concentration dependence in absorption, tissue avidity, metabolic conversion, and biliary and renal excretion of riboflavin.

3.1.4A. MALNUTRITION. Baker *et al.*[6] found the disappearance of riboflavin from plasma to be more rapid in riboflavin-deficient humans. They found a rapid half-life of 5–8 min in 5 deficient subjects, whereas that in 27 normals was 14–25 min. The slow half-life also appeared

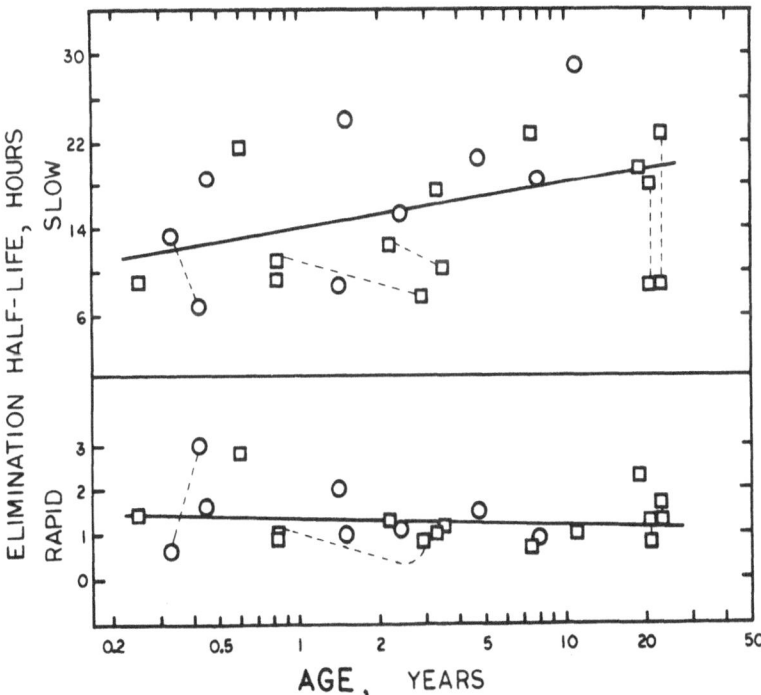

Fig. 15. Relationship between the rapid and slow half-life of elimination and age (logarithmic scale) of normal human subjects. Symbols are defined as in Fig. 4. From Jusko *et al.*[55] (Reproduced with permission of the copyright owner.)

longer in the normal subjects, and the area under the plasma level *vs.* time curve was appreciably smaller in the deficient subjects. Axelson and Gibaldi[5] measured the urinary excretion of riboflavin in riboflavin-deficient rats after parenteral doses of the vitamin (Table II). As expected, the deficient animals (*C*) retain more of the vitamin than normal rats (*G*). Riboflavin uptake into a tissue pool is thus increased in malnutrition. This fact is reflected by the more rapid disappearance of the vitamin from the plasma as well as by decreased urinary excretion. However, this pattern does not necessarily apply to cirrhotic patients with chronic hepatic debility. The lack of available protein for retention of the vitamin as flavoproteins may aggravate the riboflavin deficiency state.[60] For example, Yang and Sung[151] found that patients with severe liver disease retain much less of an 0.1 mg/kg i.m. dose of riboflavin or FAD than do normal subjects.

Fasting produces a temporary increase in urinary excretion of riboflavin. Windmueller *et al.*[142] found a mean increase of 119% in urinary riboflavin of subjects who fasted for only 24 hr. This appears to be the result of preferential utilization of labile tissue flavoproteins during negative nitrogen balance which causes the release of riboflavin and its subsequent excretion. This increased excretion is only temporary because acute starvation produces eventual depletion of riboflavin body stores, which is also reflected in urinary excretion. Consolazio *et al.*[26] recently showed that riboflavin excretion, after the early temporary increase described above, decreased from a normal level of about 400 μg/day to less than 40 μg/day within 5 days of starvation.

A number of other factors can alter the flavoprotein homeostasis in the body and thus influence the urinary excretion of riboflavin. Physiological perturbations such as work and sleep (causing decreased urinary riboflavin), and heat and bed rest (causing increased urinary riboflavin), have been investigated in man.[134]

3.1.4B. DIURESIS. Pharmacokinetic expressions have been developed by Jusko and Levy[53] for describing the renal clearance of a compound such as riboflavin which is subject to saturable tubular reabsorption. These equations predicted that the net renal clearance would be independent of urine concentration at relatively high urine and plasma concentrations of drug. However, at low concentrations of riboflavin in plasma and urine, the net renal clearance should increase with increasing urine flow rate. Studies of the renal clearance of riboflavin in the dog at varying plasma concentrations of riboflavin and urine flow rates yielded results that are in agreement with these predictions.

A direct effect of diuresis on the renal clearance of riboflavin has

TABLE XI. Effect of Diuretics on Dietary Riboflavin Excretion by Rabbits[a]

Treatment	Urine volume, ml/18 hr[b]	Amount of riboflavin excreted, μg/18 hr[b]	Statistical[c] difference
Control	32 ± 27	22 ± 20	—
Acetazolamide, 25 mg	59 ± 34	50 ± 26	$p < 0.02$
Mercaptomerin, 12.5 mg	50 ± 24	47 ± 23	$p < 0.02$

[a] From Markkanen.[82]
[b] Mean ±1 standard deviation.
[c] Method of paired comparisons (DF = 9) applied to riboflavin data.

not been demonstrated in man. However, in agreement with the above predictions, Johnson[48] found decreased urinary excretion of dietary riboflavin at urine flow rates of less than 25 ml/hr and increased excretion during diuresis of 200 ml/hr. Other studies by Tucker et al.,[134] who measured riboflavin excretion before and after severe water diuresis, were contradictory. However, Angarano and De Salvea,[2] in studies with patients receiving thiazide diuretics, showed increased riboflavin excretion during diuresis. Markkanen[82] determined the effects of acetazolamide and mercaptomerin on urinary excretion of dietary riboflavin in rabbits. Both diuretics increased riboflavin excretion in proportion to their diuretic effect (Table XI).

3.1.5. Effects of Drugs and Natural Substances

3.1.5A. GLUCOSE AND INSULIN. Glucose and insulin appear to have different effects on riboflavin excretion in animals and man. Magyar[80] maintained rats on subcutaneous doses of 400 μg/day of riboflavin and found that, during periods of injection of 250 mg glucose, riboflavin excretion decreased from 148 ± 43 μg/day to as low as 48 ± 29 μg/day ($p < 0.001$). This was explained as an inhibitory effect of glucose on phosphorylation of riboflavin. Rats given 0.1 unit of insulin exhibited no changes in riboflavin excretion. Fukuhara[36,37] found that i.v. glucose also decreased the urinary excretion of dietary riboflavin in rabbits.

Studies in man were carried out by Travia and Pelosio,[131] who showed that glucose increased the excretion rate of riboflavin given by i.m. injection. Interestingly, oral glucose, in doses of 0.76 g/kg, had a much greater effect than parenteral glucose. Fujimoto et al.[35] investigated dietary riboflavin excretion in relation to glucose levels in diabetic human subjects. Diabetics excreted more riboflavin than did normal subjects, but riboflavin excretion in the diabetics decreased with reduction of blood sugar levels. When glucose or insulin was given, riboflavin excretion increased; insulin also decreased the blood levels of riboflavin. Further details of riboflavin metabolism in diabetes are given in chapter 12.

3.1.5B. THIAMIN. Several investigators have reported an effect of thiamin on urinary excretion of riboflavin. Magyar[80] gave daily subcutaneous doses of 400 μg riboflavin to rats and found a control excretion rate of 144 ± 44 μg/day of riboflavin which was decreased to 86 ± 38 μg/day ($p < 0.001$) when 0.5- to 2-mg doses of thiamin were also given. Shinagawa[120] also found a gradual decrease in urinary excretion of dietary riboflavin when 10 mg/kg doses of thiamin were injected into rabbits. In contrast, Travia *et al.*[132] administered thiamin pyrophosphate to human subjects and obtained increased excretion of dietary riboflavin in urine, while Levy and Hewitt[45] found no effect of large oral doses of riboflavin and thiamin on their mutual excretion in man.

3.1.5C. ADENOSINE TRIPHOSPHATE. A primary source of phosphate for the formation of FMN from riboflavin is ATP. Magyar[80] found that subcutaneous administration of 5 mg ATP to rats maintained on subcutaneous doses of 400 μg/day of riboflavin increased the urinary excretion of riboflavin from 123 ± 37 to 174 ± 61 μg/day ($p < 0.005$). Fujimoto *et al.*[35] found a similar effect when ATP was administered to human diabetics. Clearance studies are required to determine if ATP enhances the renal clearance or the phosphorylation process.

3.1.5D. METABOLIC INHIBITORS. Magyar[80] maintained rats on subcutaneous doses of 400 μg/day of riboflavin and measured its daily urinary excretion. Administration of 1-3 mg iodoacetate decreased riboflavin excretion from 133 ± 49 to 60 ± 49 μg/day ($p < 0.001$), while 1-mg doses of phlorizin produced an insignificant decrease from 124 ± 38 to 103 ± 43 μg/day. It has not been established whether the effects of these compounds on riboflavin excretion into urine were metabolic or renal.

3.2. Biliary Excretion

Biliary excretion of riboflavin has been demonstrated in the rat,[99] rabbit,[91] dog,[27] and human.[76] Studies in the dog have shown that none of the free riboflavin introduced into the mesenteric circulation appears in the bile as FMN. Only a small part of FMN introduced

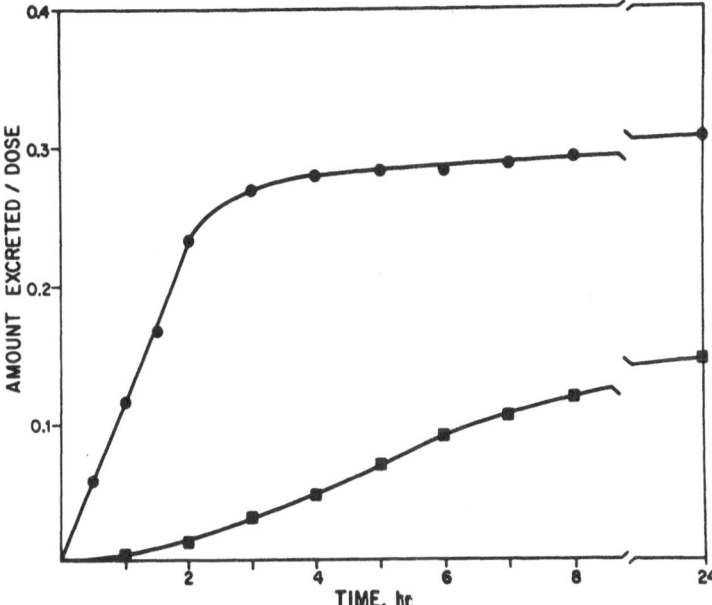

Fig. 16. Cumulative biliary excretion of riboflavin (fraction of dose) by rats with cannulated bile ducts, as a function of time after intravenous injection of about 40 μmol (●) or 0.4 μmol (■) of FMN/kg body weight. Based on data from Nogami *et al.*[99]

into the mesenteric circulation is excreted in the bile as such; the greater part is free riboflavin.[127] Similarly, parenteral administration of riboflavin, FMN, or FAD to rats resulted in the biliary excretion of free riboflavin and small amounts of FAD, but not of FMN. This fact has been attributed to the rapid hydrolysis of FMN in the blood.[99] Perfusion of riboflavin through the intact rabbit liver has resulted in the biliary excretion of 50% of the added vitamin under the experimental conditions; replacement of dehydrocholic acid in the perfusion fluid by cholic acid reduced the biliary excretion of riboflavin to 15.2%.[91]

The biliary excretion of riboflavin shows pronounced dose dependence. Parenteral administration of 0.05 mg FMN to 245- to 255-g male albino rats with cannulated bile ducts resulted in the biliary excretion of 15% of the dose; about 30% of the dose was recovered in the bile following administration of 5 mg FMN (Fig. 16). This dose dependence is also reflected in the urinary excretion of riboflavin by rats with intact and ligated bile ducts (Table II). An average of 41.3% of the dose was recovered in the urine of riboflavin deficient rats (~250 g-weight) following intraperitoneal injection of 1 mg riboflavin as FMN; the recovery in the urine increased to 72.1% in animals with ligated bile ducts. No such difference was noted when only 0.2 mg riboflavin as FMN was administered.[5] These observations show that biliary excretion contributes appreciably to the elimination of large doses of riboflavin in the rat. Nogami et al.[99] found no difference between normal and bile duct-cannulated rats in the time course of riboflavin concentrations in the blood following intravenous injection of the vitamin, suggesting that enterohepatic circulation of riboflavin was negligible under the conditions of their experiments.

The available data do not permit definitive conclusions concerning the mechanism of the dose-dependent biliary excretion of riboflavin in rats. The experimental results can be explained by assuming saturation of renal secretion, biotransformation, tissue binding, and/or biliary reabsorption processes. It will be necessary to determine the biliary *clearance* as a function of riboflavin concentration in order to determine if biliary excretion as such is a nonlinear process with respect to riboflavin.

The biliary excretion of riboflavin in man appears to be very limited. Only 0.42% of an intramuscular dose of 10 mg riboflavin (administered

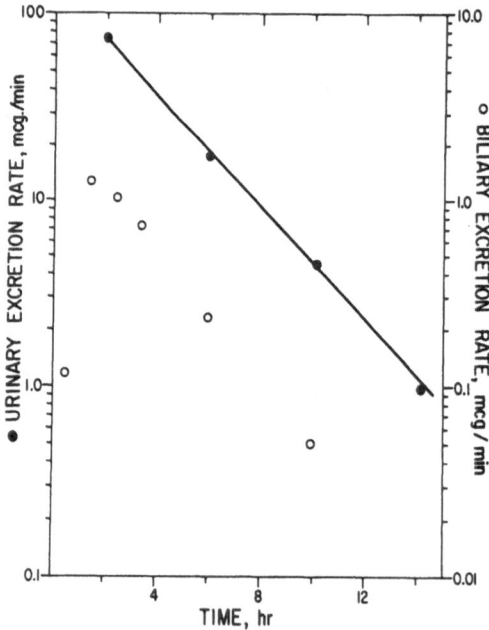

Fig. 17. Rates of urinary (●) and biliary (○) excretion of riboflavin by an 11-year-old girl with external biliary drainage, as a function of time after intramuscular injection of 17.5 mg riboflavin as FMN per square meter of body surface area. Data from Levy et al.[76]

as FMN) was recovered in the duodenal aspirate of a $3\frac{1}{2}$-year-old boy, while 95.4% was recovered in the urine. An 11-year-old girl with external biliary drainage excreted 0.97% of a 17.5 mg/m^2 dose of riboflavin (administered as FMN) in the bile and 88.7% in the urine during 24 hr after the injection.[76] The urinary and biliary excretion rates were essentially parallel (Fig. 17). The kinetics of riboflavin elimination in children with biliary obstruction does not differ from the kinetics in normal children,[59] a fact that suggests also that biliary excretion and enterohepatic circulation of riboflavin are quantitatively negligible in man. The secondary excretion rate maxima observed in man after large oral doses of FMN (which were attributed previously to enterohepatic circulation of the vitamin) are probably due to a temporary increased rate of absorption related to the discharge of bile into the intestine, but the mechanism of the absorption-enhancing effect of bile is still uncertain.

3.3. Minor Routes of Elimination

3.3.1. Milk

The nutritional importance of the B-vitamins in milk has led to comprehensive investigation of flavin secretion in human and animal milk. Funai[38] found that normal human milk from 22 mothers contained 361 ± 30 µg/liter of total flavin with the composition averaging 86% FAD, 11% FMN, and 3% FR. Colostrum, at 2 days postpartum, contains about half this total concentration. Both FAD and FMN levels in milk increase to maximum concentration at about 7 days after delivery, while the free riboflavin content remains relatively low and constant. However, Owen and Hytten[106] found an increase in free riboflavin concentration in human milk when the mothers ingested 6 mg riboflavin.

Considerable species differences occur in the flavin composition of milk. Mare and sow milk resembles human milk in that FAD is the predominant form of the vitamin. Cow, goat, ewe, and rabbit milk contains more free riboflavin than FAD and apparently has no FMN.[92]

The total flavin content of milk greatly exceeds that of blood,[38] probably due to flavin association with proteins, either as FAD in some species, or as riboflavin complexes with α- and β-casein in animals.[68]

3.3.2. Sweat

Although riboflavin is present in sweat, this route contributes negligibly to its elimination from the body in man. Subjects who were dosed with 10 mg riboflavin, as well as undosed subjects, lost an average of only 12 μg riboflavin during an hour's collection of an average of 400 ml thermally induced sweat.[129]

3.3.3. Photodegradation

Maslenikova[83] determined the effect of solar and u.v. irradiation on riboflavin levels in various organs of the rat. Exposure to the sun for about 20 hr during the course of 13 days significantly affected the total flavin concentrations in blood (25% decrease), kidneys (40% decrease), and liver (60% decrease), while urinary excretion was increased during irradiation. On the other hand, small doses of ultraviolet radiation appear to have the opposite effects on riboflavin tissue levels. The photosensitivity of riboflavin is well recognized, and the primary product formed in solution of neutral and acidic pH is lumichrome.[43]

Of interest, riboflavin pretreatment of rats has been found to decrease the subsequent toxic effects of ultraviolet irradiation of the animals by two-thirds.[138] Roth and Roth[117] recently showed that irradiation-induced changes in unprotected DNA of cultured mammalian cells were reversed by subsequent treatment of the DNA with riboflavin or FMN in the presence of visible light. These two studies suggest that flavins may have an additional physiologic function of protecting tissues from actinic radiation.

3.3.4. Intestinal Clearance

No direct evidence indicates that riboflavin is secreted through the mucosa into the lumen of the small intestine. This mechanism of elimination was suggested to occur in the rat[144] on the basis of recovery of the vitamin in the gut. One hour after injection of 17.8 mg/kg of ^{14}C-labeled riboflavin, Yagi *et al.*[149] found about 52% of the dose in the contents of the intestinal canal. This fact suggested the occurrence of either intestinal secretion or biliary excretion of riboflavin or both. However, Christensen[20] occluded the portal circulation of the rat and found a large decrease in the rate of elimination of the vitamin, which indicated indirectly that intestinal secretion does not contribute appreciably to the elimination of riboflavin. The detailed studies of Nogami *et al.*,[99] which elucidated the rapid and dose-related biliary excretion of riboflavin in the rat, explain the observations of Yagi. It is not likely that significant elimination of riboflavin by the intestinal route occurs in man because essentially all of a large parenteral dose is recovered in the urine.[124]

3.3.5. Hemodialysis

Riboflavin, like most B-vitamins, is removed from the body during hemodialysis. MacKenzie *et al.*[79] have estimated the dialysance (a parameter analogous to renal clearance) of riboflavin to be 52 ml/min. This amount is similar to body clearance values of 45 to 142 ml/min found by Jusko *et al.*[58] in two dialyzed anephric patients. The slow half-life for elimination of the vitamin from plasma in such patients is about 2 hr. This fact accounts for the need of vitamin supplementation in patients undergoing prolonged or repeated hemodialysis.

4. GENERAL PHARMACOLOGY

4.1. Summary of Pharmacokinetic Properties

The major factors that control body levels of riboflavin are summarized in Fig. 18. The pharmacokinetic properties of riboflavin are somewhat unusual in that the body tends to facilitate the maintenance of nutritionally adequate levels of the vitamin as well as the rapid elimination of excessive loads. Limited absorption of large doses of the vitamin is controlled by the easily saturated, specialized transport process of the small intestine that, on the other hand, permits the rapid and efficient absorption of small doses of riboflavin. When large amounts of the vitamin do reach the systemic circulation, the high-capacity renal

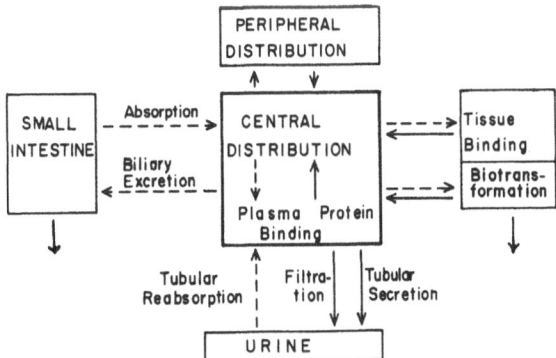

Fig. 18. General pharmacokinetic model showing the major factors which control body levels of riboflavin. The kinetics of most of the processes (arrows) depicted in the model have been found to be dose-dependent in man and/or animals.

tubular secretory process in man, and similar renal and biliary systems in the rat, cause rapid elimination of the vitamin in urine or bile. The higher the body level of the vitamin, the smaller the fraction that is either bound to plasma and tissue proteins or converted to FMN and FAD. On the other hand, very low levels of the vitamin are extensively protein-bound and metabolized, and little is excreted in the urine because of this and of extensive renal tubular reabsorption. A decrease in riboflavin intake to nutritionally suboptimal levels causes release of the vitamin from a labile tissue pool, while, at the same time, a strongly bound pool prevents tissue flavin levels from falling too low except in severe deficiency states. These general properties of riboflavin, with quantitative variations among species, make the study of its absorption and disposition both complex and fascinating.

4.2. Pharmacologic and Toxic Effects

Large doses (>0.1 mg/kg) of riboflavin and FMN produce no known pharmacologic effects in animals or man. Unna and Greslin[136] administered 40 mg/kg doses of riboflavin to cats and observed no changes in blood pressure, heart rate, and respiration and 0.1 mg/ml solutions did not alter the intestinal tone or contractions of the isolated rabbit intestine. Also, Tsutsumi[133] found no effect of FMN on similar organ systems of the rabbit. However, FAD produces a hypotensive action in rabbits which was attributed to the AMP portion of the molecule.

The toxicity of the vitamin is extremely small. The LD_{50} of riboflavin is about 560 mg/kg when given intraperitoneally to rats.[136] It was necessary to administer riboflavin in suspension, and this LD_{50} value is therefore an overestimate. Death was caused by anuria and azotemia produced by concretions of riboflavin crystals in the kidney. As might be expected from its poor gastrointestinal absorption, the LD_{50} of oral doses of riboflavin could not be measured at doses up to 10 g/kg in rats and 2 g/kg in dogs. Chronic studies with oral doses of the vitamin also failed to produce any toxic manifestations. The data of Christensen[21] indicate that plasma riboflavin concentrations must be maintained above 20 μg/ml before precipitation of riboflavin occurs in the kidneys of the rat. The water solubility of riboflavin is limited and precaution is warranted when the urine concentration of the vitamin exceeds 0.15 mg/ml.

4.3. Clinical Use of Riboflavin

The degree of clinical use of riboflavin, as it is included in multiple-vitamin preparations, is given in drug surveillance data obtained by Jick *et al.*[47] In 6312 hospitalized medical patients, vitamins were one of the most commonly prescribed items since 18% of patients were given vitamins while "vitamin depletion" was listed as an indication for such therapy in only 4.8% of patients. The subjective difficulty in clinically assessing the effects of such therapy, as well as the lack of objective measuring techniques, can be demonstrated by the fact that, when physicians were given the choice of rating the effects of drugs as: "good," "fair," "poor," or "don't know," the efficacy of multiple-vitamins was judged as "don't know" in 82% of recipient patients.

Multiple-vitamins are often used excessively for nutritional supplementation when dietary vitamin levels are questionable. On the other hand, the casual attitude toward vitamin use has resulted in their underutilization as well. It was recently found that, of 17 autopsy patients with cirrhosis of the liver, a condition where multiple-vitamin treatment is clearly indicated,[67] only 7 had received vitamins prior to death.[60]

Its low toxicity and striking, fluorescent-yellow color had led to a unique pharmacologic application of riboflavin. Vitamins are often added to intravenous infusion solutions simply as a color marker to indicate to patient-care personnel that "drugs" have been added to the bottle (personal observation). Also, riboflavin alone has been included in certain drug formulations so that patient urine can be examined under u.v. light to determine whether the prescribed drug was actually ingested.[49] The absorption characteristics of riboflavin make this method far from foolproof.

Consideration of the biopharmaceutic and pharmacokinetic properties of riboflavin provides several indications for improving the clinical use of the vitamin. The pharmaceutical dosage form must allow rapid dissolution of riboflavin so that the vitamin will be available for absorption in the proximal small intestine. In this respect, "chewable" vitamin tablets should provide better absorption than other solid dosage forms, particularly enteric-coated and sustained-release preparations. (The bioavailability of vitamins in any dosage form should be tested prior to clinical use.) Riboflavin is best absorbed in the presence of food and thus should be administered with meals. Large doses of riboflavin are wasted because of its limited gastrointestinal absorption, rapid urinary excretion, and limited capacity of tissue binding sites. Diseases affecting the intestine or liver may be accompanied by impaired absorption of riboflavin, in which cases parenteral injection of the vitamin may be warranted. In general, the continual, frequent administration of moderate doses of riboflavin is preferred to intermittent, large doses in those instances where true vitamin depletion has occurred.

5. REFERENCES

1. Ackerman, R. F., Curl, H., and Crandall, L. A., Jr. 1941. Gastrointestinal tract motility in the absence of bile, *Amer. J. Physiol.* **134**:32-36.
2. Angarano, R. M. and DeSalvea, F. 1963. Metabolic modifications induced by diuretic treatment: Urinary elimination of some vitamins of the B-complex, *Acta Vitaminol.* **17**:49-53 (*Chem. Abstr.* **59**, 15829, 1963).
3. Arakawa, T., Kagaya, A., and Inaka, Y. 1957. Effect of ursodesoxycholic acid upon the intestinal absorption of riboflavin in guinea pigs, *J. Vitaminol.* **3**:168-171.
4. Axelrod, A. E., Spies, T. D., and Elvehjem, C. A. 1941. A study of urinary riboflavin excretion in man, *J. Clin. Invest.* **20**:229-232.
5. Axelson, J. E., and Gibaldi, M. 1972. Absorption and excretion of riboflavin in the rat—An unusual example of nonlinear pharmacokinetics, *J. Pharm. Sci.* **61**:404-407.
6. Baker, H., Frank, O., Feingold, S., Gellene, R. A., Leevy, C. M., and Hutner, S. H. 1966. A riboflavin assay suitable for clinical use and nutritional surveys, *Amer. J. Clin. Nutr.* **19**:17-26.
7. Berlin, R., Dessner, L., and Wahlund, H. 1957. Can folic acid affect the absorption of riboflavine from the intestine? *Svensk. Tandlak. Tidshrift.* **50**:129-134 (*Chem. Abstr.* **55**:15725, 1961).
8. Bromberg, Y. M., Brzezinski, A., and Sulman, F. 1947. Implantation of riboflavin pellets in animals and man, *Proc. Soc. Exptl. Biol. Med.* **64**:354-357.
9. Bro-Rasmussen, F. 1958. The riboflavin requirement of animals and man and associated metabolic relations. Part II. Relation of requirement to the metabolism of protein and energy, *Nutr. Abstr. Rev.* **28**:369-386.
10. Brumfield, P. E., and Gross, H. M. 1955. Riboflavin: formulation of multivitamin parenterals, *Drug Cosm. Ind.* **77**:46-48, 120-126.
11. Brummer, P., Markkanen, T. K., and Kalliomaki, J. L. 1961. Effect of corticosteroids on urinary excretion and on the intestinal absorption of thiamine, riboflavin, nicotinic acid, pantothenic acid and biotin, *Acta Med. Scand.* **170**:183-186.
12. Brzezinski, A., Bromberg, Y. M., and Sulman, F. G. 1957. Prolonged effect of riboflavin: Aluminum monostearate suspensions in man, *J. Amer. Pharm. Assoc., Sci. Ed.* **46**:109-111.
13. Campbell, J. A., and Morrison, A. B. 1963. Some factors affecting the absorption of vitamins, *Amer. J. Clin. Nutr.* **12**:162-169.
14. Chapman, D. G., Crisafio, R., and Campbell, J. A. 1954. The relation between *in vitro* disintegration time of sugar-coated tablets and physiological availability of riboflavin, *J. Amer. Pharm. Assoc., Sci. Ed.* **43**:297-304.
15. Chen, C., and Liao, T. 1960. Histochemical study on riboflavin. *J. Vitaminol.* **6**:171-195.
16. Chen, C., and Yamauchi, K. 1960. Absorption of riboflavin in the isolated intestine of rats, *J. Vitaminol.* **6**:247-250.
17. Christensen, S. 1969a. Studies on riboflavin metabolism in the rat. I. Urinary and faecal excretion after oral administration of riboflavin-5-phosphate, *Acta Pharmacol. et Toxicol.* **27**:27-33.
18. Christensen, S. 1969b. Studies on riboflavin metabolism in the rat. II. Metabolic flavin elimination after oral or intraperitoneal administration of riboflavin-5'-phosphate, *Acta Pharmacol. et Toxicol.* **27**:34-40.
19. Christensen, S. 1969c. Studies on riboflavin metabolism in the rat. III. Disappearance rate and urinary excretion rate of flavin after intravenous infusion of riboflavin-5'-phosphate, *Acta Pharmacol. et Toxicol.* **27**:41-48.

20. Christensen, S. 1969d. Studies on riboflavin metabolism in the rat. IV. Riboflavin elimination after exclusion of the portal circulation, *Acta Pharmacol. et Toxicol.* 27:49-55.

21. Christensen, S. 1971. Renal excretion of riboflavin in the rat, *Acta Pharmacol. et Toxicol.* 29:428-440.

22. Clagett, C. O. 1971. Genetic control of the riboflavin carrier protein, *Fed. Proc.* 30:127-129.

23. Clagett, C. O., Buss, E. G., Saylor, E. M., and Girsh, S. J. 1970. The nature of the biochemical lesion in avian renal riboflavinuria: 6. Hormone induction of the riboflavin-binding protein in roosters and young chicks, *Poultry Sci.* 49:1468-1472.

24. Clarke, H. C. 1969. The relationship between whole blood riboflavine levels and results of riboflavine saturation tests in normal and pathological conditions in man, *Intern. J. Vit. Res.* 39:238-245.

25. Common, R. H., Rutledge, W. A., and Bolton, W. 1946. The influence of gonadal hormones on serum riboflavin and certain other properties of blood and tissues in the domestic fowl, *J. Endocrinol.* 5:121-130.

26. Consolazio, C. F., Johnson, H. L., Krzywicki, H. J., Daws, T. A., and Barnhart, R. A. 1971. Thiamin, riboflavin, and pyridoxine excretion during acute starvation and calorie restriction, *Amer. J. Clin. Nutr.* 24:1060-1067.

27. Cordona, N. A. 1965. The effect of 17-beta-estradiol diproprionate on the intestinal absorption of riboflavin in normal chickens, Ph.D. thesis, The Pennsylvania State University.

28. Cordona, N. A., and Payne, I. R. 1967. Absorption of riboflavin in chickens, *Poultry Sci.* 46:1176-1179.

29. DeRitter, E., Scheiner, J., Jahns, F. W., Drekter, L., and Rubin, S. H. 1955. Synthetic riboflavin-5'-phosphate, *J. Amer. Pharm. Assn., Sci. Ed.* 44:1-5.

30. Doiphode, N. G., and Bamji, M. S. 1970. Effect of aureomycin on the nutritional status of the B-vitamins in humans, *Intern. J. Vit. Res.* 40:58-63.

31. Fazekas, A. G., and Sandor, T. 1971. Flavin nucleotide coenzyme biosynthesis and its relation to corticosteroidogenesis in the rat adrenal, *Endocrinol.* 89:397-407.

32. Feldman, S., and Gibaldi, M. 1968. Effect of bile salts on gastric emptying and intestinal transit in the rat, *Gastroenterology,* 54:918-921.

33. Foye, W. O., 1961. Role of metal-binding in the biological activities of drugs, *J. Pharm. Sci.* 50:93-108.

34. Frank, O., Luisada-Opper, A. V., Feingold, G., and Baker, H. 1970. Vitamin binding by human and some animal plasma proteins, *Nutr. Rep. Intern.* 1:161-168.

35. Fujimoto, T., Tanabe, H., Uchida, M., Shiba, N., Kusano, M., Sakuyama, F., Sumoya, S., and Yoshida, Y. 1960. Riboflavin metabolism in diabetics, *Vitamin, Kyoto* 20:140-150 (*Chem. Abstr.* 61:16576, 1964).

36. Fukuhara, T. 1961a. Studies of the metabolism of riboflavin in rabbits. I. Influence of the coexistence of glucose on the intestinal absorption of riboflavin in rabbits, *Hirosaki Med. J.* 13:9-10 (*Biol. Abstr.* 38:9041, 1962).

37. Fukuhara, T. 1961b. Studies of the metabolism of riboflavin in rabbits. II. The effect of intravenous injections of glucose solution on the urinary excretion of riboflavin in rabbits, *Hirosaki Med. J.* 13:11-13 (*Biol. Abstr.* 38:9042, 1962).

38. Funai, Y. 1956. Studies on riboflavin in milk. Report 1, on riboflavin content in breast milk, *Tokushima J. Exp. Med.* 3:194-200.

39. Goldsmith, G. A. 1965. Current status of the clinical use of antibiotic-vitamin combinations, *New Engl. J. Med.* 254:165-172.

40. Greenberg, S. M., Herndon, J. F., MacDonnell, D. R., Flanagan, T. L., and Bondi, A. 1961. Human availability studies on five vitamins in sustained release form, *Amer. J. Clin. Nutr.* **9**:324-330.

41. Guttman, D. E., and Athalye, M. Y. 1960. Solubilization of riboflavin by complex formation with caffeine, theophylline, and dimethyluracil, *J. Pharm. Sci.* **49**:687-691.

42. Harbury, H. A., and Foley, K. A. 1958. Molecular interaction of isoalloxazine derivatives, *Proc. Natl. Acad. Sci.* **44**:662-668.

43. Hawler, M. 1951. The photochemistry of riboflavin and related compounds, *J. Am. Chem. Soc.* **73**:4870-4874.

44. Hayton, W. L., Levy, G., and Regardh, C-G. 1972. Effect of complex formation on drug absorption. XIV. Effect of *N,N,*-di-*n*-propylpropionamide on the intestinal absorption of certain non-steroid drugs in the rat, *J. Pharm. Sci.* **61**:473-474.

45. Hewitt, R. R., and Levy, G. 1971. Effect of viscosity on thiamine and riboflavin absorption in man, *J. Pharm. Sci.* **60**:784-786.

46. Huttenrauch, R. 1965. Hydrotroper Einfluss der Ascorbinsaure auf Riboflavin, *Die Pharmazie* **20**:243.

47. Jick, H., Miettinen, O. S., Shapiro, S., Lewis, G. P., Siskind, V., and Slone, D. 1970. Comprehensive drug surveillance, *J. Amer. Med. Assn.* **213**:1455-1460.

48. Johnson, R. E. 1946. Rate of urinary excretion of ascorbic acid, thiamine, riboflavin, and *n*-methyl-nicotinamide and the effects of diuresis, alkalosis, acidosis and ingestion of food, *Fed. Proc.* **5**:139-140.

49. Jones, I. H. 1967. Riboflavine as an indicator of drug taking behavior, *Med. J. Austral.* **1**:202-203.

50. Jusko, W. J., and Levy, G. 1967a. Absorption, metabolism, and excretion of riboflavin-5'-phosphate in man, *J. Pharm. Sci.* **56**:58-62.

51. Jusko, W. J., and Levy, G. 1967b. Effect of probenecid on riboflavin absorption and excretion in man, *J. Pharm. Sci.* **56**:1145-1149.

52. Jusko, W. J., and Levy, G. 1969. Plasma protein binding of riboflavin and riboflavin-5'-phosphate in man, *J. Pharm. Sci.* **58**:58-62.

53. Jusko, W. J., and Levy, G. 1970. Pharmacokinetic evidence for saturable renal tubular reabsorption of riboflavin, *J. Pharm. Sci.* **59**:765-772.

54. Jusko, W. J., Levy, G., Yaffe, S. J., and Gorodischer, R. 1970a. Effect of probenecid on renal clearance of riboflavin in man, *J. Pharm. Sci.* **59**:473-477.

55. Jusko, W. J., Levy, G., and Yaffe, S. J. 1970b. Effect of age on intestinal absorption of riboflavin in humans, *J. Pharm. Sci.* **59**:487-490.

56. Jusko, W. J., Khanna, N., Levy, G., Stern, L., and Yaffe, S. J. 1970c. Riboflavin absorption and excretion in the neonate, *Pediatrics* **45**:945-949.

57. Jusko, W. J., Rennick, B. R., and Levy, G. 1970d. Renal excretion of riboflavin in the dog, *Amer. J. Physiol.* **218**:1046-1053.

58. Jusko, W. J., Leonards, J. R., and Levy, G. 1970e. Riboflavin distribution and elimination in two functionally anephric human patients, *J. Pharm. Sci.* **59**:566-567.

59. Jusko, W. J., Levy, G., Yaffe, S. J., and Allen, J. E. 1971. Riboflavin absorption in children with biliary obstruction, *Amer. J. Dis. Child.* **121**:48-52.

60. Jusko, W. J., and Lewis, G. P. 1972. Effect of hepatic disease on liver flavin and protein levels. *Amer. J. Clin. Nutr.* **25**:265-268.

61. Kagaya, A. 1956. Intestinal absorption of riboflavine in malnourished dogs, *Vitamins* **11**:313-316 (*Chem. Abstr.* **51**:18165, 1957).

62. Kasper, H., 1965. Die Resorption von Cocarboxylase, Riboflavin-5'-phosphat-Natrium und Vitamin A im Colon, *Zeitschr. f. Ernahrungswiss.* **6**:54-61.

63. Katagiri, M. 1960. Phosphorylation and dephosphorylation of riboflavine. I. Phos-

phorylation of riboflavine in homogenates and mitochrondria of various organs and in the blood, *Vitamin, Kyoto* 20:70-80 (*Chem. Abstr.* 61:16556, 1964).

64. Kimberg, D. V. 1971. Hyperthyroidism: gastrointestinal tract, and hypothyroidism: gastrointestinal tract, *in*: "The Thyroid" (Werner, S. C., and Ingbar, S. H., eds.) 3rd ed., pp. 562-579 and 736-744, Harper & Row, New York.

65. Korkeila, J. 1971. Antianabolic effect of tetracyclines, *Lancet* i:974-975.

66. Kotaki, A., Kato, K., Okumura, M., Sakurai, T., and Yagi, K. 1968. Studies on riboflavin tetranicotinate. II. Some physiological and pharmacological tests, *J. Vitaminol.* 14:253-269.

67. Leevy, C. M., and Baker, H. 1970. Nutritional deficiencies in liver disease, *Med. Clin. North Amer.* 54:467-477.

68. Leviton, A., and Pallansch, M. J. 1960. Binding of riboflavin and riboflavin phosphate by the proteins of milk, *J. Dairy Sci.* 43:1713-1724.

69. Levy, G., and Jusko, W. J. 1965. Effect of viscosity on drug absorption, *J. Pharm. Sci.* 54:219-225.

70. Levy, G., and Jusko, W. J. 1966a. Factors affecting the absorption of riboflavin in man, *J. Pharm. Sci.* 55:285-289.

71. Levy, G., and Jusko, W. J. 1966b. Apparent renal tubular secretion of riboflavin in man, *J. Pharm. Sci.* 55:1322.

72. Levy, G., and Hewitt, R. R. 1971. Evidence in man for different specialized intestinal transport mechanisms for riboflavin and thiamin, *Amer. J. Clin. Nutr.* 24:401-404.

73. Levy, G., and Rao, B. K. 1972. Enhanced intestinal absorption of riboflavin from sodium alginate solution in man, *J. Pharm. Sci.* 61:279-280.

74. Levy, G., Gibaldi, M., and Procknal, J. A. 1972a. Effect of an anticholinergic agent on riboflavin absorption in man, *J. Pharm. Sci.* 61:798-799.

75. Levy, G., MacGillivray, M., and Procknal, J. A. 1972b. Riboflavin absorption in children with thyroid disorders, *Pediatrics* 50:896-900.

76. Levy, G., Mosovich, L. L., Allen, J. E., and Yaffe, S. J. 1972c. Biliary excretion of riboflavin in man, *J. Pharm. Sci.* 61:143-144.

77. Libby, D. A., Schertel, M. E., and Loy, H. W. 1965. Human bioassay techniques for determining availability of vitamins from preparations resistant to in vitro disintegration, *J. Assoc. Offic. Agri. Chem.* 48:981-985.

78. Lih, H., and Baumann, C. A. 1951. Effects of certain antibiotics on the growth of rats fed diets limiting in thiamine, riboflavin, or pantothenic acid, *J. Nutr.* 45:143-152.

79. MacKenzie, J. C., Ford, J. E., Waters, A. H., Harding, N., Cattell, W. R., and Anderson, B. B. 1968. Erythropoiesis in patients undergoing regular dialysis treatment (R.D.T.) without transfusion, *Proc. Eur. Dialysis Renal Transp. Assoc.* 5:172-178.

80. Magyar, I. 1948. Excretion of riboflavin in rats and phosphorylation, *Hung. Acta Med.* 1:37-47.

81. Markkanen, T. 1960. Studies on the urinary excretion of thiamine, riboflavin, nicotinic acid, pantothenic acid and biotin in achlorhydria and after partial gastrectomy, *Acta Med. Scand. Suppl.* 361:1-56.

82. Markkanen, T. 1965. The effect of acetazolamide and mercaptomerin on the urinary excretion of thiamine, riboflavin, and pantothenic acid, *Zeitsch. f. Vit. Horm. ü. Ferm.-forsch* 14:72-76.

83. Maslenikova, E. M. 1963. Effect of light on riboflavin metabolism, *Fed. Proc. Transl. Suppl.* 22:T605-T607.

84. Mayersohn, M., Feldman, S., and Gibaldi, M. 1969. Bile salt enhancement of riboflavin and flavin mononucleotide absorption in man, *J. Nutr.* 98:288-296.

85. Mayersohn, M., and Gibaldi, M. 1971. Drug transport. III: Influence of various

sugars on passive transfer of several drugs across the everted rat intestine, *J. Pharm. Sci.* **60**:225-230.

86. McCormick, D. B. 1961. Flavokinase activity of rat tissues and masking effect of phosphatases, *Proc. Soc. Exptl. Biol. Med.* **107**:784-786.

87. Melnick, D., Hochberg, M., and Oser, B. L. 1945. Physiological availability of the vitamins. I. The human bioassay technic. *J. Nutr.* **30**:67-79.

88. Middleton, E. J., and Grice, H. C. 1964. Vitamin absorption studies. IV. Site of absorption of C^{14}-riboflavin and S^{35}-thiamine in the rat, *Canad. J. Biochem.* **42**:353-358.

89. Middleton, E. J., Davies, J. M., and Morrison, A. B. 1964. Relationship between rate of dissolution, disintegration time, and physiological availability of riboflavin in sugar-coated tablets, *J. Pharm. Sci.* **53**:1378-1380.

90. Miyao, M., Matsuda, H., Usui, T., Tanaka, H., Kochi, T., and Yamagata, Y. 1967. Studies on the intestinal absorption of thiamine, riboflavin and calcium in liver damage, *Tokushima J. Exptl. Med.* **14**:1-12.

91. Mizuhara, S., 1950. Fates of thiamine and riboflavin in vivo. *J. Japan Biochem. Soc.* **22**:11-15 (*Chem. Abstr.* **45**:1661, 1951).

92. Modi, V. V., and Owen, E. C. 1956. Riboflavin in milk, *Nature* **178**:1120.

93. Morrison, A. B., and Campbell, J. A. 1960. Vitamin absorption studies. I. Factors influencing the excretion of oral test doses of thiamine and riboflavin by human subjects, *J. Nutr.* **72**:435-440.

94. Morrison, A. B., and Campbell, J. A. 1960. The relationship between physiological availability of salicylates and riboflavin and *in vitro* disintegration time of enteric-coated tablets, *J. Amer. Pharm. Assoc., Sci. Ed.* **49**:473-478.

95. Morrison, A. B., and Campbell, J. A., 1962. Physiologic availability of riboflavin and thiamine in "chewable" vitamin products, *Amer. J. Clin. Nutr.* **10**:212-216.

96. Morrison, A. B., Perusse, C. B., and Campbell, J. A. 1960. Physiologic availability and *in vitro* release of riboflavin in sustained-release vitamin preparations, *New Engl. J. Med.* **263**:115-119.

97. Murata, T., Eto, S., and Yamamoto, S. 1963. Effects of ursodesoxycholic acid on the amount of urinary thiamine and riboflavin from patients with pulmonary tuberculosis, *J. Vitaminol.* **9**:299-304.

98. Najjar, V. A., and Holt, L. E. 1941. A riboflavin excretion test as a measure of riboflavin deficiency in man, *Bull. Johns Hopkins Hosp.* **69**:476-481.

99. Nogami, H., Hanano, M., Awazu, S., and Iga, T. 1970. Pharmacokinetic aspects of biliary excretion. Dose dependency of riboflavin in rat, *Chem. Pharm. Bull.* **18**:228-234.

100. Ohkawa, H., Kotaki, A. and Yagi, K. 1969. Direct incorporation of orally administered riboflavin tetranicotinate into portal blood of rabbit, *J. Vitaminol.* **15**:185-186.

101. Okuda, J. 1958. Metabolism of flavin nucleotides. I. Decomposition of flavin nucleotides in digestive juice, *Chem. Pharm. Bull.* **6**:662-665.

102. Okuda, J. 1958. Metabolism of flavin nucleotides. II. Decomposition of flavin nucleotides in the small intestine, *Chem. Pharm. Bull.* **6**:665-668.

103. Okuda, J. 1959. Metabolism of flavine nucleotides. III. Distribution of enzymes in the cells of the mucosa of small intestine causing dephosphorylation of flavine mononucleotide, *Chem. Pharm. Bull.* **7**:295-296.

104. Onishi, N. 1956. Effect of ursodesoxycholic acid and adenosine on the intestinal absorption of riboflavin, *Vitamins* **11**:479-81.

105. Ostrowski, W., and Krawczyk, A. 1963. The riboflavin flavoprotein from egg yolk, *Acta Chem. Scand.* **17**:S241-S245.

106. Owen, E. C., and Hytten, F. E. 1962. Riboflavin in human milk, *Proc. Nutr. Soc.* **21**:18.

107. Palagiano, V. 1962. Riboflavinuria after parenteral loading in hyperthyroid subjects in relation to surgical intervention. *Acta Chir. Ital.* **18**:183-192, (*Biol. Abstr.* **40**:13892, 1962).

108. Pasquali, P., Bovina, C., Landi, L., and Marchetti, M. 1969. Studies on relationships between riboflavin and folate, *Experentia* **25**:1031-1032.

109. Pöntinen, J., Hyyppä, M., and Hurme, P. 1967. Hydrolysis of riboflavin-5'-phosphate by phosphatases of rat kidney, *Histochemie* **8**:283-287.

110. Ponz, F. 1944. Der Einfluss von Thyroxin auf die Resorption und Ausscheidung von Laktoflavin, *Zeitschr. f. Vitaminforsch.* **14**:213-230.

111. Rennick, B. R. 1960. Renal tubular excretion of riboflavin in the chicken, *Proc. Soc. Exptl. Biol. Med.* **103**:241-243.

112. Rhodes, M. B., Bennett, N., and Feeney, R. E. 1959. The flavoprotein-apoprotein system of egg white, *J. Biol. Chem.* **234**:2054-2060.

113. Rindi, G., and Ventura V., 1967. Phosphorylation and uphill intestinal transport of thiamine *in vitro*, *Experentia* **23**:175-177.

114. Rivlin, R. S. 1970. Riboflavin metabolism, *New Engl. J. Med.* **283**:463-472.

115. Roche Vitamin B$_2$, 1961, Hoffman LaRoche, Inc., Nutley, N.J., Publication No. 3861.

116. Roe, D. A., McCormick, D. B., and Lin, R-T., 1972. Effects of riboflavin on boric acid toxicity, *J. Pharm. Sci.* **61**:1081-1085.

117. Roth, D., and Roth, D. M., 1972. Protective action of flavins on ultraviolet irradiated DNA, *J. Invest. Dermatol.* **58**:233-237.

118. Salazar, B., Aránguiz, T., and Vargas, L. 1965. Experimentelle Undersuchungen über die Rektale Resorption von Aneurin, Riboflavin, Pyridoxin und Cyanocobalamin aus Suppositorien-Fettgrundmassen, *Mitt. Dtsch. Pharmaz. Ges.* **35**:45-59.

119. Schaefer, A. E., Sassaman, H. L., Slocum, A., and Greene, R. D. 1956. Absorption of topically applied vitamins, *J. Nutr.* **59**:171-179.

120. Shinagawa, T. 1956. Influences of the overdose of thiamine on the urinary excretion of pyridoxine and riboflavine, *Vitamin (Kyoto)* **11**:467-469 (*Chem. Abst.* **51**:14922, 1957).

121. Sorrell, M. F., Frank, O., Thomson, A. D., Aquino, H., and Baker, H. 1971. Absorption of vitamins from the large intestine *in vivo*, *Nutr. Rep. Internat.* **3**:143-148.

122. Spencer, R. P., Zamcheck, N., and Grable, H. 1961. Intestinal absorption of riboflavin by rat and hamster, *Gastroenterol.* **40**:794-797.

123. Spencer, R. P., and Bow, T. M. 1964. *In vitro* transport of radiolabeled vitamins by the small intestine, *J. Nucl. Med.* **5**:251-258.

124. Stripp, B. 1965. Intestinal absorption of riboflavin by man, *Acta Pharmacol. et Toxicol.* **22**:353-362.

125. Sugimoto, I. 1968. Studies on complexes. XII. Effect of complex formation on drug absorption from alimentary tract, *Chem. Pharm. Bull.* **16**:1098-1104.

126. Tanaka, T., Tanaka, H. and Tsubaki, T. 1969. Preparation and enzymic hydrolysis of riboflavin diesters, *J. Vitaminol.* **15**:261-265.

127. Tedeschi, G. G., 1954. Elimination of lactoflavine-phosphoric acid by way of the bile. *Boll. Soc. Ital. Biol. Sper.* **30**:663-665 (*Chem. Abstr.* **49**:1919, 1955).

128. Tedeschi, G. G., and Canali, V. 1953. Intestinal mucous-membrane permeability to the phosphoric esters of lactoflavin, thiamine, serine, and creatinine, *Ricerca Sci.* **23**:851-856 (*Chem. Abstr.* **47**:10084, 1953).

129. Tennent, D. M. and Silber, R. H. 1943. The excretion of ascorbic acid, thiamine, riboflavin, and pantothenic acid in sweat, *J. Biol. Chem.* **148**:359-364.

130. Theorell, H. 1958. Modern trends in flavoprotein research, *Proc. Fourth Int. Congr. Biochem.* **8**:167-176.

131. Travia, L., and Pelosio, C. 1948. Urinary elimination of phosphorylated lactoflavin after administration of glucose and lactoflavin in normal subjects, *Boll. Soc. Ital. Biol. Sper.* **24**:737-738 (*Chem. Abstr.* **43**:6707, 1949).

132. Travia, L., Pelosio, C., and Tecce, G. 1950. So-called antagonism between some vitamins: Thiamine-lactoflavin, *Acta Vitaminol.* **4**:148-151 (*Chem. Abstr.* **45**:6258, 1951).

133. Tsutsumi, M. 1957. The pharmacologic action of flavin adenine dinucleotide, *J. Vitaminol.* **3**:123-128 (*Biol. Abstr.* **32**:27199, 1958).

134. Tucker, R. G., Mickelsen, O., and Keys, A. 1960. The influence of sleep, work, diuresis, heat, acute starvation, thiamine intake, and bed rest on human riboflavin excretion, *J. Nutr.* **72**:251-261.

135. Turner, J. B., and Hughes, D. E. 1962. The absorption of some B-group vitamins by surviving rat intestine preparations, *Quart. J. Exptl. Physiol.* **47**:107-123.

136. Unna, K. and Greslin, J. G. 1942. Toxicity and pharmacology of riboflavin, *J. Pharmacol. Exptl. Ther.* **76**:75-80.

137. Utsumi, K. 1962. Studies on the excretion of riboflavin especially in relation to alkaline phosphatase in kidney, *Jap. J. Derm.* **72**:141-153.

138. Vacek, L. 1953. Effect of some vitamins on photodynamics, *Scripta Med. Fac. Med. Univ. Masaryk. et Palack.* **26**:1-7 (*Chem. Abstr.* **48**:3504, 1954).

139. Verzar, F. 1967. "Absorption from the Intestine" pp. 223-224, Hafner Publishing Co., New York.

140. West, D. W., and Owen, E. C. 1969. The urinary excretion of metabolites of riboflavine by man, *Brit. J. Nutr.* **23**:889-898.

141. Wilson, T. H. 1962. "Intestinal Absorption" p. 44, W. B. Saunders Co., Philadelphia.

142. Windmueller, H. G., Anderson, A. A., and Mickelson, O. 1964. Elevated riboflavin levels in urine of fasting human subjects, *Amer. J. Clin. Nutr.* **15**:73-76.

143. Winter, W. P., Buss, E. G., Clagett, C. O., and Boucher, R. V. 1967. The nature of the biochemical lesion in avian renal riboflavinuria. II. The inherited change of a riboflavin-binding protein from blood and eggs, *Comp. Biochem. Physiol.* **22**:897-906.

144. Yagi, K. 1954. Destination of injected vitamin B_2. II. Emigration of vitamin B_2 to intestinal canal through intestinal mucosa, *Vitamin* **7**:36-38.

145. Yagi, K., and Okuda, J. 1958. Phosphorylation of riboflavin by transferase action, *Nature* **181**:1663-1664.

146. Yagi, K., Harada, M., Fujimoto, S., and Yamamoto, H. 1961a. Destination of injected riboflavin. V. Excretion of riboflavin in the urine when FAD and FMN were injected, *Vitamin* **22**:294-297.

147. Yagi, K., Yamamoto, Y., and Okuda, J. 1961b. Hydrolysis of fatty acid esters of riboflavin by pancreatic lipase, *Nature* **191**:174-175.

148. Yagi, K., Okuda, J., and Matsubara, T. 1964. Studies on fatty acid esters of flavins. IV. Fate of injected fatty acid esters of riboflavin in rabbits. *J. Vitaminol.* **10**:275-283.

149. Yagi, K., Nagatsu, T., Nagatsu-Ishibashi, I, and Ohashi, A. 1966. Migration of injected ^{14}C-labelled riboflavin into rat tissues, *J. Biochem.* **59**:313-315.

150. Yagi, K., Yamada, M., and Okuda, J. 1969. Studies on fatty acid esters of flavins. VI. Incorporation of riboflavin part of riboflavin tetrabutyrate-2-^{14}C into flavin nucleotides in the organs of rat, *J. Vitaminol.* **15**:155-159.

151. Yang, W-K, and Sung, J-L. 1966. Riboflavin metabolism in liver diseases. II. Flavin adenine dinucleotide loading in liver diseases, *J. Form. Med. Assn.* **65**:210-214.

5

METABOLISM OF RIBOFLAVIN

Donald B. McCormick

1. TISSUE UPTAKE, STORAGE, AND DISTRIBUTION OF FLAVINS AND FLAVIN COENZYMES

More particular details of natural occurrence and absorption of flavins in animals are considered in preceding and succeeding chapters, respectively. However, as both quantitative and qualitative aspects of the metabolism of the different forms of riboflavin (vitamin B_2) require some understanding of the intake and output of the vitamin, as well as its alteration by an organism, it is helpful to integrate some of this information here.

1.1. Uptake and Storage

Some of the initial information on the gross rate and extent of flavin intake by mammals was obtained in the 1930s by those German and Swiss scientists who were responsible for elucidating the chemical nature of vitamin B_2, the structural formula for which is given as follows:

DONALD B. McCORMICK—Section of Biochemistry, Molecular and Cell Biology, and Division of Nutritional Sciences, Cornell University, Ithaca, New York 14853.

Riboflavin

Kuhn et al.[73] examined the levels of flavin in liver and muscles from normal, partially repleted, and riboflavin-deficient rats. Though the liver was found to be sensitive to depletion, nearly half of the normal flavin content appeared to be maintained up to death of the animal. Depletion in the muscles was measured to be more extensive. An excess of riboflavin in the diet leads to the storage of only a slightly higher than normal level in the liver, since such capacity is largely limited to the amount of total flavoproteins present.

Prerequisite to knowing the riboflavin requirement of humans, as well as experimental animals, concomitant studies on the former were also made, usually of blood and urinary levels of the vitamin. Najjar et al.[103] had observed that a reduction in riboflavin intake by older subjects reduced the urinary riboflavin to a minimal level. An investigation of the minimal riboflavin requirement of the 6- to 9-kg infant by Snyderman et al.[135] led to the suggestion that 0.4–0.5 mg per day served to maintain adequate blood levels and to keep the urinary excretion at the upper limit of the zone of minimal excretion, and is not associated with clinical evidences of deficiency. Similar studies also have almost exactly delineated the amount of riboflavin that must be taken in by the adult to at least balance against excretory loss.

In recent years, Levy and Jusko[75] and Jusko and Levy[52] have shown that riboflavin and the 5′-phosphate are absorbed from the gastrointestinal tract of man by a site-specific and saturable specialized transport process rather than by passive diffusion

As techniques for assay of tissue flavin improved, understanding of the relationship between intake and storage became clearer. Bessey et al.[8] measured the concentration of riboflavin (free and bound) in the liver and the rest of the carcass of weanling rats that had been maintained for 3–5 weeks with 0–160 µg of riboflavin per day. In general agreement with the earlier findings of Kuhn et al.,[73] levels of the vitamin in animals given no dietary riboflavin were found to fall to a little less than half the initial value by the end of 3 weeks and remain stationary.

Maximal riboflavin concentrations are obtained with intakes of about 40 μg per day, while maximal growth rates are obtained with about 75% of this. Male rats grow faster than females, even with suboptimal tissue flavin. Hence, tissues from male animals were found to contain less riboflavin than females with a given suboptimal intake. Approximately the same expenditure of riboflavin is required by the growing as the nongrowing rat to maintain a given tissue concentration when allowance is made for flavin deposited in or released from the tissues. When only gross intakes are compared, however, a rapidly growing rat may require up to three times as much riboflavin per gram as a nongrowing rat to maintain a specific tissue level.

Most of the flavin taken in by an organism is stored as coenzymes, which are largely in association with specific proteins with which they function catalytically in numerous biological oxidation–reduction reactions. Burch et al.[14] measured the changes in levels of xanthine oxidase, D-amino acid oxidase, glycolic acid oxidase, riboflavin, and protein in livers and (except for glycolic acid oxidase) in kidneys of rats from birth to weaning at 21 days of age, and in normal adult males and females. From birth to 21 days, riboflavin increases 60% in liver and 120% in kidney with respect to protein which, itself, increases 29% and 65% respectively. Increases over the same period are twelve-, five-, and fivefold, respectively, for xanthine oxidase, D-amino acid oxidase, and glycolic acid oxidase in liver; levels increased thirteen- to fivefold in kidney for xanthine oxidase and D-amino acid oxidase, respectively. The hepatic and renal values for xanthine oxidase at 21 days are only 60% and 20%, respectively, of those found in the adult, whereas the oxidases for D-amino acids and glycolic acid are near the adult levels by this time. D-Amino acid oxidase is low in maternal liver at parturition. Hepatic glycolic acid oxidase is twice as high in adult male as compared to female rats.

The relationship that exists between protein intake, with the consequent change in protein level of tissues, and the intake and storage of riboflavin has been well quantitated. Kawai et al.[63] measured the activities of the same enzymes in the livers from rats as did Burch and colleagues in the before-mentioned study relating to age. However, Kawai et al. followed the changes as a direct function of protein offered in the diet at levels of 0, 7, 25, and 40%. Xanthine oxidase activity, largely present in the supernatant fraction of cells, was scarcely detected in the liver of rats fed the protein-free diet; maximal activity was observed with a dietary protein content of 25%. Oxidase activities for glycolic acid, D-amino acid, and glycine remain, to some extent, in the liver of rats fed on the protein-free diet and give maximal values in the case of the 7% protein diet. These latter enzymes are found in both mitochondrial and supernatant fractions. A comparison of these results with those obtained in riboflavin deficiency also indicates that the activities of these latter oxidases are mainly sensitive only to the flavin content of the tissue. However, xanthine oxidase is affected not only by riboflavin content, but also by protein uptake.

Expectedly, the quality, as well as quantity, of the protein in the diet also affects riboflavin metabolism, partly through an effect on the ability to store the vitamin in forms suitable for physiological function. Askarov[5] has examined the effect of feeding 18% animal (casein) or vegetable (gluten) protein, with and without supplementation with limiting essential amino acids, on uptake, storage, and excretion of riboflavin in male rats. The growth parameters measured (trunk length and weight) were poor with gluten alone but as satisfactory with gluten, adequately supplemented with lysine, tryptophan, and methionine, as with casein. Less riboflavin was consumed and less was stored in the livers of gluten-fed rats. Also, urinary excretion of flavin decreased gradually in this group but increased when casein was fed. Thus, in rats fed gluten, regardless of a sufficient supply of dietary riboflavin, endogenous riboflavin deficiency develops as a result of the inadequate amounts of three essential amino acids in the protein.

1.2. Distribution

Most of the early literature on flavins has to do with establishing how much of the vitamin occurs in diverse natural materials rather than what particular forms have the 7,8-dimethyl-10-(1'-D-ribityl) isoalloxazine[1] structure incorporated within themselves. It was fairly quickly realized in the 1930s that, besides small amounts of the free vitamin, the actual "physiologically active" (or coenzyme) forms that predominate in living tissues, or preparations carefully derived therefrom, are mainly flavin adenine dinucleotide (FAD) and, somewhat less commonly, flavin mononucleotide (FMN).[2] The structural formulas for these coenzymes are as follows:

---

[1] The numbering system used herein is that now most widely accepted, viz., the atoms within the heterocyclic rings are numbered consecutively from the pyrimidinoid nitrogen 1, and the side chain positions from proximal to distal relationship to the rings are designated with a prime superscript.

[2] FMN is D-riboflavin 5'-phosphate, and FAD is the 5'-(adenosine 5'-pyrophosphoryl) derivative of the vitamin.

Flavin mononucleotide

Flavin-adenine dinucleotide

More recently, other less common but nonetheless important forms, such as glycosides and peptides, of flavins are being found.

1.2.1. Predominant Forms

An early study of the distribution of vitamin B_2, largely in the animal body, was made by György et al.[37] For bioassay of materials, these investigators regarded the amount of B_2, which elicited a 40 g increase of weight in deficient rats over 30 days, as B_2 unity. One such unit of activity was found in about 0.2-0.4 g (fresh weight) liver and kidney, and in 0.5-1.0 g yeast. Bovine cardiac muscle contains high amounts of B_2, more than five times that measured in cross-striated skeleton muscle. Leg muscle from chickens contains about two times higher amounts of B_2 than breast muscle. The B_2 activity measured decreases in the following order: beaf heart; veal heart; chicken leg; veal, beef, and chicken breast. Differences in B_2 content of such muscle tissue were noted with variations in age, as well as species, of animals. It was also found that B_2 is present in beef thymus, pancreas, and milt. Even at this early date, it was noted that not all vitamin B_2 activity could be extracted by boiling natural products, but that the B_2 extracted by such means is dialyzable. This was certainly a prelude to our present realization that peptide-linked forms of the vitamin are widespread.

Succeeding investigations often were aimed at distinguishing the different molecular types of vitamin B_2, as well as quantitating these. Some studies were undertaken to resolve more adequately flavin from contaminating compounds in natural materials. For example, Wagner-Jauregg and Wollschitt[170] separated flavin from the yellow urochrome fraction in urine by absorption on fuller's earth or Frankonit KL. By the mid-1930s, it became increasingly apparent that most cellular flavin must be in phosphorylated forms. Euler and Adler had already shown that beef liver contains flavin in a high-molecular weight, nondialyzable form. Most of this we now recognize is flavin in coenzyme form but tightly associated with protein enzymes. The free flavin was isolated by Karrer and co-workers. Theorell found that the flavin-enzyme material from yeast consists of flavin phosphate and protein. Both Theorell and Karrer, and their colleagues,[162] then began purification and delineation of the phosphate components within the flavin fraction from beef liver. Rather soon it was found that the simple orthophosphate ester of riboflavin, FMN, represented but the lesser part of phosphorylated flavin extracted. For instance, Karrer and Meerwein[53] proved that some of the flavin phosphate from liver was accompanied by adenine nucleotide, which must be a constituent part. Such work as this, the work of Warburg, and the subsequent finding and confirmation of the principal flavin coenzyme, FAD, had been well reviewed by others, such as Sebrell and Harris[126] and Beinert.[7]

The strong fluorescence of flavin compounds has permitted accurate assessment of their presence in extracts from numerous materials. Burch et al.[13] have reported fluorometric measurements of riboflavin, FMN, and FAD in small quantities of blood, serum, and cells. Data on 13 adult humans, presumably adequately nourished, were given. The average (as $\mu g/100$ ml sera) for free riboflavin plus FMN is 0.8 and for FAD is 2.4. Together, white cells and platelets contain 252, and red cells 22.4, $\mu g/100$ ml. The potential use of blood flavin assays as a means to assess riboflavin adequacy, already suggested in the earlier work of Snyderman et al.,[135] was underscored by a parallel study of the relationship between riboflavin in the diet and that in serum, red cells, white cells, and urine from rats. Shortly following this work, Bessey et al.[9] further developed the fluorometric assay in conjunction with differential excretion of the free versus phosphorylated forms of the vitamin; the latter account for practically all the flavin of animal tissue. Riboflavin is distinguished from FMN and FAD by the much greater partition coefficient for the vitamin in benzyl alcohol. The measurement of the dinucleotide, which accounts for 70–90% of total tissue flavin, is based on the fact that it has less than a fourth the fluorescence of riboflavin or FMN, which are essentially the same, and can be readily hydrolyzed to FMN. Pearson[120] has reviewed some of the useful modifications of these techniques of benzyl alcohol extractions with and without hydrolysis before fluorometric measurements, which are currently used to quantitate the predominant forms of natural flavins.

After further study of the influences of flavin concentration, ionic strength, and different ions on the fluorescence of riboflavin, FMN, and FAD, Cerletti and Ipata[16] worked out a method for the extraction and separate determination of these compounds from animal tissues. A summary of average results obtained by these investigators for flavin extractable by potassium phosphate buffers with heating is given in Table I. Another few percent of flavin, largely FAD, can be obtained after digestion with such proteolytic enzymes as trypsin and chymotrypsin. Heart muscle is especially rich in such FAD-peptide material, with approximately 10% of the total in such form.

The more recent use of radioactive riboflavin has allowed a more exact quantitation of the kinetics of flavin distribution. Yagi et al.[185] injected, subcutaneously, rather large amounts, physiologically (17.8 mg/kg), of riboflavin-2-^{14}C into rats and found highest radioactivity in kidney, small intestine, and liver after 1 hr. In view of the large amount of radioactivity injected (about six times the daily requirement), these data appear to be more complex in that migration and excretion of flavin, more than incorporation and distribution, may predominate. Intra-abdominal injection gives a similar distribution, but flavin in liver becomes especially high. Partitioning of radioactivity 24 hr after injection of more nearly physiological levels (55 µg) of the ^{14}C-labeled vitamin into 170-g, male Sprague-Dawley rats has been reported by Yang and McCormick.[190] Some of the results are given in Table II. About 81%

TABLE I. *Salt-Dissociable Flavin Composition of Rat Tissues*[a]

| Tissue | Wet weight, µg/g | | |
	FAD	FMN	Riboflavin
Liver	59.0	8.4	0.8
Kidney	46.2	13.5	1.6
Heart	35.5	2.0	0.1
Spleen	9.9	0.2	1.1
Brain	6.0	0.9	0.2

[a] Homogenates (12.5%) were extracted thrice by stirring for 12 min in potassium chloride-phosphate buffers (pH 6.8) at 80° C followed by centrifugations.

TABLE II. Tissue Distribution of Radioactivity a Day after Administration of Riboflavin-2-^{14}C to Rats[a]

Tissue	Percent	$dpm \times 10^3/g$
Liver	27.86	375
Kidney	4.32	261
Small intestine	4.57	84
Cecum and large intestine	1.82	63
Blood	0.02	—
Rest of carcass	40.30	33.6

[a]Radioactivity injected intraperitoneally as 67.3×10^3 dpm/g rat with values given as the average from three rats.

of the radioactivity injected was retained in the body, most of it being in the liver and "rest of the carcass." On the basis of disintegrations per minute per gram fresh weight of tissue, the values are high in liver and kidney, being 375,000 and 261,000 dpm/g, respectively, as compared with the 67,400 dpm/g administered. The values in the intestines are about the same level as those administered, whereas the value for the "rest of carcass" is only half that of the administered level, and the radioactivity in the contents of intestines is low. The radioactivity in the blood is extremely low. Distribution of organ radioactivity, only a fraction of the total injected, indicates, with respect to time after injection, that riboflavin must be converted sequentially to FMN and the latter, in turn, to FAD. Liver and kidney have a higher ratio of radioactive FAD than FMN, and small intestine has more as the free vitamin than in coenzyme forms. Specific activities are always riboflavin > FMN > FAD. As pointed out by Yagi and co-workers, a higher ratio of FMN radioactivity to FAD than riboflavin to FMN suggests that the rate-limiting step in mammalian biosynthesis of FAD is FMN to FAD, rather than the preceding riboflavin to FMN.

Quite obviously, the route by which compounds are taken into an organism often affects their momentary distribution. Flavins are no exception. As previously noted, both the means by which riboflavin is administered, as well as the quantity given, influence the amounts present in specific tissues at specific times. Nagatsu-Ishibashi et al.[102] examined the quantities of flavin in rat brain after injection of each of the three principal natural forms. The animals (100 g) were injected intraabdominally with 20 mg/kg (calculated as riboflavin); 1 hr later, a blood sample was taken from the carotid artery and the brain removed after decapitation. While controls receiving no additional flavin were reported to contain 3.32 μg/g wet weight of brain (lower than the values reported by Cerletti and Ipata[16]; see Table I), values for those rats that received riboflavin, FMN, or FAD were 5.18, 3.73, and 3.75, respectively. An even larger injection of riboflavin (50 mg/kg) led to a value of 7.37. Increases of flavins in blood at 1 hr after administration to each animal were almost the same for the three types of flavins, being less than 1 µg/ml. Since the brain contains about 24 µl blood per gram, the increase of flavins due to the blood content was about 0.02 µg/g. Hence, flavins penetrate the blood-brain barrier with riboflavin crossing more easily than FMN or FAD. Confirmation and more exact quantitation of these results were then obtained with peripheral administration of riboflavin-2-^{14}C by Nagatsu et al.[100] About 0.05% of total radioactivity was found in brain 1 hr after injection. By 15 hr, the radioactivity in blood could not be detected, but the level in brain remained the same. Marked radioactivities were observed in FMN and FAD.

The transport and storage of ^{14}C-riboflavin in the retina and liver of normal and deficient rats was investigated by Foley et al.[28] because the free vitamin had been reported to exist, in significant amounts, in parts of the eyes of some animals (some amphibia, a lemur, and so forth), and an unusual flavin had been found in cat eyes. Liver, on the other hand, is well known to contain mainly the coenzyme forms. Deficient rats retain slightly less of an injected amount of ^{14}C-riboflavin per unit weight of liver than do controls, but levels in retina were similar for the two groups. A possible small preferential decrease in flavoproteins of liver, but not of retina, is suggested. No significant difference in rate of uptake by these tissues of the two groups was found after the 2-week depletion period. Riboflavin in the retinas of albino rats exists predominantly as FAD and FMN, with free riboflavin levels comparable to those found in liver.

In connection with problems of flavin transport in nonmammalian species, Blum[10] has made a series of detailed studies on riboflavin metabolism in the laying hen. As soon as ovarian activity begins, and under the action of estrogens, a new serum protein appears. This protein is capable of complexing free riboflavin that comes from either the diet or tissue reserves. It is incorporated progressively into the yolk during the growth of the ovocyte. The protein that complexes the riboflavin of albumen is synthesized in situ in the magnum. It is probable that this latter riboflavin-binding protein is enriched in the vitamin, without becoming saturated, at the expense of the labile flavoproteins of this organ. The riboflavin-binding protein of serum intervenes only to reconstitute the labile flavoproteins.

Another source of animal tissue that has been reported by Needham[105] to contain a relatively high concentration of the vitamin is the chloragogen tissue of the earthworm. The chloragogue cells, which surround the digestive tract and dorsal blood vessel of annelida, can synthesize urea and are, therefore, thought to have an excretory function. The function of flavin in this capacity may be similar to that of the flavin in the Malphigian tubules of such insects as the cockroach or even in the kidneys of mammals where there is also a high content of flavin, mainly FAD.

Several other studies have been made of the normal distribution of the predominant flavin forms in nature. Some of these have been concerned with plant as well as animal tissues, e.g., that of Mitsuda *et al.*[94] Others, e.g., Kawai *et al.*[62] and Treadwell[163] have examined only plant material.

Alterations in the distribution of flavins as a result of numerous factors have been observed. As is obvious and has previously been noted, a deficit of riboflavin in animals, which require it, leads to some redistribution of the available amount. Burch *et al.*[15] analyzed four tissues of rats on four different dietary regimens for FMN and FAD, and for six enzymes. In normal tissues, liver is richest in FAD, reduced nicotinamide adenine dinucleotide (NADH)[3] dehydrogenase, xanthine oxidase, and glycolic acid oxidase. Kidney is richest in FMN, D- and L-amino acid oxidases, and glycine oxidase (largely synonymous with D-amino acid oxidase). Brain is lowest in all these enzymes; it contains only a tenth as much NADH dehydrogenase as liver, even though its oxygen consumption is at least as great. During depletion there are large differences in the rates at which coenzymes and enzymes fall. Changes are negligible in the brain. In liver, FMN is lost more rapidly than FAD, and some enzymes show rapid and large decreases. Changes are much smaller in kidney and heart. NADH dehydrogenase has the highest activity in all tissues and is significantly decreased only in severe deficiency. In order of their decreasing sensitivity to riboflavin deficiency, hepatic oxidases are: those that act on glycolate, D-amino acids, glycine, xanthine, L-amino acids, and NADH. Xanthine oxidase decrease parallels FAD fall in liver, whereas decreases in oxidases for D-amino acid and glycolate during deficiency follow the decrease of FMN. The large decrease in these enzymes does not occur in weight-control animals. Hence, it was suggested that dietary riboflavin has some special role in formation or maintenance of these latter enzymes. Rapid regeneration of FAD, glycolic acid oxidase, D-amino acid oxidase, and xanthine oxidase

---

[3] The currently preferred names for the nicotinamide coenzymes are: nicotinamide adenine dinucleotide (NAD), which was formerly called diphosphopyridine nucleotide (DPN); and nicotinamide adenine dinucleotide phosphate (NADP), formerly called triphosphopyridine nucleotide (TPN). The natural reduced forms are indicated by adding a hydrogen to the abbreviation, e.g., NADH or NADPH.

occurs in liver upon alleviation of riboflavin deficiency. FMN, L-amino acid oxidase, and glycine oxidase come back more slowly. Weight-control animals on restricted food intake with ample riboflavin show lower than normal activity for a number of enzymes in both liver and kidney. This, again, stresses the interrelationship of protein intake.

Age, too, has an effect on the content of flavin coenzymes within tissues. Quarto di Palo et al.[122] noted that there is a reduction, variable from organ to organ, in old rats. FAD is more remarkably reduced, while the FMN content does not show any appreciable change between adult and old age.

Unnatural chemicals can affect flavin content. Sung and Yang[137] found that the content of riboflavin and of FAD is much lower in hepatomas induced by p-dimethylaminoazobenzene than in normal liver.

Genetic effects also have been related to the overall flavin metabolism of certain species. Clagett and his colleagues have studied the nature of the biochemical lesion in avian renal riboflavinuria. Winter et al.[183] compared a strain of single-comb, white Leghorn chickens, carrying the recessive riboflavinuria alleles (rdrd), to the heterozygote (Rdrd) and to the normal genotype (RdRd). The effect of the mutant gene was observed to cause a deficiency of riboflavin-binding protein in the albumen and yolks of eggs and in the blood serum. The phenotypic expression of this mutant gene is almost exactly 2(RdRd):1(Rdrd):0(rdrd) in terms of riboflavin-binding proteins in the albumen and yolk. (See Chapter 4.)

1.2.2. Less Common Forms

Whitby[178] observed the formation of a previously unknown flavin during incubation of riboflavin with homogenates or acetone powders of rat liver. Paper chromatography in five solvent systems excluded FMN, FAD, lumiflavin, and lumichrome. Since lumiflavin could be prepared from the unknown, the alteration must be in the flavin side chain. Lack of phosphorus excluded an altered nucleotide. Lyxoflavin, claimed (probably erroneously) by Pallares and Garza[119] to have been isolated from human heart tissue, also seemed unlikely. Further studies by Whitby[179] led to identification of the compound as 7,8-dimethyl-10-(5'-[α-D-glucopyranosyl]-D-ribityl)isoalloxazine (riboflavinyl glucoside), with an elemental composition of $C_{23}H_{30}O_{11}N_4$. It was suggested that the glucosidic linkage in this compound is of the α-configuration. The structural formula for this compound is as follows:

CH_2OH

H_3C, H_3C, O, N, NH, O

Riboflavinyl glucoside

Preliminary investigations indicated that an enzyme catalyzes a transglycosidation of D-glucose from maltose or glycogen to riboflavin. This reaction was studied in more detail by Whitby,[180] who recognized that the liver enzyme catalyzes synthesis of several isoalloxazine derivatives, many of which are antivitamin B_2. Maltose, maltulose, and turanose serve as glucosyl donors with relative rates of 10:9:6. The reaction of riboflavin plus maltose to yield the riboflavinyl α-D-glucoside is competitively inhibited by α-D-glucose-l-phosphate. The enzyme may have glucosidase, as well as transglucosidase, activity. As the solubility of riboflavinyl glucoside is much greater than riboflavin, it was suggested that this may be a natural derivative of importance in the transport of the vitamin.

Numerous other riboflavinyl glycosides and oligosaccharides of riboflavin, and the enzymes responsible,[146] have been described more recently by Japanese workers. Transglucosidases that catalyze formation of riboflavinyl glucoside were found in *Aspergillus oryzae* by Tachibana and Katagiri,[154] in *Escherichia coli* by Katagiri et al.,[54] in *Leuconostoc mesenteroides* by Suzuki and Katagiri,[139] and in cotyledons of pumpkin (*Cucurbita pepo*) and sugar beet (*Beta vulgaris*) by Tachibana.[151] The formation of 5'-D-riboflavin-β-D-galactoside by *C. acetobutyricum* and by *A. oryzae* when incubated with lactose and riboflavin was reported by Tachibana.[142,143] Transfructosidations from sucrose and, to a lesser extent raffinose, by enzymes detected in *E. coli*, *A. oryzae*, and *C. acetobutyricum* have similarly been described by Tachibana[142] and by Katagiri et al.[56,60] As for oligosaccharides of riboflavin, the isomaltoside, dextrantrioside, and dextrantetraoside were noted by Katagiri et al.[55] to be formed by prolonged incubation with extracts from *E. coli*. Glucosyl derivatives up to a pentaoside were identified by Suzuki and Uchida[140,141] using *L. mesenteroides*. Riboflavinyl galactobioside and galactotrioside were noted by Katagiri et al.[57] to be formed by prolonged incubations with *E. coli* preparations. The isolation and properties of some of these riboflavinyl glycosides have been recently summarized by Whitby[181] and by Tachibana.[151]

Cyclic nucleotide forms of flavine have been isolated from natural materials, but there is often a question as to whether or not such compounds are artifacts. During the isolation of FAD from various tissues, Dimant *et al.*[22] observed the presence of an unidentified flavin nucleotide, which they named FAD-X. This substance was later identified as a cyclic form of FAD, since, upon enzymatic hydrolysis with nucleotide pyrophosphatase, Huennekens *et al.*[48] found that it yielded riboflavin 4',5'-cyclic phosphate and AMP. As pointed out by Huennekens,[46] FAD-X has no known coenzymatic activity and may well be an artifact resulting from the exposure of FAD to basic solutions, for example, pyridine, during the isolation procedure. Such behavior is well known for other phosphorylated polyhydroxy compounds. On the other hand, the ready susceptibility of phosphorylated compounds to assume a cyclic phosphodiester structure under the influence of chemical reagents may suggest the occurrence of a corresponding reaction under enzymic control.

Tachibana[149] claims that he and his co-workers have isolated at least three riboflavin phosphates, other than FMN and FAD, from cultures of molds. Tachibana and Katagiri[155] isolated a riboflavin diphosphate (presumably cyclic) produced by *A. oryzae*. A riboflavinyl glucoside mononucleotide and riboflavin cyclic 2',5'-mononucleotide were isolated by Tachibana[144,145] from *Rhizopus oryzae*. The mononucleotide of riboflavinyl glucoside is produced from the glucoside and is distinguishable from earlier known flavins by paper chromatography in several solvent systems. Upon hydrolysis with sulfuric acid, an FMN-like substance is produced and glucose released. The enzymatic cleavage of this new compound by the phosphomonesterase in Takadiastase produces riboflavinyl glucoside and phosphate. The one mole of glucose and of phosphate in the compound were identified chemically; the absorption spectrum is similar to FMN. Interestingly, flavinyl glucoside mononucleotide was reported by Tachibana's group[147,149,153] not to stimulate growth of *Lactobacillus casei*, but it will after acid hydrolysis. The same was found to be true for both the flavin cyclic diphosphate and the flavin cyclic 2',5'-mononucleotide. Presumably, *L. casei* lacks phosphatases for such forms. Some of the characteristics of the flavin cyclic mononucleotide were given by Tachibana,[159] along with details of the effects of inorganic salts on production of this compound from both *R. oryzae*[160] and *R. javanicus*.[158] Both chemical and enzymatic evidence certainly verify the cyclic structure and differentiate this "natural" compound from the well-known riboflavin 4',5'-cyclic monophosphate that predominates from alkaline treatment of FMN. The natural cyclic FMN has different mobilities upon paper chromatography and electrophoresis, consumes only 1 mol periodate to give a product different from that obtained by similar treatment of FMN, and is more stable against hydrolysis catalyzed by 5'- or 3'-nucleotidase or by the cell-free extracts of *A. oryzae*. Tachibana *et al.*[156,157] reported that the fluorescence–pH profile of the cyclic mononucleotide is somewhat different from that of riboflavin or FMN but not as markedly quenched as FAD toward more nearly neutral pH values. The cyclic compound also is less able than FMN to act as a photosensitizer in dye-sensitized polymerization of acrylamide or even to cause photolysis of its own side chain. These results suggest that there must be less efficient conversion of absorbed light energy into excited states of the flavin because of the presence of the phospho-diester link at what would most reasonably be the 2'-position of the ribityl chain. The presumed structural formula for this natural cyclic FMN is as follows:

Riboflavin 2',5'-cyclic phosphate

Tachibana[148,150] has also found a synthetase from *Rhizopus*, which most effectively uses guanosine 5'-triphosphate to produce flavin cyclic 2',5'-mononucleotide.

The diversity of peptide-linked forms of flavins is rapidly being made more apparent. Green and co-workers[36] noted that fragments of the mitochondrial respiratory chain liberate appreciable amounts of flavin material that is not extractable by acidification or boiling. The source of at least most of this tightly bound flavin turned out to be succinate dehydrogenase, since purified, soluble preparations of the enzyme were found by Kearney and Singer[67] to liberate flavin only upon proteolytic extraction. About the same time, Boukine[11] observed that a variety of plant and animal tissues, particularly those rich in succinate dehydrogenase, liberate their total flavin content only after proteolytic treatment. King *et al.*[69] determined that the acid–nonextractable flavin in beef heart, which is solubilized after proteolysis and measured spectrophoto-metrically, represents 0.11-0.12 μmol/gram of protein for both a Keilin-Hartree preparation or isolated mitochondria. Depending upon the extent of proteolysis of succinic dehydrogenase, FAD peptides of varying chain length are released, as found by Kearney and Singer[67] and by Wang et al.[174] A hexapeptide was isolated in pure form by Kearney.[65]

The partial characterization of such peptides was accomplished by Singer et al.,[130] Wang et al.,[175] and Singer and Kearney.[129] One characteristic property of the flavin peptides from succinic dehydrogenase is the fluorescence-pH profile. Although the covalently attached flavin at the monophosphate or riboflavin level exhibits the same level of fluoresence at pH 3.2-3.4 as free FMN or riboflavin in this pH range, the flavin peptides have insignificant fluorescence at pH 7, where the fluorescence of FMN and riboflavin is maintained. This unusual depen-dence of fluroescence of pH of the flavin from succinate dehydrogenase has been utilized in the fluorometric determination of flavin peptides developed by Singer et al.[128] Similar procedures were evolved by Cerletti et al.[17] and by Wilson and King.[182]

The point of attachment of the peptide to the flavin moiety of FAD from succinate dehydrogenase has been ascertained after the efforts of several different groups. Since alkaline photolysis, resulting in removal of the N(10)-side chain, was shown by Kearney[65] not to liberate the peptide from the flavin, attachment must be to the isoalloxazine ring system. Alkaline hydrolysis was shown by Chi et al.[20] to remove urea rather than a ureido peptide. Hence, the substitution cannot be in the 1, 2, or 3 position of the flavin; positions 4 and 5 can be excluded on the basis of lability. With synthetic flavins, Dudley and Hemmerich[25] showed that such substituents as OR, NR_2, and SR are split easily from position 4 by acid, as well as alkaline, hydrolysis. Hydrogen, as well as alkyl and even aryl, residues can be removed from position 4 by photooxidation, yielding, again, "normal" flavin, as shown by Müller and Hemmerich,[98] Müller et al.,[99] and Bamberg et al.[6] The removal of alkyl substituents from N(5), on the other hand, was shown by Walker et al.[171] to occur easily in acid medium. No transformation of succinate dehydrogenase flavin into nonpeptide-linked flavin occurs under similar hydrolytic and/or oxidative conditions. There is consider-able chemical reactivity of the 8-methyl group of usual lumiflavin and riboflavin types, though, as evidenced by the formation of "biflavins" under alkaline, anhydrous conditions reported by Hemmerich et al.,[42] by facile deuteration as reported by Bullock and Jardetzsky,[12] or by bromination and subsequent oxidation as found by McCormick.[84] An investigation of the hyperfine structures of the electron spin resonance

(ESR) spectra of the semiquinone of acid-hydrolyzed succinate dehydro-genase flavin and of its alkaline photoderivative led Hemmerich et al.[41] to conclude that attachment of peptide was, indeed, at the 8α-position of the flavin. This assignment was confirmed by Walker et al.[173] using the ENDOR technique. The generalized structural formula for such a flavin peptide is as follows:

Flavin peptide

More recent advances have led Singer et al.[131] to conclude that actual linkage of the flavin to the peptide is via a ring nitrogen of a histidine residue. This has been verified, through chemical synthesis of the spectroscopically identical histidinyl flavin peptide, by Ghisla et al.[33] The sequence of a flavin-appended, histidyl-containing pentapeptide from the active center of succinate dehydrogenase now has been established by Kenny et al.[68] as ser-ɪɪis (flavin)-thr-val-ala.

Another covalently attached flavin occurs in animal amine oxidases. Nara et al.[104] pointed out that the flavin within beef liver mitochondrial monoamine oxidase is not released by treatment even with trichloroacetic acid. Igaue et al.[49] also showed that the flavopeptide is FAD-like, but it is inactive in activating apo-D-amino acid oxidase. Walker et al.[172] then succeeded in proving that the FAD of hepatic monoamine oxidase is linked through the 8α-methylene, as with succinate dehydrogenase, but to the thioether sulfur from a cysteinyl residue within a peptide, which was determined as ser-gly-gly-cys (flavin)-tyr. Interestingly, the fluorescence properties of this covalently attached flavin, at the riboflavin or FMN level, resemble the vitamin rather than histidyl riboflavin.

The flavin of *Chromatium* cytochrome c-552 has been reported by Hendriks and Cronin[43] to be another peptide-linked FAD, probably also with covalent attachment through the 8α-methylene, but clearly not of a histidyl flavin type. As with the thioether flavinyl peptide from hepatic monoamine oxidase, the riboflavinyl peptide from *Chromatium* also exhibits a fluorescence behavior rather similar to free riboflavin.

Still other covalently attached flavins occur in nature. There is some evidence, published by Frisell and MacKenzie[31] that part of the covalently bound flavin of mammalian liver mitochondria may originate from dimethylglycine dehydrogenases. Chelkowski[19] estimates that up to 7% of the total flavin content of pig liver, yeasts, propionibacteria, and wheat is comprised of flavin peptides.

Finally, among the presently known natural, but less abundant flavins, one that has yet to be elucidated structurally is nekoflavin, found by Matsui[76] in extracts from the choroid of cat eye. This yellowish-green, fluorescent substance is distinguishable from riboflavin, its nucleotides, glucoside, and known photodecomposition products. The ocular manifestations of riboflavin deficiency in the human have been known for some time, as, for example, in the "Shibi-Gattchaki" disease described by Irinoda and Sato. [51]

2. INTERCONVERSIONS OF FLAVINS, FLAVIN GLYCOSIDES, AND FLAVIN COENZYMES

Some understanding of the interconversion processes among flavins has been gained through investigating the alteration in the distribution pattern of all the flavins after uptake of a given flavin. For example, the increase in the FMN content of tissue from a riboflavin-deficient animal to which the vitamin has been administered may be initially more rapid than the rise in level of FAD, although the final concentration of this latter coenzyme is usually much greater. This fact suggests the sequence for formation *in vivo* of the predominant coenzyme forms from riboflavin must be first FMN and then FAD. Within most tissues, however, are not only enzymes that are responsible for syntheses of flavin coenzymes, but, also, there are phosphatases and nucleotidases that are capable of catalyzing the hydrolysis both of FAD to yield FMN and of the latter to yield riboflavin. In broken-cell preparations, often the activities of the degradative enzymes mask, and under some conditions may even overwhelm, those involved in biosynthesis of flavin coenzymes. Hence, findings from such measurements *in vitro* must always be carefully reconciled with what actually is found in the intact organism.

2.1. Interconversions of Flavins and Flavin Glycosides

Much of the work that has led to our knowledge of flavin glycosides was cited within the earlier section on distribution of the less common forms of flavins. It is appropriate here to consider more details concerning the enzymes responsible for these reactions.

After his discovery of the first flavin glycoside, 5'-D-riboflavin α-D-glucopyranoside, Whitby[180] found that preparations from mammalian (rat) liver possess the ability to transglucosidate several isoalloxazines (e.g. L- and D-araboflavin, L-lyxoflavin, and isoriboflavin) that bear polyhydroxy side chains at position 10.

The characteristics of several other known transglucosidases that form riboflavinyl glucoside have been summarized recently by Whitby.[181] Among those described is the enzyme from *E. coli* reported by Katagiri et al.;[54] this enzyme has a pH for optimal activity near 6.8, as does the liver enzyme, and retains activity well above the temperature optimum of 30° C. The enzyme from *A. oryzae* found by Tachibana and Katagiri[154,155] shows optimal activity near pH 5 and catalyzes increasing production of riboflavinyl glucoside up to 50° C. By contrast, the enzyme in *L. mesenteroides* reported by Suzuki[138] has an optimal pH of 5.3 with activity falling off sharply above 30° C. The enzyme from *Ashbya gossypii* was found by Onozaki and Takakuwa[109] to have maximal activity at pH 4 and 20° C.

The specificity of such enzymes for the glucose donor varies with the source and the degree of purification. Taking into account the large number of carbohydrates and derivatives that have been found incapable of acting as glucose donors, it may be concluded that the enzymes in rat liver and *E. coli* require the disaccharide maltose or one of its higher homologs, or a limited number of oligosaccharides containing an α-glucopyranosyl residue and possessing a free reducing group. By contrast, the dextran sucrose from *L. mesenteroides* shows a high specificity for sucrose as glucose donor in the synthesis of riboflavinyl glucoside. Besides inadequate purification of a given enzyme, some of the inconsistent results in the earlier experiments with microorganisms on the glycose-donor specificity may have been due to failure to exclude light during prolonged incubations, especially at acid pH, since photochemical formation of flavin glycosides in aqueous solutions of glucose, fructose, and galactose has been observed by Katagiri et al.[61] However, as reviewed by Tachibana,[151,152] it is clear that lower and higher plant forms contain enzymes that catalyze transglycosidations with flavins of a rather broad scope.

Overall, interconversions of flavin glycosides as catalyzed by transglycosidases may be depicted as in the following equation:

$$\text{Flavin} + (\text{hexose})_n \rightleftharpoons \text{flavin glycoside} + (\text{hexose})_{n-1}$$

Whitby[181] has pointed out that the natural occurrence of such flavin glycosides has not been demonstrated for any species. Certainly, no significant amount of any flavin glycoside has been isolated from fresh animal tissue carefully extracted to account for approximately all flavin-like compounds. Although this obviously does not exclude trace quantities functioning in some transient role such as transport, it does seem unlikely that an essential function will be found for flavin glucosides, at least in higher animal forms.

2.2. Interconversions of Flavins with Flavin Phosphates

It became increasingly apparent during the 1930s that the active forms of vitamin B_2 were phosphorylated, since these were not only isolated from the most enzymatically active preparations then available, but also caused greater stimulation of activity than the vitamin when added to such preparations initially resolved from flavin material. Kuhn and Rudy[74] chemically phosphorylated riboflavin and found, in a biological test, that methylene blue was decolorized more rapidly by the synthetic riboflavin phosphate than by riboflavin.

2.2.1. Formation of Flavin Phosphates from Flavins

Rudy[123] noted that the first stage in the synthesis of "yellow enzyme" (flavoproteins) in an organism might be the esterification of riboflavin with phosphoric acid. Flavin mononucleotide was formed when glycerinated extracts from rat intestine were incubated with riboflavin at 37° C and pH 7.2 in 0.1 M phosphate. If the extracts were first heat-inactivated, no phosphorylation occurred. Later work, such as by Yagi,[184] also suggested that intestinal mucosa is an important site for this conversion within the mammal.

Nonspecific (trans)phosphorylation of flavin catalyzed by alkaline phosphatase, such as that which occurs in intestinal mucosa, was then firmly established for certain animal tissues. Yagi and Okuda[186] demonstrated that the intestinal alkaline phosphatase (a phosphomonoesterase) can catalyze such transphosphorylations as between a chemically rather stable (low group-transfer potential) phosphate donor, such as β-glycerophosphate, and riboflavin to produce an equilibrium mixture also containing glycerol and riboflavin 5'-phosphate. This can be indicated for the general case as:

Flavin + phosphate ester $\xrightarrow{\text{phosphatase}}$ flavin phosphate + alcohol

Domján[23] found that homogenates from chick embryo brain can also catalyze an effective phosphate transfer from β-glycerophosphate to riboflavin. Formation of FMN *in vitro* can reach a maximum value of about 70%. The intensity of the FMN synthesis under the experimental conditions used increases considerably during the course of the ontogenetic development, when based on wet weight of tissue, but is considerably less when the calculation is based on 100 mg of tissue protein.

The more specific phosphorylation of flavin catalyzed by certain phosphokinases has been recognized and received increasing attention in the last couple of decades. Kearney and England[66] were the first to coin the name "flavokinase" for an enzyme, which they isolated in partially purified form from brewer's yeast (*Saccharomyces carlsbergensis*). The yeast enzyme is apparently activated by Mg^{2+}, as well as certain other divalent cations, such as Zn^{2+}. It preferentially uses adenosine 5'-triphosphate (ATP) as phosphate donor, though the 5'-diphosphate (ADP) is somewhat effective with impure preparations. Also, the absolute specificity of yeast flavokinase for flavins was reasonably well documented in this report. Kearney[64] then enlarged upon the relative specificity of the yeast kinase for different flavins. The partially purified enzyme acts on riboflavin, dichloroflavin [7,8-dichloro-10-(1'-D-ribityl)isoalloxazine], and D-araboflavin [7,8-dimethyl-10-(1'-D-arabityl)isoalloxazine], but not on isoriboflavin [6,7-dimethyl-10-(1'-D-ribityl)isoalloxazine] or derivatives of isoalloxazines that have hexityl chains at position 10. The reaction for the general case can then be indicated as:

$$\text{Flavin} + \text{ATP} \xrightarrow[\text{Mg}^{2+} \text{ (or Zn}^{2+})]{\text{kinase}} \text{flavin phosphate} + \text{ADP}$$

The occurrence of flavokinase in other microorganisms has been noted. Giri and Krishnaswamy[34] also studied a flavokinase from yeast. The production of FMN from riboflavin and ATP in preparations from several bacteria was reported by Haley and Lambooy,[38] Snoswell,[134] and Katagiri *et al.*[58]

In addition to the earlier work that indicated intestinal mucosa can phosphorylate riboflavin rather nonspecifically as catalyzed by alkaline phosphatase, England[26] demonstrated the probable occurrence of an ATP-dependent flavokinase in this tissue. However, the presence of phosphatases, which can degrade FMN, the product of the kinase reaction, has often made an assessment of flavokinase activity difficult. This problem was pointed out clearly by McCormick,[77] who demonstrated that flavokinase can be detected in several rat tissues, but the level of apparent activity is markedly suppressed by phosphatases, most of which are maximally active near pH 5. In supernatant solutions from tissue homogenates, specific activities of the kinase measured with riboflavin, ATP, and Zn^{2+} in phosphate buffer at pH 8 were found to be liver > kidney > brain > spleen > intestine.

The first flavokinase from animal tissue to be partially purified and characterized was the rat liver enzyme reported by McCormick.[79,80] This enzyme, purified over eighty-fold by fractionation with ammonium sulfate and by column chromatography over diethylaminoethyl (DEAE-) cellulose, was found to be localized to the true supernatant solution (cell sap) from isotonic homogenates. The rate of reaction *in vitro* is zero order for over 1 hr at 37° C. with enzyme and near optimal concentrations of riboflavin, ATP, and Zn^{2+}, which is somewhat superior to Mg^{2+} as activating divalent cation. The Michaelis–Menten constant (K_m) for riboflavin is 1.2×10^{-5} M. A temperature optimum near 50° C was found for a 30-min incubation; the pH optimum is 8.

A preliminary investigation by McCormick[79,80] of flavin substrate specificity indicated that the requirements of the liver kinase appear similar for those analogs of vitamin B_2 that were tested for the yeast kinase. More detailed studies with variously substituted flavin analogs were undertaken. McCormick and Butler[89] presented the outlines of the apparent requirements in flavin structure for interaction with flavo-kinase. A closer examination by specific alteration of certain portions of the flavin structure then followed. McCormick *et al.*[88] studied the effects from substitution in the ring system of D-ribitylisoalloxazines. Then, Chassy *et al.*[18] investigated the effects from variations in length and degree of hydroxylation of the 10-side chains in 7,8-dimethylisoal-loxazines. From such studies, the relative substrate efficiencies of flavins with liver flavokinase could be summarized, as given by McCormick[86] and presented in Table III.

With sufficient information on the tolerances in structures of flavins for binding with flavokinase, Arsenis and McCormick[3,4] synthesized flavin–cellulose compounds as biochemically specific absorbents for "affinity" chromatographic purification of the enzyme. For this, 7-amino-10-(1'-D-ribityl)isoalloxazine (a synthetic substrate) or 8-amino-7,-10-dimethylisoalloxazine (a synthetic competitive inhibitor) was reacted with chlorocarbonylmethyl cellulose prepared from carboxymethyl cellu-lose. Use of substrate flavin–cellulose and inhibitor flavin–cellulose permitted marked purification of liver flavokinase from the stage of a dialysate of an ammonium sulfate fraction with a specific activity of approximately 20 nmol of FMN, formed per milligram of protein per hour under defined conditions, to a specific activity of 3750.

Importantly, an understanding of the reactivity with the kinase system of flavin analogs, some of which are antivitamin in behavior, allows

TABLE III. Substrate Efficiencies of Flavins with Flavokinase from Rat Liver

Substituent changes in D-riboflavin[a]	Relative efficiency for phosphorylation
None	100
10-Substituent:	
D-Erythrityl	33
D-Allityl	26
D-Arabityl	25
2'-Deoxy-D-ribityl	18
7,8-Substituents	
Dichloro	94
Dibromo	51
Diiodo	47
Diethyl	40
7-Methyl-8-fluoro	38
Dimethoxy	2
8-Substituent	
Amino	31
7-Substituent	
Methyl	24
7-Methyl-9(N)-pyrido	22
Chloro	20
Ethyl	16
Ethoxy	13
Methoxy	11
Amino	11
2-Substituent	
Thio	62[b]
Imino	31
Benzylazino	31
Methylmercapto	9
Deoxy	4

[a] 7,8-Dimethyl-10-(1'-D-ribityl)isoalloxazine.
[b] Partially decomposes to riboflavin during incubation.

some understanding of how certain of these compounds act in living organisms. The experimental comparison of such such information was made by Yang et al.,[188] who examined the activities of several flavin derivatives in riboflavin-dependent cultures of Lactobacillus casei and with rat liver flavokinase. As examples, 7,8-diethyl-, 7-methyl-, and 2'-deoxyriboflavin are phosphorylated in the flavokinase system and serve as sole sources of flavin for the growing microbe. D-Erythroflavin, 7,8-dihaloriboflavins, and other flavins substituted only in position 7 or 8, are poor replacers of riboflavin for growth. Certain of these latter analogs, such as D-erythroflavin or a flavin not substituted (preferably with a methyl) in position 7 or 8, are poorly phosphorylated and may also act as riboflavin antagonists (competitive inhibitors, specifically) at high concentrations. The dichlororiboflavin is readily phosphorylated but does not function properly as a coenzyme.

Much of such work relating the activity or inactivity of flavins in enzyme systems to their behavior as oxidation–reduction coenzymes in the living organism has led to a fuller understanding of which portions of the molecular architecture of the vitamin are essential for which functions. These findings have actually evolved over several decades. Within a few years following the elaboration of the structure of riboflavin, a sizable number of analogs were synthesized in the laboratories of Kuhn and Karrer for chemical and biological tests intended to circumscribe the behavior of this vitamin. Reviews on their work, as well as that of others, have been published by Wagner-Jauregg[169] and by Beinert.[7] The syntheses and testing *in vivo* of riboflavin analogs continued with Lambooy (see Chapter 10) and later McCormick, who, as previously pointed out, also began to ascertain just which enzyme systems were involved. Some of the primary considerations of how pseudovitamins may partially replace and interfere with vitaminic functions, especially in mammals, has been synoptically discussed with examples from the flavin literature by McCormick.[81]

The occurrence of flavokinases in higher plants has also been well documented. Giri *et al.*[35] established the presence of the kinase in the bean, *Phaseolus radiatus*. Mitsuda *et al.*[95] then found that flavokinase activity is widespread in the green leaves of plants. As with most extracts from animal tissues, those from plant leaves also contain considerable degradative activity for the flavin product, FMN. Again, such enzymes are mainly phosphatases. The presence of potassium fluoride in trishydroxymethylaminomethane- (Tris-) buffered incubations was found to prevent the phosphatase-catalyzed hydrolysis of FMN. In Tris buffer, the pH optimum for partially purified kinase is between 8.5 and 9.0. Among divalent cations tested, Mg^{2+} appeared to be the best activator with considerable stimulation also afforded by Zn^{2+}. ADP, as well as ATP, is effective in the preparations examined, perhaps due to contaminating 5'-adenylate kinase; AMP is a competitive inhibitor. Sadasivam and Shanmugasundaram[124] detected another leaf flavokinase in *Solanum nigrum* L. with properties very similar to others. Maximal activity is achieved at pH 8.6 and between 40° and 45° C over 1 hr. The K_m for riboflavin is around 10^{-5} M. Mg^{2+} activates over a rather wide range of concentrations, whereas Zn^{2+} and Mn^{2+} activate at lower (10^{-4} M) and inhibit at higher (10^{-3} M) concentrations.

The most extensive purification of a plant flavokinase was reported by Mitsuda and colleagues[96] for the soybean enzyme. Through extraction, dialysis, protamine sulfate treatment, fractionation with ammonium sulfate, and chromatography on DEAE-cellulose, they obtained a kinase preparation with a specific activity of 80 mμmol of FMN formed per milligram of protein per hour at 30° C. It was claimed that this preparation did not contain phosphatase activity and behaved as a nearly homogeneous system upon electrophoresis and ultracentrifugation. The optimum pH is around 9, and the optimum temperature is about 40° C. ATP is the specific phosphate donor; Mg^{2+} is the most effective divalent cation. As with most reported flavokinases, the K_m value for riboflavin is near 1.3×10^{-5} M.

Tachibana[144,145] claimed that a mononucleotide of riboflavinyl glucoside is formed from the glucoside by *Rhizopus* extracts, but the nature of an enzyme responsible for this phosphorylation has not been revealed. Also, as mentioned before, Tachibana discovered a new flavin phosphate, the cyclic 2',5'-mononucleotide of riboflavin, which he found to be formed by extracts from *R. oryzae*. Tachibana[148,149] reported isolation of a crude synthetase from the fraction precipitated by 70-80% saturated ammonium sulfate. Several characteristics of this enzyme, more recently reported by Tachibana[150] to occur in numerous species of *Rhizopus*, distinguish it from the more conventional flavokinase. In the first place, GTP ($K_m = 10^{-4}$ M), rather than ATP, is the preferred phosphate donor to riboflavin. UTP and ITP are active at higher concentrations. The enzyme preparation contains neither flavokinase nor any phosphotransferase for which usual phosphate donors can serve. At 37° C, the optimal pH is around 5.5; conversely, the apparent temperature optimum is 37°C at pH 5.5. The K_m for riboflavin is 1.5 $\times 10^{-5}$ M. Both Mg^{2+} ($K_m = 2.5 \times 10^{-5}$ M) and Mn^{2+} are effective as divalent cations for activation. Importantly, an additional cofactor, as yet unidentified, is required for the reaction. Boiled cell-free extracts from *Rhizopus* contain this thermo-stable factor. As presently understood, then, this reaction can be indicated as:

$$\text{Riboflavin} + \text{GTP} \xrightarrow[\text{Mg}^{2+}\text{(or Mn}^{2+}\text{)}]{\text{synthetase}} \text{riboflavin } 2',5'\text{-cyclic phosphate} + \text{ADP}$$

2.2.2. Hydrolysis of Flavin Phosphate to Flavins

As previously pointed out, most extracts from both animal and plant tissues contain phosphomonoesterases capable of catalyzing hydrolysis of FMN. Prior to investigations of flavokinases, however, little was known of those enzymes that "mask" FMN formation. In only a few instances, such as reported by Tsuboi and Hudson[167] for acid phosphatases and by Garen and Levinthal[32] for alkaline phosphatase, had FMN been included among those organic phosphate esters tested as potential substrates for fairly well-characterized phosphatases.

Studies on the transphosphorylative synthesis of FMN catalyzed by alkaline phosphatases should not obscure knowledge about the simply hydrolytic action of these enzymes; that is, where water (HOH) replaces an alcohol (ROH) in the reaction with FMN, riboflavin and inorganic orthophosphate rather than an organic phosphate ester result:

$$FMN + H_2O \xrightarrow{\text{phosphatase}} riboflavin + P_i$$

This can be seen with the enzymes reported to be active with FMN at alkaline pH values; namely, those from small intestinal mucosa,[186] brain,[23] and E. coli.[32]

Although Tsuboi and Hudson[167] observed that acid phosphatases from erythrocytes, as well as yeast, can catalyze hydrolysis of FMN, the first detailed investigation of phosphatases from animal tissues most active on FMN at acid pH were made by McCormick and Russell.[90] In this work, a comparative survey of the tissues from several animals showed that phosphatases that hydrolyze FMN are widespread. In vertebrates, the greatest activities are found in liver, kidney, and spleen; among invertebrates, the gastropod, Limax, and the protozoan, Tetrahymena, contain high activities. The pH optima are generally near 5. Extracts from Tetrahymena and Limax exhibit a second optimum for phosphatase activity at pH 3-4. The liver enzyme has a temperature optimum near 40°C. and is apparently more active with FMN than other usual physiological substrates tested, although the synthetic substrates, p-nitrophenylphosphate and o-carboxyphenylphosphate, are readily hydrolyzed. p-Chloromercuribenzoate and p-chloromercuriphenylsulfonate are potent inhibitors, and their effect is reversed by reduced glutathione. This fact points to the essentiality of cysteinyl sulfhydryl functions within the phosphatase. Also, several heavy metal ions are inhibitory unless chelated by ethylene diamine tetraacetate. Phosphate, a product, somewhat suppresses the liver enzyme activity by competitive inhibition.

Mitsuda et al.[97] studied the enzymatic hydrolysis of FMN catalyzed by acid phosphatase from green leaves. In spinach, the activity of cytoplasmic enzyme is about 1000 times more active than flavokinase measured in vitro. However, hydrolysis of FMN is extremely retarded by nucleotide, inorganic phosphate, and some metal ions, such as Zn^{2+}.

The optimal pH is near 5.5 and markedly decreases above 7. The K_m for FMN is 2×10^{-4} M.

Tachibana[144,145] has observed that preparations of Takadiastase contain a phosphatase that can catalyze the hydrolysis of the phosphate moiety from riboflavinyl glucoside mononucleotide.

2.3. Interconversions of Flavin Mononucleotide with Flavin Adenine Dinucleotide

2.3.1. Formation of FAD from FMN

Schrecker and Kornberg[125] were the first to report partial purification and properties of an FAD pyrophosphorylase (ATP:FMN adenylyltransferase), which they obtained from fractionation of autolysates of dried beer yeast. The reaction, optimal near pH 7.5, proceeds according to the following equation:

$$\text{FMN} + \text{ATP} \underset{\text{Mg}^{2+}}{\overset{\text{pyrophosphorylase}}{\rightleftharpoons}} \text{FAD} + PP_i$$

Dissociation constants, determined with enzyme purified about ninety fold from the autolysate, were 1.4×10^{-6} M for FMN, 1.2×10^{-5} M for ATP, and $< 5.3 \times 10^{-6}$ M for FAD. Neither metaphosphate nor inorganic orthophosphate replaces pyrophosphate with this yeast enzyme. However, the best preparations obtained still contained nucleotide pyrophosphatase and inorganic pyrophosphatase, so that specific inhibitors were employed to avoid their interference in balance studies of FAD synthesis and pyrophosphorolysis.

Other microorganisms also have been shown to have FAD-synthesizing systems that, at least in some cases, can form analogs. Snell et al.[133] found that L-lyxoflavin promotes maximum growth of Lactobacillus lactis in the absence of riboflavin but cannot do so with L. casei. The nucleotide forms of lyxoflavin were then isolated from L. lactis grown on the analog by Huennekens et al.[47] Katagiri et al.[59] studied the biosynthetic reaction to form FAD in a partially purified preparation from E. coli. A typical pyrophosphorylase, which requires FMN and ATP in the forward direction and pyrophosphate for the breakdown of FAD is involved. The pH range for optimal activity is between 7.8 and 8.2. Activation by Mg^{2+} is optimal at 3×10^{-3} M. Culture broths from mutant strains of Brevibacterium ammoniagenes and Micrococcus glutamicus have been found by Tanaka and Nakamura[161] to contain considerable quantities of FAD. Biosynthesis of FAD, as well as FMN and riboflavin, in the mycelia of *Eremothecium ashbyii* is also well recognized. For instance, the formation of the radioactive coenzyme from ^{14}C-formate with this mold was reported by Nagatsu *et al.*[101]

The enzyme system responsible for formation of FMN from FAD in mammalian tissue may be somewhat different from the one found in microorganisms and perhaps higher plants. Ochoa and Rossiter[106] had observed the synthesis *in vivo* and rapid restoration of normal levels of FAD in heart, liver, and blood following the injection of riboflavin into flavin-deficient rats. Klein and Kohn[70] then showed a slow but definite synthesis *in vitro* of the dinucleotide from riboflavin in human blood cells. The synthesis of FAD in tissue slices from liver, brain, kidney, heart, and intestine was reported by Trufanov.[164] Siliprandi and co-workers[127] reproduced their earlier synthesis *in vivo* of FAD in normal and alloxan-diabetic rats by a study with intact cells isolated by selective centrifugation of rat liver homogenates. DeLuca and Kaplan[21] then proceeded to delineate the mammalian system *in vitro*. A synthetase, which catalyzes formation of FAD from FMN and ATP, is localized in the soluble or supernatant fraction from cells of animal tissues. This activity is widespread but especially high in liver. Whole-tissue homogenates show little ability to form FAD because of the presence of an enzyme (or enzymes) in the particulate fraction that cleave(s) the dinucleotide. The synthetase from rat liver was separated from FAD-destructive activities by column chromatography on powdered cellulose using a gradient elution with decreasing concentrations of ammonium sulfate. However, the partially purified enzyme does not seem to catalyze a pyrophosphorolysis of FAD as does the yeast enzyme, although other characteristics are generally similar. The pH optimum is approximately 7.5 in Tris buffer; Mg^{2+} at an optimal concentration of 10^{-3} M is the preferred activator; near optimal concentrations of FMN and ATP are 5×10^{-4} M each.

McCormick[82] demonstrated that the rat liver enzyme has an apparent absolute specificity for ATP but only a relative specificity for flavin phosphate. This latter finding has been summarized by McCormick[87] and is indicated by the data in Table IV. Under the conditions used, isoriboflavin 5'-phosphate is an even better substrate than the natural one, FMN. As had been demonstrated by McCormick,[79] and McCormick and Butler,[89] isoriboflavin 5'-phosphate is not formed in the mammalian flavokinase reaction and does not inhibit the normal phosphorylation of riboflavin. However, McCormick[83] found that free isoriboflavin does inhibit FAD pyrophosphorylase. Also, it had been shown earlier that isoriboflavin is an effective antagonist to riboflavin *in vivo* and, as reported

TABLE IV. Substrate Efficiencies of Flavin Phosphates with FAD Synthetase
from Rat Liver

Flavin monophosphate	Relative efficiency for formation of flavin adenine dinucleotide
Riboflavin 5'-phosphate	100
Isoriboflavin 5'-phosphate	280
7-Methylriboflavin 5'-phosphate	73
7,8-Dibromoriboflavin 5'-phosphate	31
D-Araboflavin 5'-phosphate	12
D-Erythroflavin 4'-phosphate	12
2',3',4'-Trideoxyriboflavin 5'-phosphate	21
2'-Deoxyglyceroflavin 3'-phosphate	10

by Kearney,[64] inhibits the binding of FMN to NADPH cytochrome
c reductase *in vitro*. Taken altogether, these findings suggest that
isoriboflavin may displace FMN, both as substrate for FAD pyrophosphorylase and as coenzyme. There are other known cases of riboflavin
analogs that neither are phosphorylated by flavokinase nor competitively
inhibit phosphorylation of riboflavin, but do have an antagonistic action
in vivo. An example is offered by a study on the effects of galactoflavin
and the synthetic 6'-phosphate by Prosky *et al.*[121] Other flavins can
be adequately converted to flavin coenzyme forms but may not be entirely
adequate as such. This latter seems to be the case with 7,8-
diethylriboflavin, which additionally was reported by Aposhian and
Lambooy[2] to retard growth of the Walker Rat Carcinoma 256.

Hormonal control is exerted on the biosynthesis of flavin coenzymes
within the mammal. Kókai and Domján[71] found that the FAD contents
in the livers of thyroidectomized rats decrease as compared with the
normal. As further noted by Kókai and Domján,[24] treatment of such
thyroidectomized rats with thyoxine prevents such a decrease. Hence,
thyroxine plays a role in maintaining the normal FAD level. This and
other features of hormonal control will be discussed by Rivlin in Chapter
12.

2.3.2. Hydrolysis of FAD to FMN

As already mentioned, the presence of enzymes that catalyze cleavage
of FAD, especially nucleotide pyrophosphatase, has been noted by most
investigators who were attempting to measure FAD synthesis in crude
preparations. In some instances, however, attempts have been made

to consider quantitatively the levels of such enzymes, which may be involved in the degradation of FAD.

Mitsuda[93] has pointed out the factors affecting levels of flavin coenzymes in higher plants, such as spinach leaves. In general, the hydrolyzing enzymes operate at more acidic pH values, under which condition their optimal activities far surpass those of the biosynthesizing enzymes. Also, the presence of adenine nucleotides suppresses the hydrolyses. FAD bound to protein is much more resistant to nucleotide pyrophosphatase than is the free coenzyme.

Krishnan[72] has recently investigated FAD-hydrolyzing enzymes that he obtained from fish and sheep livers. The one from sheep liver was purified over 200-fold and found to hydrolyze FAD to FMN plus AMP optimally at pH 9.7 and to be inhibited by AMP in a sigmoidal fashion. NAD and NADP are also hydrolyzed by this nucleotide pyrophosphatase. The enzyme from liver of a fresh-water fish (*Wallago attu*) hydrolyzes FAD best at pH 4.5 and 80° C. This latter preparation is not inhibited by AMP or inorganic phosphate and appears to be different from the rat lysosomal enzyme.

In the rat liver, carcinoma induced by *p*-dimethylaminoazebenzene leads to hydrolytic activity, reported by Yang and Sung[193] to be ten fold higher than normal. Yang and Sung[194] have also found an elevation of enzymic activity for the hydrolysis of FAD in the serum from human patients with liver diseases (see also Chapter 14).

3. EXCRETION AND BREAKDOWN OF RIBOFLAVIN

Certain aspects of the urinary excretion of riboflavin, particularly in the human, will be taken up by Jusko and Levy in Chapter 4. A broader survey of some literature dealing with loss as related to overall metabolism of the vitamin is intended here.

3.1. Turnover and Displacement

3.1.1. Natural Flavins

One of the more serious early attempts to assess loss, as well as replacement, in the economy of riboflavin in an experimental animal was the study on rats by Bessey et al.[8] These investigators erroneously attributed much of the rat "maintenance requirement" of riboflavin to loss through decomposition within the body. That most of the actual loss was via excretion in this animal was demonstrated by Faulkner and Lambooy,[27] but these authors, too, reported a considerable "rate of destruction" of riboflavin, estimated to be -1.26 ± 0.21 μg per day per rat. This rate may be compared to their calculation of 1.94 ± 0.28 μg per day for the rate of accumulation, which they estimated to be approximately equal to the rate of fecal excretion. This latter could be superimposed on a relatively constant riboflavin content of the tissues and excretion of riboflavin in the urine.

Innami et al.[50] administered large amounts of riboflavin orally to rats and collected feces periodically. Half a dozen fluorescent products, presumably formed from flavin by intestinal bacteria, were then detected following paper chromatography. Also, decomposition of the vitamin was found after incubations with feces in vitro.

A study by Yagi et al.[185] using ^{14}C-labeled riboflavin helped emphasize the stability of this vitamin in rat tissue homogenates. Approximately half of a subcutaneously injected dose of 17.8 mg/kg (much above a "physiological" level of intake) was found in the contents of the intestinal canal as riboflavin. Radioactivity collected in the urine reached 20% after 1 hr and was found to be 97% riboflavin and 3% FMN.

Since most of this earlier work was undertaken with either deficiency or overdosage of the vitamin, Yang and McCormick[189,190] carefully reassessed the degradation and excretion of more physiological amounts of the accurately detected 2-^{14}C-riboflavin in the rat. In this study, samples were not only counted directly but were also acidified and extracted with chloroform to assess the less-polar radioactive catabolites, principally lumichrome, as assessed by chromatographic mobilities and by absorption and fluorescence spectra. Typical recoveries of radioactivity after intraperitoneal injection into normal male rats can be seen in Table V. In all cases, relatively high recoveries were obtained. The distribution pattern of ^{14}C-compounds in urine, feces, and carcass are somewhat related to body size, as well as to the amount of riboflavin administered. Generally, higher body retentions of ^{14}C-compound are observed for experiments with larger animals and with lower levels of ^{14}C-riboflavin administration. The quantity of [14]CO$_2$ exhaled was detectable but much less than 1% of the ^{14}C administered. The chloroform-soluble values range from 2 to 5% for feces, whereas for urinary and carcass samples the values are in the same range as that for the control of chloroform-extracted ^{14}C-riboflavin solution. In the aqueous phases of the samples of urine, feces, and carcass, no degradative product

TABLE V. Recovery of Radioactivity After Administration of 2-^{14}C-Riboflavin to Rats

(Number) and average weight of animals, g	(3) 110		(3) 170		(3) 104		(2) 165	
^{14}C-Riboflavin administered, μg	80 (5 μCi)		55 (5 μCi)		55 (5 μCi)		83 (7.5 μCi)	
Length of experiment, hr	24		24		72		100	
	%	%CSC[a]	%	%CSC[a]	%	%CSC[a]	%	%CSC[a]
Recovery in								
Urine	26.2	0.23	10.2	0.68	19.2	0.43	24.6	0.61
Feces	5.8	5.50	2.9	3.23	12.8	1.72	20.4	2.27
Carcass	62.4	0.12	80.8	0.31	65.6	0.26	50.5	0.09
^{14}CO$_2$					tr		tr	
Total	94.4		93.9		97.6+		95.5+	

[a] Chloroform-soluble compounds.

was detected, though the presence of trace amounts was not ruled out. The dietary effects on the chloroform-soluble fraction are indicated in Table VI. For rats maintained with a riboflavin-supplemented diet for 2 weeks, the percent chloroform-soluble compound (CSC) in feces was found to be 10% as compared with a value of 3% for rats fed a standard laboratory ration. On the other hand, for the rats fed a riboflavin-supplemented diet for the first week and an additional 1% succinylsulfathiazole for the second week, the percent CSC was reduced to 4%. This fact strongly suggests the intestinal microfloral origin of these flavin catabolites. A similar relationship was also observed for the contents of cecum and large intestine. The percent CSC values of other samples are very low and in the range for the ^{14}C-riboflavin solution. In all cases, the percent CSC values in the contents of the cecum and large intestine are higher than those of the cecal and large intestinal tissues of the rat. Hence, it appears that the site of degradation is, indeed, in the contents, which contain bacteria capable of degrading the flavin side chain, mainly to lumichrome. Overall, a half-life of 16 days for tissue riboflavin was determined and is in good agreement with that reported by Amos et al.[1] The turnover rate is directly affected by the level of the dietary riboflavin. A much slower turnover rate was reported by Faulkner and Lambooy[27] for rats fed a riboflavin-deficient diet. Assuming a body concentration of 400 μg of flavin for a 100-g rat, the depletion rate of 0.043 observed by Yang and McCormick[190] corresponds to an excretion rate of 17.2 μg of riboflavin daily. This amount is very close to that required to maintain tissues of a growing rat. Thus, the loss of riboflavin from a growing rat, under normal physiological conditions, is due mainly to excretion rather than to decomposition. A recent appraisal of the overall economy of flavins in this experimental animal has been written by McCormick.[85]

The work of Owen and his associates has enlarged our understanding of the metabolic fate of riboflavin in ruminants, rabbits, and also man. However, as these efforts have centered around identification of the small amounts of certain catabolites resultant from bacterial degradation of the flavin side chain, they will be discussed in Section 3.2.1.

3.1.2. Effect of Analogs

The biological activities of some derivatives of riboflavin, as affecting turnover and displacement of the vitamin, will be considered in more detail in other places in this book, notably in Chapter 10. However, a couple of studies have been aimed rather directly at quantitating the rate and extent of excretion of flavin analogs, which spare, to some

TABLE VI. *Effect of Riboflavin-Enriched Diet and Succinylsulfathiazole on Percentage of Chlorofororm-Soluble Compound(s) (CSC)*[a]

Diet	Laboratory ration	Laboratory ration + riboflavin (15 µg/g diet)	Laboratory ration + riboflavin + 1% succinyl-sulfathiazole
(Number) and average weight of animals, g	(2) 110	(3) 110	(3) 110
^{14}C-Riboflavin administered, µg	110 (10 µCi)	110 (10 µCi)	110 (10 µCi)
	%CSC	%CSC	%CSC
Recovery in			
Urine	0.25	0.32	0.21
Feces	3.10	9.91	4.45
Cecum and large intestine (minus contents)	0.25	0.39	0.20
Contents of cecum and large intestine	1.50	3.20	1.36
Rest of carcass	0.36	0.56	0.46

[a] Each experiment was carried out for 50 hr.

extent, the normal excretion of the vitamin. Ogunmodede and McCormick[107,108] showed that analogs of riboflavin in which the 1'-D-ribityl substituent in position 10 is replaced by ω-hydroxyalkyl chains of two through six carbons in length can be excreted in the urine in place of the vitamin, but are not able to function as such, since they cannot be converted to coenzyme forms. By supplying increasing amounts of such analogs in the place of decreasing amounts of riboflavin to the diets of growing rats, it could be shown that a major portion of the daily dietary intake of the vitamin is wasted via excretion (mainly urinary) and can be largely "spared" by ω-hydroxyalkyl analogs given up to about three-fourths of the maintenance requirement of the vitamin.

Tu and McCormick[168] also investigated the biological activity and excretion of 7,8-dimethyl-10-(ω-carboxyalkyl)isoalloxazines, that is, cases in which the terminal position on an aliphatic side chain is a carboxylic acid function. These compounds weakly antagonize the utilization of suboptimal amounts of riboflavin in growing rats rather than exert a sparing action. The 5'-^{14}C-carboxypentylflavin is readily excreted in the urine, and small and trace amounts of radioactivity appear in feces and CO_2, respectively. The minor breakdown of the side chain of this analog by intestinal microflora is decreased by succinylsulfathiazole.

3.2. Bacterial Degradation

An article by Tsai and Stadtman[166] indicates the three known pathways by which riboflavin is degraded by bacteria. These can be summarized by the scheme shown on page 187.

3.2.1. Flavin Side Chain

One pathway for bacterial degradation of riboflavin is that to lumichrome, which was demonstrated by Foster,[29,30] who isolated an organism, *Pseudomonas riboflavina,* from riboflavin-supplemented enrichment cultures. Yanagita and Foster[187] then showed that the lumichrome is formed by a hydrolytic cleavage of the riboflavin side chain to produce ribitol as the other product, which is further oxidized. The broader flavin specificity of the hydrolase system was studied by Yang and McCormick.[191,192] The relative substrate activities of flavins are given in Table VII. The significant, but decreased, activities of iso- and dichlororoboflavin point up the preference for the 7,8-dimethylisoalloxazine structure of the natural vitamin. Also, the system is more reactive toward a D-ribityl side chain, as shown by the lower substrate activities of the polyhydroxyl chains of L-lyxo- and D-araboflavin and the ω-hy-

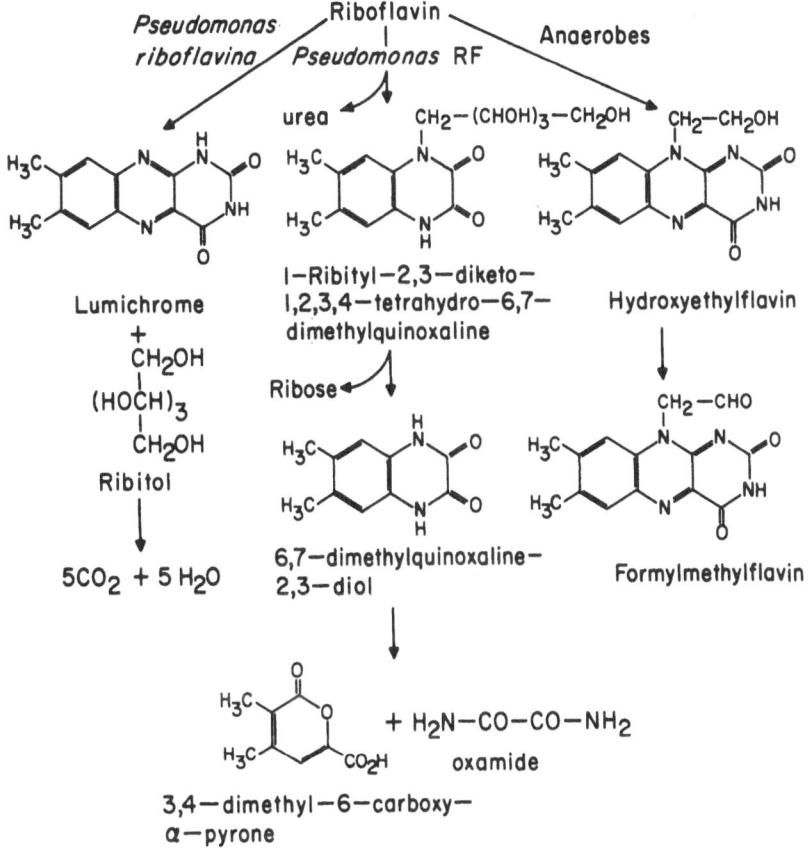

Bacterial Degradation of Riboflavin

droxyalkyl chains of 5'-hydroxypentyl- and 4'-hydroxybutylflavin. Lumichrome also has been identified by Stadtman[136] as the major end product from riboflavin metabolism by a species of *Nocardia*. Moreover, certain of the bacteria present in the intestines of animals can produce lumichrome or compounds very easily converted to lumichrome, as was shown by Yang and McCormick.[189,190]

A second pathway for partial degradation of the side chain of riboflavin was found by Miles and Stadtman.[92] This system, demonstrated to occur in anaerobic enrichment cultures, involves cleavage of the ribityl side chain between carbons 2' and 3' to produce 7,8-dimethyl-10-(2'-hydroxyethyl)isoalloxazine, which accumulates as a green quinhydrone-like complex consisting of a mole each of half-reduced and oxidized forms. The urinary excretion of hydroxyethylflavin by goats was noted by Owen et al.[111] Its secretion into milk was also

TABLE VII. *Substrate Efficiencies of Flavins with Riboflavin Hydrolase from Pseudomonas riboflavina*

Flavin	Relative efficiency for formation of lumichrome
D-Riboflavin	100
Isoriboflavin	31
Dichlororiboflavin	16
3-Methylriboflavin	2
L-Lyxoflavin	26
L-Deoxylyxoflavin	8
D-Lyxoflavin	3
D-Araboflavin	13
D-Galactoflavin	4
D-Sorboflavin	1
D-Dichlorosorboflavin	3
D-Alloflavin	5
D-Erythroflavin	6
DL-Glyceroflavin	5
6'-Hydroxyhexylflavin	9
5'-Hydroxypentylflavin	14
4'-Hydroxybutylflavin	17
3'-Hydroxypropylflavin	7
2'-Hydroxyethylflavin	6
Formylmethylflavin	5
Lumiflavin	7

observed by Owen.[110] Owen and his colleagues,[112-117] e.g., Hobson,[44] then examined the bacterial formation of this catabolite excreted by ruminants. Owen et al.[118] found that hydroxyethylflavin is produced in the cecum of conventional, but not germfree, rabbits as well. Owen and West[115] also found that the 7,8-dimethyl-10-formylmethylisoalloxazine also accompanied the hydroxyethyl compound as had been suspected.[176] Both hydroxyethyl- and formylmethylflavins, plus other riboflavin metabolites, have been shown by West and Owen[177] to be present in human urine. Recently, Owen and West[116,117] have summarized their procedures for isolation and identification of hydroxyethylflavin and formylmethylflavin.

3.2.2. Isoalloxazine Ring System

The third pathway by which riboflavin is known to be catabolized involves complete degradation of the isoalloxazine ring. Stadtman and his co-workers detailed the intermediates and enzymes involved, as has been reviewed by Tsai and Stadtman.[166] The principal organism investigated, *Pseudomonas* RF, converts riboflavin to acetate, propionate, butyrate, CO_2, oxamide, urea, and 3,4-dimethyl-6-carboxy-α-pyrone. The main steps in the catabolic sequence outlined above were elucidated by the studies of Smyrniotis et al.,[132] Miles et al.,[91] Tsai et al.,[165] and Harkness et al.[39,40]

Hotta and Ando [45] also reported the isolation of 1-ribityl-2,3-diketo-1,2,3,4-tetrahydro-6,7-dimethylquinoxaline as a degradation product of riboflavin in plant tissues. Apparently, though, such cleavages of the isoalloxazine ring of flavins do not occur to any real extent in animal tissues.

4. REFERENCES

1. Amos, W. H., Jr., Balaghi, M., Ramirez, O., Jr., and Sauberlich, H. E. 1966. Metabolism of ¹⁴C-riboflavin in the rat, *Fed. Proc.* **25**:245.
2. Aposhian, H. V., and Lambooy, J. P. 1951. Retardation of growth of Walker Rat Carcinoma 256 by administration of diethyl riboflavin, *Proc. Soc. Exptl. Biol. Med.* **78**:197-199.
3. Arsenis, C., and McCormick, D. B. 1964. Chromatographic purification of flavokinase by means of ES and EI complexation on flavin-cellulose compounds, *Fed. Proc.* **23**:534.
4. Arsenis, C., and McCormick, D. B. 1964. Purification of liver flavokinase by column chromatography on flavin-cellulose compounds, *J. Biol. Chem.* **239**:3093-3097.
5. Askarov, K. A. 1966. Riboflavine metabolism in albino rats on a diet containing vegetable and animal proteins, *Vopr. Pitaniya* **25**:57-60.
6. Bamberg, P., Hemmerich, P., and Erlenmeyer, H. 1960. Studien in der Lumiflavin-Reihe. VII. Zur Kenntnis der 4-Desoxyflavine und der Struktur von Flavin-Metall-chelaten, *Helv. Chim. Acta* **43**:395.
7. Beinert, H. 1960. Flavin coenzymes, *in:* "The Enzymes" (P. D. Boyer, H. Lardy, and K. Myrback, eds.), Vol. 2 (part A), pp 339-416, Academic Press, New York.
8. Bessey, O. A., Lowry, O. H., Davis, E. B., and Dorn, J. L. 1958. The riboflavin economy of the rat, *J. Nutrition* **4**:185-202.
9. Bessey, O. A., Lowry, O. H., and Love, R. H. 1949. The fluorometric measurement of the nucleotides of riboflavin and their concentration in tissues, *J. Biol. Chem.* **180**:755-769.
10. Blum, J.-C. 1967. Le Métabolisme de la Riboflavine chez la Poule pondeuse, Documentation Roche.
11. Boukine, V. N. 1955. *Cong. Intern. Biochim. 2ᵉ Résumés des Communications* **61**, Societé Belge de Biochemie, Liege, Belgium.
12. Bullock, F. Y., and Jardetzsky, O. 1965. An experimental demonstration of the nuclear magnetic resonance assignments in the 6,7-dimethylisoalloxazine nucleus, *J. Org. Chem.* **30**:2056-2057.
13. Burch, H. B., Bessey, O. A., and Lowry, O. H. 1948. Fluorometric measurements

of riboflavin and its natural derivatives in small quantities of blood and serum and cells, *J. Biol. Chem.* **175**:457-470.

14. Burch, H. B., Lowry, O. H., DeGubareff, T., and Lowry, S. R. 1958. Flavin enzymes in liver and kidney of rats from birth to weaning, *J. Cell. Comp. Physiol.* **52**:503-510.

15. Burch, H. B., Lowry, O. H., Padilla, A. M., and Combs, A. M. 1956. Effects of riboflavin deficiency and realimentation on flavin enzymes of tissues, *J. Biol. Chem.* **223**:29-45.

16. Cerletti, P., and Ipata, P. 1960. Determination of riboflavin and its coenzymes in tissues, *Biochem. J.* **75**:119-124.

17. Cerletti, P., Strom, R., and Giordano, M. G. 1963. Flavin peptide in tissues: The prosthetic group of succinic dehydrogenase, *Arch. Biochem. Biophys.* **101**:423-428.

18. Chassy, B. M., Arsenis, C., and McCormick, D. B. 1965. The effect of the length of the side chain of flavins on reactivity with flavokinase, *J. Biol. Chem.* **240**:1338-1340.

19. Chelkowski, J. 1971. Flavine peptides and flavines in biological material, *Bull. Acad. Pol. Sci., Ser. Sci. Biol.* **19**:153-160.

20. Chi, T.-F. Wang, Y.-L., Tsou, C.-L., Fang, Y.-C., and Wu, C. H. 1965. Studies on succinic dehydrogenase. V. The linking between the flavin prosthetic group and the apoenzyme, *Scientia Sinica* **14**:1193.

21. DeLuca, C., and Kaplan, N. O. 1958. Flavin adenine dinucleotide synthesis in animal tissues, *Biochim. Biophys. Acta* **30**:6-11.

22. Dimant, E., Sanadi, D. R., and Huennekens, F. M. 1952. The isolation of flavin nucleotides, *J. Am. Chem. Soc.* **74**:5440-5444.

23. Domján, G. 1966. *In vitro* biochemical examination of FMN synthesis with the brain homogenate of developing chicken embryo, *Enzymologia* **31**:1-8.

24. Domján, G., and Kókai, K. 1966. The flavin adenine dinucleotide (FAD) content of the rat's liver in hypo:.yroid state and in the liver of hypothyroid animals after *in vivo* thyroxine treatment, *Acta Biol. Hung.* **16**:237-241.

25. Dudley, K. H., and Hemmerich, P. 1967. Stabile dihydroflavine und quartäre Flaviniumsalze, *Helv. Chim. Acta* **50**:355-363.

26. Englard, S. 1952. Enzymatic phosphorylation of riboflavin to flavin mononucleotide in animal tissues. *Federation Proc.* **11**:208.

27. Faulkner, R. D., and Lambooy, J. P. 1961. Intestinal synthesis of riboflavin in the rat, *J. Nutrition* **75**:373-378.

28. Foley, B., MacKenzie, R. E., and McCormick, D. B. 1967. Transport and storage of ^{14}C-riboflavin in the retina and liver of rats, *Proc. Soc. Exptl. Biol. Med.* **126**:715-718.

29. Foster, J. W. 1944. Microbiological aspects of riboflavin. I. Introduction. II. Bacterial oxidation of riboflavin to lumichrome, *J. Bacteriol.* **47**:27-41.

30. Foster, J. W. 1944b. Microbiological aspects of riboflavin. III. Oxidation studies with *Pseudomonas riboflavina*, *J. Bacteriol.* **48**:97-111.

31. Frisell, W. R., and MacKenzie, C. G. 1962. Separation and purification of sarcosine dehydrogenase and dimethylglycine dehydrogenase, *J. Biol. Chem.* **237**:94-98.

32. Garen, A., and Levinthal, C. 1960. A fine-structure genetic and chemical study of the enzyme alkaline phosphatase of *E. coli*, *Biochim. Biophys. Acta* **38**:470-483.

33. Ghisla, S., Hartman, U., and Hemmerich, P. 1970. The synthesis of succinate-dehydrogenase riboflavin, *Angew. Chem., Intern.* Ed. **9**:642-643.

34. Giri, K. V., and Krishnaswamy, P. R. 1956. Circular paper chromatography. Part X. Separation, identification and quantitative estimation of riboflavin and flavin compounds. *J. Indian Inst. Sci.* (A) **38**:232-244.

35. Giri, K. V., Krishnaswamy, P. R., and Rao, N. A. 1958. Studies on plant flavokinase, *Biochem. J.* **70**:66-71.

36. Green, D. E., Mii, S., and Kohout, P. M. 1955. Studies on the terminal electron transport system. I. Succinic dehydrogenase. *J. Biol. Chem.* **217**:551-561.

37. György, P., Kuhn, R., and Wagner-Jauregg, T. 1934. Verbreitung des Vitamins B$_2$ im Tierkörper, *Hoppe-Seyler's Z. für Physiol. Chem.* **223**:21-27.

38. Haley, E. E., and Lambooy, J. P. 1954. Synthesis of D-riboflavin-d-C^{14} and its metabolism by *Lactobacillus casei*, *J. Am. Chem. Soc.* **76**:2926-2929.

39. Harkness, D. R., and Stadtman, E. R. 1965. Bacterial degradation of riboflavin. VI. Enzymatic conversion of riboflavin to 1-ribityl-2,3-diketo-1,2,3,4-tetrahydro-6,7-dimethylquinoxaline, urea, and carbon dioxide, *J. Biol. Chem.* **240**:4089-4096.

40. Harkness, D. R., Tsai, L., and Stadtman, E. R. 1964. Bacterial degradation of riboflavin. V. Stoichiometry of riboflavin degradation to oxamide and other products, oxidation of C^{14}-labeled intermediates and isolation of the pseudomonad effecting these transformations, *Arch. Biochem. Biophys.* **108**:323-333.

41. Hemmerich, P., Ehrenberg, A., Walker, W. H., Eriksson, L. E., Salach, J., Bader, P., and Singer, T. P. 1969. On the structure of succinic dehydrogenase flavocoenzyme, *Federation European Biochem. Soc. Ltrs.* **3**:37-40.

42. Hemmerich, P., Prijs, B., and Erlenmeyer, H. 1959. Studien in der Lumiflavin-Reihe. V. Spezifische Reaktivität 8-ständiger Substituent am Isoalloxazine-Kern; Flavin-Dimere, *Helv. Chim. Acta* **42**:2164-2177.

43. Hendriks, R., and Cronin, J. R. 1971. The flavin of *Chromatium* cytochrome c-552, *Biochem. Biophys. Res. Commun.* **44**:313-318.

44. Hobson, P. N., Summers, R., Owen, E. C., Spencer, J. C., and West, D. W. 1969. A study of cultures of rumen anaerobic bacteria in the presence of excess riboflavine (vitamin B$_2$), *Proc. Nutr. Soc.* **28**:53A.

45. Hotta, K., and Ando, O. 1961. The occurrence of riboflavin degradation product in plant tissues, *J. Vitaminol.* **7**:196-201.

46. Huennekens, F. M. 1956. Flavin nucleotides and flavoproteins, *Experientia* **12**:1.

47. Huennekens, F. M., Felton, S. P., and Snell, E. E. 1957. Lyxoflavin nucleotides, *J. Am. Chem. Soc.* **79**:2258-2261.

48. Huennekens, F. M., Sanadi, D. R., Dimant, E., and Shepartz, A. Q. 1953. The occurrence of a new flavin dinucleotide (FAD-X), *J. Am. Chem. Soc.* **75**:3611-3612.

49. Igaue, I., Gomes, B., and Yasunobu, K. T. 1967. Beef mitochondrial monoamine oxidase, a flavin dinucleotide enzyme, *Biochem. Biophys. Res. Commun.* **29**:562-567.

50. Innami, S., Kawachi, T., and Oizumi, H. 1965. Decomposition of riboflavin in rat intestine, *Japanese J. Nutrition* **23**:117-122.

51. Irinoda, K., and Sato, S. 1954. Contribution to the ocular manifestation of riboflavin deficiency, *Tohoku J. Exp. Med.* **61**:93-104.

52. Jusko, W. J., and Levy, G. 1967. Absorption, metabolism, and excretion of riboflavin 5'-phosphate in man, *J. Pharm. Sci.* **56**:58-62.

53. Karrer, P., and Meerwein, H. 1936. Zur Konstitution der Lactoflavinphosphorsäure aus Leber, *Helv. Chim. Acta* **20**:79-83.

54. Katagiri, H., Yamada, H., and Imai, K. 1957. On the transglycosidation relating to riboflavin by *Escherichia coli*. I. Formation of riboflavinyl glucoside, *J. Vitaminol.* **3**:264-273.

55. Katagiri, H., Yamada, H., and Imai, K. 1958. On the transglycosidation relating to riboflavin by *Escherichia coli*. II. Formation of riboflavin compounds of oligosaccharides, *J. Vitaminol.* **4**:126-131.

56. Katagiri, H., Yamada, H., and Imai, K. 1959. On the transglycosidation relating to riboflavin by *Escherichia coli*. VI. Preliminary investigations on transfructosidation, *J. Vitaminol.* **5**:298-303.

57. Katagiri, H., Yamada, H., and Imai, K. 1959. On the transglycosidation relating to riboflavin by *Escherichia coli*. IV. Formation of galactosyl compounds of riboflavin, *J. Vitaminol.* **5**:8-13.

58. Katagiri, H., Yamada, H., and Imai, K. 1959. Biosynthesis of flavin coenzymes by microorganisms. I. Bacterial flavokinase, *J. Vitaminol.* **5**:129-133.

59. Katagiri, H., Yamada, H., and Imai, K. 1959. Biosynthesis of flavin coenzymes by microorganisms. II. Enzymatic synthesis of flavin-adenine dinucleotide by *Escherichia coli, J. Vitaminol.* **5**:307-311.

60. Katagiri, H., Yamada, H., and Imai, K. 1960. Transglycosidation relating to riboflavin by *Escherichia coli*. VII. The characteristics of transfructosidase, *J. Vitaminol.* **6**:94-97.

61. Katagiri, H., Yamada, H., and Imai, K. 1960. Transglycosidation relating to riboflavine by *Escherichiacoli*. VIII. Photochemical glucosidation of riboflavine, *J. Vitaminol.* **6**:98-102.

62. Kawai, F., Miyoshi, T., and Mitsuda, H. 1960. Studies on flavin. III. Confirmation of flavin compounds and the other fluorescent substances in wheat seedling, *Vitamins* **19**:133.

63. Kawai, F., Tonomura, B., and Mitsuda, H. 1960. Studies on flavin. IV. Relationship between protein content in diet and activities of flavin enzymes in rat liver. Vitamins **21**:157.

64. Kearney, E. B. 1952. The interaction of yeast flavokinase with riboflavin analogues, *J. Biol. Chem.* **194**:747-754.

65. Kearney, E. B. 1960. Studies on succinic dehydrogenase. XII. Flavin component of the mammalian enzyme, *J. Biol. Chem.* **235**:865-877.

66. Kearney, E. B., and England, S. 1951. The enzymatic phosphorylation of riboflavin, *J. Biol. Chem.* **193**:821-834.

67. Kearney, E. B., and Singer, T. P. 1955. On the prosthetic group of succinic dehydrogenase, *Biochim. Biophys. Acta* **17**:596-597.

68. Kenney, W. C., Walker, W. H., Kearney, E. B., Zeszotek, K. E., and Singer, T. P. 1970. Amino acid sequence at the active center of succinate dehydrogenase, *Biochem. Biophys. Res. Commun.* **41**:488-491.

69. King, T. E., Howard, R. L., Wilson, D. F., and Li, J. C. R. 1962. The partition of flavins in the heart muscle preparation and heart mitochondria, *J. Biol. Chem.* **237**:2941-2946.

70. Klein, J. R., and Kohn, H. J. 1940. The synthesis of flavin-adenine dinucleotide from riboflavin by human blood cells *in vitro* and *in vivo, J. Biol. Chem.* **136**:177-189.

71. Kókai, K., and Domján, G. 1965. The flavine adenine dinucleotide (FAD) contents of the rat's liver as affected by thyroidectomy, *Biologiai Kozlem.* **13**:127-129.

72. Krishnan, N. 1971. Metabolism of water soluble vitamins: Studies on enzymes from sheep liver and from livers of fresh water fishes (*Wallago attu*) that hydrolyze nucleotides. Ph.D. thesis, Department of Biochemistry, Indian Institute of Science, Bangalore 12, India.

73. Kuhn, R., Kaltschmitt, H., and Wagner-Jauregg, T. 1935. Über den Flavingehalt der Leber und Muskulatur von gesunden and B_2-avitaminotischen Ratten, *Hoppe-Seyler's Z. für Physiol. Chem.* **232**:36-40.

74. Kuhn, R., and Rudy, H. 1935. Synthetische Vitamin-B_2-Phosphosäure, *Ber. dtsch. chem. Ges.* **68**:383-386.

75. Levy, G., and Jusko, W. J. 1966. Factors affecting the absorption of riboflavin in man, *J. Pharm. Sci.* **55**:285-289.

76. Matsui, K. 1965. Nekoflavin, a new flavin compound, in the choroid of cat's eye, *J. Biochem. (Japan)* **57**:201-206.

77. McCormick, D. B. 1961. Flavokinase activity of rat tissues and masking effect of phosphatases, *Proc. Soc. Exptl. Biol. Med.* **107:**784-786.

78. McCormick, D. B. 1961. Purification and properties of flavokinase from rat liver, *Fed. Proc.* **20:**447.

79. McCormick, D. B. 1962. The intracellular localization, partial purification, and properties of flavokinase from rat liver, *J. Biol. Chem.* **237:**959-962.

80. McCormick. D. B. 1962. Substrate specificity of liver flavokinase, *Fed. Proc.* **21:**239.

81. McCormick, D. B. 1962. Biochemical advances in vitamin research. Partial replacement and interference of vitaminic functions by pseudovitamins, *N. Y. State J. Med.* **62:**2842.

82. McCormick, D. B. 1964. Specificity of flavin adenine dinucleotide pyrophosphorylase for flavin phosphates and nucleoside triphosphates, *Biochem. Biophys. Res. Commun.* **14:**493-497.

83. McCormick, D. B. 1964. Inhibition of flavin adenine dinucleotide pyrophosphorylase by isoriboflavin, *Nature* **201:**925-926.

84. McCormick, D. B. 1970, Flavin derivatives via bromination of the 8-methyl substituent, *J. Heterocyclic Chem.* **7:**447-450.

85. McCormick, D. B. 1970. The fate of riboflavin, *in:* "Problems of Assessment and Alleviation of Malnutrition in the United States" (R. G. Hansen and H. N. Munro, eds.), Proceedings of Workshop, Vanderbilt University, Nashville, Tenn.

86. McCormick, D. B. 1971. Flavokinase (ATP:riboflavin 5'-phosphotransferase, EC 2.7.1.26) from rat liver, *in:* "Vitamins and Coenzymes, Methods in Enzymology," (D. B. McCormick and L. D. Wright, eds.), Vol. 18C, p. 544-548, Academic Press, New York.

87. McCormick, D. B. 1971. Specificity of FAD pyrophosphorylase (ATP:FMN adenyl-transferase, EC 2.7.7.2) from rat liver, *in:* "Vitamins and Coenzymes, Methods in Enzymology" (D. B. McCormick and L. D. Wright, eds.), Vol. 18B, p. 555-557, Academic Press, New York.

88. McCormick, D. B., Arsenis, C., and Hemmerich, P. 1963. Specificity of liver flavokinase for 9-(1'-D-ribityl)isoalloxazines variously substituted in positions 2, 6 and 7, *J. Biol. Chem.* **238:**3095-3099.

89. McCormick, D. B., and Butler, R. C. 1962. Substrate specificity of liver flavokinase, *Biochim. Biophys. Acta* **65:**326-332.

90. McCormick, D. B., and Russell, M. 1962. Hydrolysis of flavin mononucleotide by acid phosphatases from animal tissues, *Comp. Biochem. Physiol.* **5:**113-121.

91. Miles, H. T., Smyrniotis, P. Z., and Stadtman, E. R. 1959. Bacterial degradation products of riboflavin. III. Isolation, structure determination and biological trans-formations of 1-ribityl-2,3-diketo-1,2,3,4-tetrahydro-6,7-dimethylquinoxaline, *J. Am. Chem. Soc.* **81:**1946-1951.

92. Miles, H. T., and Stadtman, E. R. 1955. Isolation and characterization of 6,7-dimethyl-9-(2'-hydroxyethyl)isoalloxazine as a bacterial fermentation product of riboflavin, *J. Am. Chem. Soc.* **77:**5746-5747.

93. Mitsuda, H. 1966. Factors affecting levels of the flavin coenzymes in higher plants, *Proc. Japan Acad.* **42:**940.

94. Mitsuda, H., Kawai, F., and Miyoshi, T. 1958. Studies on flavin. I. Distribution and forms of flavin in animal and plant tissues, *J. Agr. Chem. Soc. (Japan)* **32:**847-851.

95. Mitsuda, H., Kawai, F., Nakayama, Y., and Tomozawa, Y. 1963a. Studies on plant flavokinase. I. Occurrence of flavokinase in green leaves, *J. Vitaminol.* **9:**136-141.

96. Mitsuda, H., Tomozawa, Y., and Kawai, F. 1963b. Studies on plant flavokinase. II. The purification and some properties of bean flavokinase, *J. Vitaminol.* **9:**142-148.

97. Mitsuda, H., Tomozawa, Y., Tsuboi, T., and Kawai, F. 1964. On the enzymatic

hydrolysis of FMN in green leaves, *Vitamin (Japan)* **30**:157-164

98. Müller, F., and Hemmerich, P. 1966. Thione, Imine, Oxime und Azine des Riboflavins Nucleophile Substitutionsreaktionen am Flavinkern, *Helv. Chim. Acta* **49**:2352-2364.

99. Müller, F., Massey, V., Heizmann, C., Hemmerich, P., Lhoste, J. M., and Gould, D. C. 1969. The reduction of flavins by borohydride:3,4-dihydroflavin. Structure, absorption and luminescence, *Eur. J. Biochem.* **9**:392-401.

100. Nagatsu, T., Nagatsu-Ishibashi, I., Okuda, J., and Yagi, K. 1967. Incorporation of peripherally administered riboflavine into flavine nucleotides in the brain, *J. Neurochem.* **14**:207-210.

101. Nagatsu, T., Nagatsu-Ishibashi, I., and Yagi, K. 1963. Biosynthesis of C^{14}-labelled flavin adenine dinucleotide by *Eremothecium ashbyii*, *J. Biochem. (Japan)* **54**:152-155.

102. Nagatsu-Ishibashi, I., Nagatsu, T., and Yagi, K. 1961. Changes of quantity of flavin in the brain after peripheral administration of flavins, *Nature* **190**:728.

103. Najjar, V. A., Johns, G. A., Mediary, G. C., Fleischmann, G., and Holt, L. E. 1944. The biosynthesis of riboflavin in man, *J. Am. Med. Assoc.* **126**:357-358.

104. Nara, S., Igaue, I., Gomes, B., and Yasunobu, K. T. 1966. The prosthetic groups of animal amine oxidases, *Biochem. Biophys. Res. Commun.* **23**:324-328.

105. Needham, A. E. 1966. The chloragogen-pigment of earthworms, *Life Sciences* **5**:33-39.

106. Ochoa, S., and Rossiter, R. J. 1939. Flavin-adenine-dinucleotide in rat tissues, *Biochem. J.* **33**:2008-2016.

107. Ogunmodede, B., and McCormick, D. B. 1966. Sparing of riboflavin by 6,7-dimethyl-9-(ω-hydroxyalkyl)isoalloxazines, *Fed. Proc.* **25**:246.

108. Ogunmodede, B., and McCormick, D. B. 1966. Sparing of riboflavin in rats by 6,7-dimethyl-9-(ω-hydroxyalkyl)isoalloxazines, *Proc. Soc. Exp. Biol. Med.* **122**:845.

109. Onozaki, H., and Takakuwa, T. 1963. Biosynthesis of riboflavinylglucoside by *Ashbya gossypii*, *Vitamins* **28**:45-48.

110. Owen, E. C. 1962. The characterization of riboflavin metabolite (RMl) as 9-(2'-hydroxyethyl)-6,7-dimethylisoalloxazine, *Biochem. J.* **84**:96P.

111. Owen, E. C., Montgomery, J. P., and Proudfoot, R. 1961. Properties of a metabolite of riboflavin, *Biochem. J.* **82**:8P.

112. Owen, E. C., Proudfoot, R., and West, D. W. 1966. Riboflavine metabolism in the newborn kid, *Proc. Nutr. Soc.* **25**:XI.

113. Owen, E. C., Proudfoot, R., and West, D. W. 1966. Metabolism of riboflavine, *Proc. Nutr. Soc.* **25**:X.

114. Owen, E. C., and West, D. W. 1968. Bacterial degradation of riboflavin, *J. Chem. Soc.* (C), 34-36.

115. Owen, E. C., and West, D. W. 1970. Metabolites of riboflavine in milk, urine and tissues of animals in relation to alimentary symbiotic bacteria, *Brit. J. Nutr.* **24**:45-60.

116. Owen, E. C., and West, D. W. 1971. Isolation and identification of 7,8-dimethyl-10-(2'-hydroxyethyl)isoalloxazine from natural sources, *in:* "Vitamins and Coenzymes, Methods in Enzymology," (D. B. McCormick and L. D. Wright, eds.), Vol. 18B, p. 574-579, Academic Press, New York.

117. Owen, E. C., and West, D. W. 1971. Isolation and identification of 7,8-dimethyl-10-formylmethylisoalloxazine as a product of the bacterial degradation of riboflavin, *in:* "Vitamins and Coenzymes, Methods in Enzymology," (D. B. McCormick and L. D. Wright, eds.), Vol. 18B, p. 579-581, Academic Press, New York.

118. Owen, E. C., West, D. W., and Coates, M. E. 1970. Metabolism of riboflavine in germ-free and conventional rabbits, *Brit. J. Nutr.* **24**:259-267.

119. Pallares, E. S., and Garza, H. M. 1949. Isolation of lyxoflavine from the human myocardium, *Arch. Biochem.* **22**:63-65.
120. Pearson, W. N. 1967. Riboflavin, *in:* "The Vitamins," (P. György and W. N. Pearson, eds.), Vol. 8, p. 99, Academic Press, New York.
121. Prosky, L., Burch, H. B., Bejrablaya, D., Lowry, O. H., and Combs, A. M. 1964. The effects of galactoflavin on riboflavin enzymes and coenzymes, *J. Biol. Chem.* **239**:2691-2695.
122. Quarto di Palo, F. M., Gastaldi, L., and Mombelli, L. E. 1965. Le modificazioni con l'invecchiamento nel contenuto in coenzimi nicotinici e flavinici di alcuni tessuti del ratto, *Giorn. Geront.* **13**:347.
123. Rudy, H. 1935. Enzymatische Phosphorylierung des Lactoflavins, *Naturwiss.* **23**:286-287.
124. Sadasivam, S., and Shanmugasundaram, E. R. B. 1966. Studies on the flavokinase of *Solanum nigrum* L., *Enzymologia* **4**:203-208.
125. Schrecker, A. W., and Kornberg, A. 1950. Reversible enzymatic synthesis of flavin-adenine dinucleotide, *J. Biol. Chem.* **182**:795-803.
126. Sebrell, W. H., Jr., and Harris, R. S., eds. 1954. Riboflavin *in* "The Vitamins," Vol. 3, pp. 300-402, Academic Press, New York.
127. Siliprandi, N., Navazio, F., and Fioretti, P. 1955. The formation of flavin-adenine dinucleotide in liver cells prepared from normal and alloxan diabetic rats, *Experientia* **11**:497.
128. Singer, T. P., Hauber, J., and Kearney, E. B. 1962. Fluorometric determination of the succinate dehydrogenase content of respiratory chain preparations, *Biochem. Biophys. Res. Commun.* **9**:146-149.
129. Singer, T. P., and Kearney, E. B. 1959. In: "Vitamin Metabolism," (W. Umbreit and H. Molitor, eds.) p. 209, Macmillan, London.
130. Singer, T. P., Kearney, E. B., and Massey, V. 1956. Observations on the flavin moiety of succinic dehydrogenase, *Arch. Biochem. Biophys.* **60**:255-257.
131. Singer, T. P., Salach, J., Hemmerich, P., and Ehrenberg, A. 1971. Flavin peptides, *in:* "Vitamins and Coenzymes, Methods in Enzymology" (D. B. McCormick and L. D. Wright, eds.), Vol. 18B, p. 416-427, Academic Press, New York.
132. Smyrniotis, P. Z., Miles, H. T., and Stadtman, E. R. 1958. Isolation and structure proof of 3,4-dimethyl-6-carboxy-α-pyrone as a bacterial degradation product of riboflavin, *J. Am. Chem. Soc.* **80**:2541-2545.
133. Snell, E. E., Klatt, O. A., Briuns, H. W., and Cravens, W. W. 1953. Growth-promotion by lyxoflavin. II. Relationship to riboflavin in bacteria and chicks, *Proc. Soc. Exptl. Biol. Med.* **82**:583-590.
134. Snoswell, A. M. 1957. Flavokinase of *Lactobacillus arabinosus* 17.5, *Australian J. Exptl. Biol. Med. Sci.* **35**:427-436.
135. Snyderman, S. E., Ketron, K. C., Burch, H. B., Lowry, O. H., Bessey, O. A., Guy, L. P., and Holt, E., Jr. 1949. The minimum riboflavin requirement of the infant, *J. Nutr.* **39**:219-232.
136. Stadtman, E. R. 1958. The biosynthesis and degradation of riboflavin. Symposium XI. Vitamin metabolism, *Proc. 4th Intern. Congr. Biochem., Vienna.*
137. Sung, J.-L., and Yang, W.-K. 1967. Riboflavin metabolism in liver diseases. III. Flavine contents of liver and other tissues of *p*-dimethylaminoazobenzene-fed rats and humans, *Taiwan I-Hsueh-Hui Tsa-Chih* **65**:242 (*Chem. Abstr.* **22**:897).
138. Suzuki, Y. 1965. Studies on dextransucrase. III. Isolation and properties of the

enzyme of *Leuconostoc mesenteroides* producing riboflavinylglucoside, *J. Vitaminol.* 11:95-101.

139. Suzuki, Y., and Katagiri, H. 1963. Studies on dextransucrase. I. Formation of riboflavinylglucoside in dextran-producing cultures of *Leuconostoc mesenteroides*, *J. Vitaminol.* 9:285-292.

140. Suzuki, Y., and Uchida, K. 1967. Studies on dextransucrase. VII. Formation of riboflavin compounds of glucosyl oligosaccharide by *Leuconostoc mesenteroides*, *Vitamins* 35:27-30.

141. Suzuki, Y., and Uchida, K. 1967. Studies on dextransucrase. VIII. Isolation and identification of riboflavin compounds of glucosyl oligosaccharides, *Vitamins* 35:31-37.

142. Tachibana, S. 1955. Transglycosidation by *Clostridium acetobutyricum*, *Vitamins* 8:363-365.

143. Tachibana, S. 1955. Sugar compounds of riboflavine. II. Biosynthesis of riboflavin-ylgalastoside by *Aspergillus oryzae*, *Vitamins* 9:119-124.

144. Tachibana, S. 1961. New type flavine nucleotide. I. Biosynthesis of riboflavinyl glucoside mononucleotide, *Vitamins* 22:291.

145. Tachibana, S. 1961. Studies on a new type of flavin nucleotide. I. Biosynthesis of riboflavinylglucoside mononucleotide, *J. Vitaminol.* 7:294-298.

146. Tachibana, S. 1962. Occurrence of new enzymes, flavin-inactivating enzymes, *Vitamins* 29:209.

147. Tachibana, S. 1962. On the microbial activities of the new flavin phosphates, *Vitamins* 29:534.

148. Tachibana, S. 1966. Discovery of a new flavin phosphate synthetase which requires guanosine-t'-triphosphate, *Vitamins* 33:533-535.

149. Tachibana, S. 1967. The formation of new flavin phosphates by molds, *J. Vitaminol.* 13:70-79.

150. Tachibana, S. 1967. Discovery of anew flavin phosphate synthetase which requires guanosine-5'-triphosphate, *J. Vitaminol.* 13:89-92.

151. Tachibana, S. 1971. Isolation of riboflavin glycosides, *In:* "Vitamins and Coenzymes, Methods in Enzymology," (D. B. McCormick and L. D. Wright, eds.), Vol. 18B, p. 413-416, Academic Press, New York.

152. Tachibana, S. 1971. GTP-Dependent flavin phosphate synthetase, *in:* "Vitamins and Coenzymes, Methods and Enzymology." (D. B. McCormick and L. D. Wright, eds.), Vol. 18B, p. 553-555, Academic Press, New York.

153. Tachibana, S., and Mihi, K. 1967. On the effects of zinc and cadmium ions on the new flavin phosphate-producing activity of *Rhizopus javanicus*, *J. Vitaminol.* 13:64-69.

154. Tachibana, S., and Katagiri, H. 1955a. Sugar compounds of riboflavine. I. Biosynthesis of riboflavinyl glucoside by *Aspergillus oryzae*, *Vitamins* 8:304-308.

155. Tachibana, S., and Katagiri, H. 1955b. Biosynthesis of a new riboflavine phosphate by *Aspergillus oryzae*, *Vitamins* 8:309-314.

156. Tachibana, S., Nojiri, Y., Shiode, J., and Ota, Y. 1964. Photochemical properties of the new flavin phosphate of *Rhizopus*, *Vitamins* 31:154-158.

157. Tachibana, S., Nojiri, Y., Shiode, J., and Ota, Y. 1967. Photochemical properties of the new flavin phosphate of *Rhizopus*, *J. Vitaminol.* 13:52-56.

158. Tachibana, S., Oosaki, T., and Shiode, J. 1967. On the microbial activities of the new flavin phosphates, *J. Vitaminol.* 13:57-63.

159. Tachibana, S., Shiode, J., and Matsuno, S. 1963. On a new flavine mononucleotide produced by *Rhizopus oryzae*, *J. Vitaminol.* 9:197-200.

160. Tachibana, S., Takenaka, H., and Shiode, J. 1963. On the effects of inorganic salts

on the new flavin phosphate producing activity of *Rhizopus oryzae*, *Vitamins* 30:247-250 (I), 251-254 (II), 255-258 (III).

161. Tanaka, M., and Nakamura, N. 1966. Flavine adenine dinucleotide by fermentation, *Chem. Abstr.* 65:16029.

162. Theorell, H., Karrer, P., Schöpp, K., and Frei, P. 1935. Flavinphosphorsäure aus Leber, *Helv. Chim. Acta* 18:1022-1026.

163. Treadwell, G. E., Jr., and Metzler, D. E. 1972. Development and application of methods for the study of free flavins in plant tissues, *Anal. Biochem.*, 46:261.

164. Trufanov, A. V. 1942. Enzymic synthesis of flavin-adenine-nucleotide, *Biokhimiya* 7:188 (*Chem. Abstr.* 38:131, 1944).

165. Tsai, L., Smyrniotis, P. Z., Harkness, D., and Stadtman, E. R. 1963. Bacterial degradation products of riboflavin. IV. Oxidative cleavage of 1-ribityl-2,3-diketo-1,2,-3,4-tetrahydro-6,7-dimethylquinoxaline to 6,7-dimethylquinoxaline-2,3-diol and ribose, *Biochem. Z.* 338:561-581.

166. Tsai, L., and Stadtman, E. R. 1971. Riboflavin degradation, *in:* "Vitamins and Coenzymes, Methods in Enzymology," (D. B. McCormick and L. D. Wright, eds.), Vol. 18B, p. 557-571, Academic Press, New York.

167. Tsuboi, K. K., and Hudson, P. B. 1956. Acid phosphatase. VI. Kinetic properties of purified yeast and erythrocyte phosphomonoesterase, *Arch. Biochem. Biophys.* 61:197-210.

168. Tu, S.-C., and McCormick, D. B. 1969. Biological activity and excretion of the riboflavin analogues, 6,7-dimethyl-9-(ω-carboxyalkyl)-isoalloxazines in rats, *J. Nutr.* 97:307-310.

169. Wagner-Jauregg, T. 1954. Riboflavin chemistry, *in:* "The Vitamins," (W. H. Sebrell, Jr., and R. H. Harris, eds.), Vol. 3, p. 325, Academic Press, New York.

170. Wagner-Jauregg, T., and Wollschitt, H. 1934. Bemerkungen zu einer Mitteilung "Über Urochrom und die Teilnahme von Lyochromen an der Zellatmung," *Naturwiss.* 22:107.

171. Walker, W. H., Hemmerich, P., and Massey, V. 1967. Studien in der Flavinreihe. 15. Reduktive photoalkylierung des flavinkerns und flavinkatalysierte photodecarboxylierung von phenylacetat, *Helv. Chim. Acta* 50:2269-2279.

172. Walker, W. H., Kearney, E. B. Seng, R., and Singer, T. P. 1971. Sequence and structure of a cysteinyl flavin peptide from monoamine oxidase, *Biochem. Biophys. Res. Commun.* 44:287-289.

173. Walker, W. H., Salach, J., Gutman, M., Singer, T. P., Hyde, J. S., and Ehrenberg, A. 1969. ENDOR studies on the covalently bound flavin at the active center of succinate dehydrogenase, *Federation European Biochem. Soc. Lett.*, 5:237-240.

174. Wang, T. Y., Tsou, C. L., and Wang, Y. L. 1956. Studies on succinic dehydrogenase. I. Isolation, purification, and properties, *Scientia Sinica* 5:73.

175. Wang, T. Y., Tsou, C. L., and Wang, Y. L. 1958. Studies on succinic dehydrogenase. II. Further observations on the properties of the enzyme and its prosthetic group, *Scientia Sinica* 7:65-74.

176. West, D. W., and Owen, E. C. 1968. Metabolism of riboflavine in goats with a cecal fistula, *Proc. Nutr. Soc.* 27:39A.

177. West, D. W., and Owen, E. C. 1969. The urinary excretion of metabolites of riboflavine by man, *Brit. J. Nutr.* 23:889-898.

178. Whitby, L. G. 1950. Enzymic formation of a new riboflavin derivative, *Nature* 166:479-480.

179. Whitby, L. G. 1952. Riboflavinyl glucoside: a new derivative of riboflavin, *Biochem. J.* 50:433-438.

180. Whitby, L. G. 1954. Transglucosidation reactions with flavins, *Biochem. J.* 57:390-396.

181. Whitby, L. G. 1971. Glycosides of riboflavin, *in:* "Vitamins and Coenzymes, Methods in Enzymology," (D. B. McCormick and L. D. Wright, eds.), Vol. 18B, p. 404–413, Academic Press, New York.

182. Wilson, D. E., and King, T. E. 1964. The determination of the acid–nonextractable flavin in mitochondrial preparations from heart muscle, *J. Biol. Chem.* **239**:2683–2690.

183. Winter, W. P., Buss, E. G., Clagett, C. O., and Bouchers, R. V. 1967. The nature of the biochemical lesion in avian renal riboflavinuria. II. The inherited change of a riboflavin-binding protein from blood and eggs, *Comp. Biochem. Physiol.* **22**:897–906.

184. Yagi, K. 1954. Distribution of riboflavin nucleotides in rat organs influenced by the administration of flavin compounds, *J. Biochem. (Japan)* **41**:757–762.

185. Yagi, K., Nagatsu, T., Nagatsu-Ishibashi, I., and Ohashi, A. 1966. Migration of injected C^{14}-labelled riboflavin into rat tissues, *J. Biochem. (Japan)* **59**:313–315.

186. Yagi, K., and Okuda, J. 1958. Phosphorylation of riboflavin by transferase action, *Nature,* **181**:1663–1664.

187. Yanagita, T., and Foster, J. W. 1956. A bacterial riboflavin hydrolase, *J. Biol. Chem.* **221**:593–607.

188. Yang, C. S., Arsenis, C., and McCormick, D. B. 1964. Microbiological and enzymatic assays of riboflavin analogues, *J. Nutr.* **84**:167–172.

189. Yang, C. S., and McCormick, D. B. 1967. Degradation of riboflavin in the rat, *Fed. Proc.* **26**:305.

190. Yang, C. S., and McCormick D. B. 1967. Degradation and excretion of riboflavin in the rat, *J. Nutr.* **93**:445–453.

191. Yang, C. S., and McCormick, D. B. 1967. Substrate specificity of riboflavin hydrolase from *Pseudomonas riboflavina, Biochim. Biophys. Acta* **132**:511.

192. Yang, C. S., and McCormick, D. B. 1971. Riboflavin hydrolase (EC 3.5. 99.1) from *Pseudomonas riboflavina, in:* "Vitamins and Coenzymes, Methods in Enzymology," (D. B. McCormick and L. D. Wright, eds.), Vol. 18B, p. 571–573, Academic Press, New York.

193. Yang, W.-K. and Sung, J.-L. 1966. Riboflavin metabolism in liver diseases. IV. Enzymic splitting and synthesis of flavine adenine dinucleotide in the *p*-dimethylamin-oazobenzene-induced rat liver carcinoma tissue, *Taiwan I-Hsueh-Hui Tsa-Chih* **65**:299 (*Chem. Abstr.* **66**:63474, 1967).

194. Yang, W.-K. and Sung, J.-L. 1966. Riboflavin metabolism in liver diseases. V. Clinical studies on the enzymic splitting of flavine adenine dinucleotide in serum, *Taiwan I-Hsueh-Hui Tsa-Chih* **65**:306 (*Chem. Abstr.* **66**:63475, 1967).

NUTRITIONAL INTAKE OF RIBOFLAVIN

Sara M. Hunt

1. HISTORICAL PERSPECTIVES

Feeding experiments employed in early nutritional investigations very quickly forced recognition of the fact that experimental diets containing purified protein and carbohydrate plus butterfat and a good salt mixture were lacking some "essential" necessary for animal growth. The investigators found that this nutritional essential could be met by the feeding of yeast. Furthermore, they discovered that this essential was the same substance that prevented or cured beri-beri. As a result of the discovery, the customary procedure in laboratory feeding experiments was to use yeast as a source of vitamin B and to attribute to the antineuritic substance (or thiamine) whatever "vitaminic" values yeast was found to have.[37] Some years later, however, it became apparent that yeast must contain some heat-resistant growth factor in addition to the heat-labile antineuritic substance, since heated yeast was still nutritionally significant in its action. The heat-stable growth factor, discovered first in yeast, was found to be present also in milk in quantities even greater than those for thiamine. Furthermore, egg whites that contain only a trace of thiamine proved a significant source of the heat-stable splinter of the B vitamin.

SARA M. HUNT—Department of Community Health and Nutrition, Georgia State University, Atlanta.

The common factor in yeast, milk, and egg white was lactoflavin, a greenish-yellow water-soluble natural coloring matter first isolated from milk. Lactoflavin, whether obtained from milk, egg white, or yeast, proved to be chemically the same and to have similar nutritional effects. It was synthesized in the laboratory and, with the establishment of its chemical nature, its name was changed to riboflavin in order to suggest its chemical structure. Further investigation showed that riboflavin was widely distributed in food and was identical with the growth essential whose relative amount in food had previously been expressed as "Bourquin-Sherman Units of Vitamin G."[37]

Because of the historically close association between riboflavin and thiamin, early estimates for riboflavin requirements and/or recommended intake were based upon those for thiamin with the assumption that the need for riboflavin—like that of thiamin—increased as caloric consumption and expenditure increased. The first recommended dietary allowances were published in 1943, and at that time the allowances for riboflavin were set at a ratio of 3:2 in comparison with the allowances for thiamin, since these proportions reflected the relative need for the two vitamins in growing experimental animals.[9] Although results of excretion studies in intervening years caused a downward revision in the recommended absolute amount of both thiamin and riboflavin, the same proportion between intakes of riboflavin and thiamin remained in the 1945 recommended allowances.[10]

The human requirement for riboflavin has been estimated traditionally through excretion studies, since there is a high correlation between intake and urinary excretion. Horwitt[19] showed that adult men maintained on 2200 kcal daily and receiving 1.1 mg riboflavin would excrete approximately 10% of the vitamin intake, while an ingestion of 1.6 mg riboflavin increased the urinary loss to 30% of intake. The point at which urinary losses rise sharply is designated as the critical point of excretion and indicates an intake at which the body is using the vitamin efficiently. This critical point of excretion coincides with optimum requirement or tissue "saturation" only in rapidly growing children and pregnant women who remain in positive nitrogen balance for long periods of time.[1,2]

Minimum requirements for riboflavin during early life are determined as the level necessary for growth (this level is indicated by the critical level of excretion), but for the adult minimum requirements must be determined by signs of riboflavin deficiency. For man the limits within which the adult minimum requirements seem to lie—0.25 and 0.27 mg/1000 kcal—are approximately one-half of those levels required to produce the critical point of excretion.[2]

Various investigators have approached calculation of the level of

TABLE I. *Evolution of Recommended Dietary Allowances for Riboflavin in Adult Man*[a]

Year	Weight, kg	Age, yr	Level of activity	Kilocalories	Protein, g	Basis for riboflavin recommendation	RDA for riboflavin, mg
1943	70	No specification	"Very active"	4500	70	Calorie expenditure and relation to thiamin needs	3.3
1945	70	No specification	"Very active"	4500	70	Calorie expenditure (0.6 mg/1000 kcal)	2.6
1948	70	No specification	"With heavy work"	4500	70	Body weight (20 mg/kg + safety factor)	1.8
1953	65	25	"Fairly active"	3200	65	Recommended protein intake (65 g × 0.025 mg/g)	1.6
1958	70	25	"Moderate physical activity"	3200	70	Recommended protein intake (65 g × 0.025 mg/g)	1.8
1964	70	25	"Moderately active"	2900	70	Caloric expenditure (0.6 mg/1000 kcal)	1.7
1968	70	22	"Light activity"	2800	65	Metabolic body size (0.07 mg/kg.[75])	1.7
1974	70	23–50	"Normal activity"	2700	56	Caloric expenditure (0.6 mg/1000 kcal)	1.6

[a] After Food and Nutrition Board, 1943–1968.

efficient use (or optimum requirement in the case of rapidly growing children and pregnant women) of riboflavin by different methods, and the variety of methods employed have been reflected in revisions of the NRC Recommended Allowances (Table I), which have appeared every 3 to 5 years since the first edition in 1943.[9-15a]

Pearson[34] compared in all age groups of children the Recommended Dietary Allowances for riboflavin based upon protein requirement[13] with those levels calculated from the amount of riboflavin needed per 1000 kcal[32,39] and/or per kilogram of body weight.[40] All figures were in rather good agreement regardless of the approach to riboflavin need. For example, in the 10- to 12-year-old age group, riboflavin intake required for tissue saturation was 1.75 mg when calculated on a calorie basis, 2.00 mg when figured on a weight basis, and 1.8 mg when related to protein need.

The very fact that many different bases have been practicable for estimating the human need for riboflavin reflects the close relationship that must exist between riboflavin adequacy and body metabolism in general. In the 1968 edition of the Recommended Dietary Allowances,[15] requirement for riboflavin was based upon body metabolism as predicted by metabolic body size, which is body weight in kilograms taken to the 0.75 power.[24] In the younger age groups, the Recommended Dietary Allowances for riboflavin calculated through use of metabolic body size did not differ markedly from the 1964 kilocalorie-based allowances, but the recommendations were somewhat higher in the older age groups since a decline in metabolic body size is not considered to occur with age. Nevertheless, for practical purposes the riboflavin allowance in the 1974 edition of the Recommended Dietary Allowances was once again computed on the basis of calories.[15a]

The increased need for riboflavin exhibited during pregnancy is apparently related solely to the concomitant elevation of metabolic activity, since utilization of the vitamin by normal pregnant women does not seem to differ from that in the nonpregnant.[21,33] The riboflavin allowance recommended for nonpregnant females (1.5 mg/24 hr) is increased during pregnancy by 0.3 mg daily in order to compensate for the estimated increase in metabolic body size induced by growth of the fetus and accessory tissue.[15,15a]

2. FARMING AND RIBOFLAVIN INTAKE

The fact that riboflavin as a component of coenzymes is involved in tissue oxidation and respiration assures the presence of the vitamin

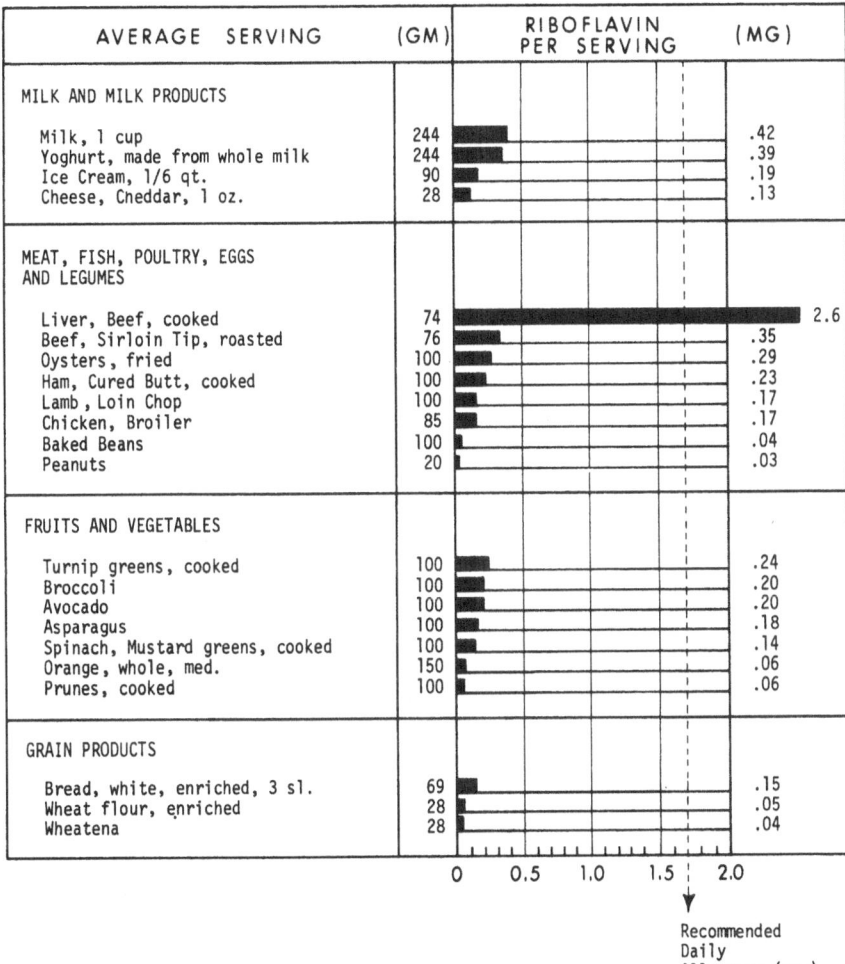

AVERAGE SERVING	(GM)	RIBOFLAVIN PER SERVING	(MG)
MILK AND MILK PRODUCTS			
Milk, 1 cup	244		.42
Yoghurt, made from whole milk	244		.39
Ice Cream, 1/6 qt.	90		.19
Cheese, Cheddar, 1 oz.	28		.13
MEAT, FISH, POULTRY, EGGS AND LEGUMES			
Liver, Beef, cooked	74		2.6
Beef, Sirloin Tip, roasted	76		.35
Oysters, fried	100		.29
Ham, Cured Butt, cooked	100		.23
Lamb, Loin Chop	100		.17
Chicken, Broiler	85		.17
Baked Beans	100		.04
Peanuts	20		.03
FRUITS AND VEGETABLES			
Turnip greens, cooked	100		.24
Broccoli	100		.20
Avocado	100		.20
Asparagus	100		.18
Spinach, Mustard greens, cooked	100		.14
Orange, whole, med.	150		.06
Prunes, cooked	100		.06
GRAIN PRODUCTS			
Bread, white, enriched, 3 sl.	69		.15
Wheat flour, enriched	28		.05
Wheatena	28		.04

0   0.5   1.0   1.5   2.0

Recommended
Daily
Allowance (men)

Fig. 1. Riboflavin in average servings of foods classified in the four food groups. (Adapted from H. S. Mitchell et al.[28])

to some degree in virtually all naturally occurring foodstuffs. The foods that contain the greatest amount of the vitamin are shown in Fig. 1. As can be noted, certain cholorophyll-containing plants such as broccoli, asparagus, and greens of various kinds contain a considerable amount of riboflavin. The vitamin is formed during the growth process of the plant, and in this age of extreme interest in organic farming the question of whether or not mode of cultivation has an effect upon the vitamin content of growing plants naturally arises.

To answer this question, it is necessary to review briefly the nature of plant growth.[1] Plants are autotropic; that is, they need no organic molecules to survive, no previously incorporated carbon sources from which to derive energy. Plants exist entirely on inorganic compounds: carbon dioxide from the atmosphere, hydrogen and oxygen from water, and minerals from the soil. Therefore, the only element used in the synthesis of riboflavin that comes from the soil is nitrogen, which can be supplied by nitrate or ammonia. Furthermore, neither the fertility of the soil nor the type of fertilizer used seems to have any effect upon the vitamin content of the plant. In poor soil the yield of crops is decreased, but those plants that are able to obtain sustenance and grow in this soil contain approximately that nutrient level dictated by their particular genetic makeup.

Thus, organic farming apparently would be expected to have little or no effect upon improving riboflavin content of plant food, since plants cannot use organic molecules and their nutrient content is dictated by their genes rather than by their nourishment. Jukes[22] points out that hydroponics in which plants are grown inorganically without any soil leads to the production of vegetables and fruits with the same protein, carbohydrate, vitamin, and mineral content as when the same strains of plants are grown with lots of manure.

Manure and compost do have great value, however, in their contribution of organisms necessary for decomposition of biological residues and the resulting solubilization of minerals for plant nourishment and good crop production. Artificial fertilizers, of course, also provide plant nourishment, but the minerals are presented in an already soluble form. Use of organic materials for improvement of soil quality is an excellent practice for the small-scale farmer and/or gardener and should be encouraged for these groups, but the public should understand that the importance of fertilizer is related to improved crop production and not improved nutritional value of the crops thus produced.

Unlike crops, animals must consume riboflavin and, therefore, animal sources of the vitamin can be affected by the level of riboflavin ingested. For example, milk contains more riboflavin during spring and early summer when cattle are grazing on young green grass than when they must depend entirely on dry feed with its lower riboflavin content. The muscle, liver, and eggs of the fowl can be affected by its riboflavin intake. Although the influence of vitamin intake on muscle content of riboflavin is only slight, altered intake can bring about an appreciable change in the liver and eggs. In addition to the riboflavin contributed

[1] Personal communication with A. J. R. Guttay, Professor of Agronomy and Head of Plant Science Department, University of Connecticut, Storrs, Connecticut.

by feed, fowl may obtain a considerable amount of the vitamin from their feces, to which they usually have access.[3]

3. PROCESSING AND HANDLING OF RIBOFLAVIN FOOD SOURCES

Although the method by which crops are produced seems to have little effect upon their nutrient content, the handling and processing of crops from their source until time of consumption can greatly affect their nutrient content.

The properties of specific nutrients dictate correct handling for their preservation, and special care must be exercised in the handling of foods that contribute the greatest proportion of the various nutrients to the diet. The contribution of riboflavin to diet in the United States by the various food groups is given in Fig. 2.

Although most of the riboflavin consumed in the United States and in Europe is supplied by milk, meat, fish, and eggs, the principal sources of the vitamin in developing countries are either cereals or starchy roots and tubers.[5] In Africa, fruits and vegetables may also contribute significant amounts of riboflavin. It is important, therefore, to consider

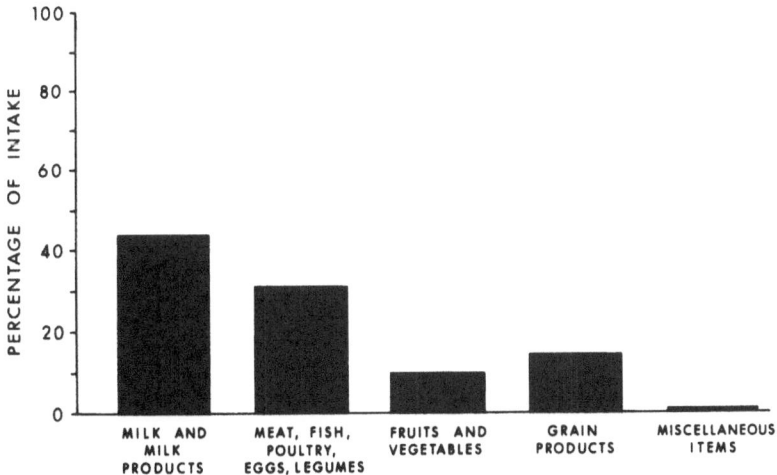

Fig. 2. Contribution of major food groups to riboflavin available for civilian consumption, 1967. (Adapted from 1968 "Outlook Issue," National Food Situation, NFS-122, Economic Research Service, United States Department of Agriculture, November 15, 1967.)

the effect of handling and processing upon riboflavin content in all groups of food, since every group appears to be an important source of the vitamin in some part of the world.

In the following discussion concerning the handling and processing of food and their effect upon the possible destruction or retention of riboflavin, the following chemical properties of the vitamin must be kept in mind: solubility in water, resistance to oxidation and to an acid pH, stability in dry form to heat, and sensitivity to alkali and light.

3.1. Milk and Milk Products

The pasteurization of milk causes only minimal losses of riboflavin (approximately 5%), but exposure of milk to direct sunlight can cause in a period of 4 hr a destruction of 71% of the vitamin. The use of brown glass bottles and paper cartons as containers has done much to protect milk against destruction of its riboflavin.

Evaporation and dehydration processes affect only negligibly the riboflavin content of milk, but evaporated milk stored at high temperatures can cause as much as 37% loss of the vitamin within a year's time. About 23% of the riboflavin present in milk is retained in the production of cheddar cheese and no further diminution of content is caused by the ripening process.[46]

3.2. Meat, Fish, Poultry, Eggs, and Legumes

The riboflavin content of processed meat products is similar, per unit of protein, to that of unprocessed cuts of meat. In the United States, canning, freezing, dehydration, and irradiation apparently have little effect upon the riboflavin content of meat, fish, or poultry.[36] On the other hand, dehydration by sundrying as practiced in tropical countries can be quite detrimental to the riboflavin content of fish.[5] Slow freezing as opposed to rapid freezing may change texture of foods so that loss of water-soluble factors can occur in the leakage of liquids during and after defrosting. Riboflavin lost in the thaw juices of beef is estimated at approximately 10%.

Methods by which foods within the meat group are prepared for consumption can be important in the conservation of riboflavin. Very little riboflavin is destroyed in the roasting of meat, fish, and poultry, particularly when low temperatures are used (around 300° F).[7] However, since riboflavin is water soluble, much of the vitamin can be found in meat juices and in liquids used in moist-heat cookery. To ensure minimum losses of riboflavin in meat cookery, all of the accompanying juices should be used either as gravies or as seasonings for other dishes such as soups.

Noble[31] studied the effects of stewing and braising upon riboflavin retention in variety meats and found that the kind of meat as well as the type of cookery could affect the amount of riboflavin retained. More riboflavin was retained when meats were stewed, but the highest percentage of retention (75%) was found in heart from veal, lamb, beef, or pork, while the least amount of the vitamin (55%) was retained by beef kidney. The cooking liquid contained 13-22% of the riboflavin originally present in the raw sample.

In some instances, there has been an apparent increase of riboflavin during the cooking and holding of meat. The explanation for the increase is not known, but it is theorized that certain derivatives of riboflavin are broken up during the cooking process and become available to the microorganisms used in the assay.[29]

Cold storage of eggs can cause a reduction in riboflavin content. Approximately 14-18% of the vitamin is lost upon storage from 3 to 12 months.[29] Exposure to light during the cooking process is also important in promoting destruction of riboflavin in eggs. Open-pan scrambling has been shown to cause a riboflavin destruction as high as 48%, while only a 22% decrease in riboflavin occurred when cooking was done in a closed pan. Baking of the eggs permitted complete retention of the vitamin.[29] The type of oven used for baking, be it an electronic range or the conventional electric oven, seems to make no significant difference in the retention of riboflavin.[45]

Since riboflavin is sensitive to alkali, the practice of using baking soda to soften dried beans and peas for quick cooking destroys much of the vitamin contained in these legumes.

3.3. Fruits and Vegetables

Foods of plant origin are often blanched before they are frozen or canned. Apparently, very little riboflavin is lost in the process if high temperature, short-time blanches are used. Nor does the canning or freezing of fruits and vegetables have much effect upon the riboflavin content of these foods.[6] Modern methods of dehydration also preserve the original riboflavin content in plant foods, but sun drying of fruits and vegetables as practiced in tropical countries causes a considerable destruction of the vitamin due to the sensitivity of riboflavin to light.

Riboflavin is retained to the extent of 60-90% in boiled vegetables, and retention of the vitamin does not appear to be influenced by the volume of cooking water.[30] Use of a small amount of cooking water has practical value, however, because if the vegetable cooking water can be utilized in some way such as in a sauce or in soup, there is no riboflavin lost from the vegetable. When the riboflavin content of cooking water is combined with that found in the prepared vegetable, the total equals the vitamin value of the raw plant. Although riboflavin is not easily destroyed in cooking, the holding of warm vegetables after preparation and/or the addition of baking soda to green vegetables for color enhancement can cause considerable destruction of the vitamin.

3.4. Grain Products

Milling of grain products drastically reduces their content of riboflavin because much of the vitamin is contained in the germ and bran. The polishing of rice illustrates the stepwise process by which riboflavin is lost in the milling. Polished rice contains approximately 59% of the riboflavin originally present in brown rice, with 20% lost during the first hulling, 10% in the second hulling, and 11% in the final polishing.[4]

Parboiling or "converting" the rice before it is polished can, however, increase the riboflavin content of the polished product. For centuries it has been the practice in India to steep rough rice in water, steam it, and dry it in the sun before milling it. This process is called "parboiling." "Converting" rice is a modified method of "parboiling" in which vacuum and pressure are used. In both processes, the steeping and steaming treatments carry water-soluble nutrients of the germ and aleurone layers into the starchy part of the endosperm. The brief steaming gelatinizes the starch in the outer layers of the endosperm, helping to hold the nutrients inside and to strengthen the kernel, thus leading to a considerable reduction in breakage during the milling process. Reduction in breakage is important since riboflavin is apparently not easily destroyed in unbroken grain under normal conditions of storage. Conservation of vitamins effected by parboiling is sufficient to protect populations subsisting only on parboiled polished rice from developing the vitamin deficiency symptoms observed in those people living on nonparboiled polished rice.

Although enrichment of rice is mandatory in certain countries such as Puerto Rico and the Phillipines, the enrichment premix contains no riboflavin because of its yellow color, which when imparted to rice makes the product apparently unacceptable to the population.[38]

A standard white flour, which is of approximately 70% extraction, contains only about 35% of the riboflavin found in whole wheat.[4]

Although the milling of wheat does decrease its content of riboflavin, enriched refined flour has a higher concentration of the vitamin than does the whole wheat itself.[16] During World War II, federal legislation made it mandatory that all bread sold throughout the United States be enriched. Although this federal regulation is no longer in effect, state laws have been responsible for the continued enrichment of approximately 80-90% of all white bread and all-purpose flour sold in the United States.

Products labeled enriched and sold in interstate commerce must meet standards of identity set by the Food and Drug Administration. These standards require that enriched flour contain thiamin, riboflavin, niacin, and iron at levels between a set minimum and maximum. The riboflavin content of enriched flour is set at a minimum level of 1.2 mg and a maximum of 1.5 mg/lb, while that of enriched bread must fall between 0.7 mg and 1.6 mg/lb. When the enrichment program began, the policy was to add vitamins and minerals to flour and bread in the amounts that would be found in whole wheat products. In the case of riboflavin, however, the assay method used for determining the riboflavin content of whole wheat yielded a value higher than that actually present; therefore, more riboflavin was added to enriched products than was initially intended. Even when better analytical methods became available, the enrichment standard for riboflavin, although high, was never changed because of the relatively low riboflavin intake by certain population groups in this country.

On December 3, 1971, the Food and Drug Administration proposed in the *Federal Register*[8] the improvement of the nutritional quality of enriched wheat flour and related products such as enriched self-rising flour, enriched farina, and enriched bread and rolls. The main purpose of the proposal was to increase the iron supplementation of these products, but the vitamins thiamin, riboflavin, and niacin would also be increased above the levels currently in use. Instead of the minimum and maximum standards previously specified, the new proposal suggested requirements of only one level that were close to the existing maximum level standards. No action, however, has been taken on this proposal because of the objections raised by many physicians against the increase in iron supplementation; therefore, the future of a new maximum standard supplementation of riboflavin in enriched flour and cereal products is uncertain.

Degermed grits and meal are both highly refined products, containing only one-third to one-half of the riboflavin found in whole corn.[38] Whenever these products are enriched, riboflavin can be included in the premix, since a yellow color does not decrease the acceptability of corn products to the consumer as it does in the case of rice.

4. INTAKE OF RIBOFLAVIN

Determination of intake of nutrients in a population group is a difficult task because the tools suitable to a nutrition survey can give only rough measurements. Krehl and Hodges[26] point out that the ideal way to obtain information regarding dietary intake of any nutrient is to measure the quantity of nutrient actually ingested through analysis of a select meal or meals. Such a method, unfortunately, is not applicable to group surveys.

The tools most often used to determine nutrient intake consist of household group consumption surveys and dietary histories or records. In addition, certain pertinent biochemical measurements may be employed to estimate the adequacy of nutrient intake.

The household consumption survey[42] records "food available for consumption" and includes plate waste, food fed to pets, and the like. Average per-person intake can be calculated by dividing the household food supply equally among all persons who are eating. Although the food consumption survey covers a 7-day period, the average intake per person must necessarily be a very gross estimate.

A dietary record may be a retrospective recall of food eaten in the past 24 hr. Such a record, because it depends upon memory, is of necessity defective. Another type of dietary record or history is the meal-by-meal reporting of food intake, the duration of which may range from 1 to 7 days. Amounts of food recorded are most often only approximations of the amount of food actually eaten. Furthermore, the fact that one is recording his food intake can make him deviate from his normal eating habits. Finally, there is the pitfall of depending too heavily upon the reliability of food composition tables. Food tables prepared by the U.S. Department of Agriculture represent an average of values obtained from various laboratories in the United States and cannot take into full account all of the genetic factors of various food sources nor the environmental and processing factors that can markedly change the nutrient value of certain foods. Although the hazards of placing too much weight on nutrient intake data are easily recognized, these data can nevertheless be useful as a guide for estimating nutrient intake of various population groups.[25]

Urinary levels of riboflavin have provided the primary biochemical measurement of adequacy of intake.[35] Urinary vitamin excretions per gram of creatinine have been used as an index of intake in most nutrition surveys. Survey experience with vitamin-to-creatinine ratios reveals that the ratios suitable for adults cannot be used with children. A child on a given intake of riboflavin will excrete considerably more riboflavin per gram of creatinine than will an adult under the same conditions because the child is excreting less creatinine than the adult. This observation has forced the use of a sliding interpretive scale for urinary vitamin excretion.

Using the minimum requirement of 0.25 mg riboflavin/1000 kcal,[20] Pearson[34] prepared a tentative guide for the interpretation of riboflavin excretion (μg/g creatinine) by children. By using the NRC Recommended Allowances for kilocalories, he estimated daily intakes of riboflavin at different levels per 1000 kcal (Deficient <0.25; Low 0.25 to 0.49; Acceptable 0.50 to 0.70; High >0.70) for various age groups. No modification was made for age per se, since Stearns[40] found no age influence on children's requirement for riboflavin when need was based on body weight. Assuming an excretion of 10% on a deficient intake and 20% on all other intakes, Pearson[34] then predicted urinary excretions. These predictions were used for determination of adequacy of riboflavin intake in the recently completed Ten-State Nutrition Survey in the United States.[41]

Interpretation of urinary riboflavin excretion in casual urine samples is made very difficult because of the many physiological and environmental factors unrelated to riboflavin intake which may affect riboflavin excretion. For example, the effect of fasting, heavy labor, and a thiamine-deficient diet may be cited. Fasting can cause a marked increase in riboflavin excretion accompanied by large losses of nitrogen but stable creatinine levels. The consequently elevated ratio of riboflavin to creatinine would indicate an adequate intake of the vitamin when actually the intake at that particular time is zero.[47] A diet deficient in thiamine can cause an increased urinary excretion of riboflavin, while hard labor will decrease excretion of the vitamin.[23] Factors affecting the excretion of riboflavin are discussed further in Chapter 4.

A recent study by Lewis et al.[26] has raised a serious question about the use of casual urine samples for estimation of riboflavin intake, since excretion of creatinine and riboflavin showed so much variation in samples collected over a 24-hr period. So great was the variation in creatinine and riboflavin that a subject's riboflavin excretion could be considered deficient or high depending upon which voiding sample during the 24-hr period was used for determination. Furthermore, there appears to be no consistency in the time of the high and low peaks.

Determination of riboflavin intake within a population group must presently of necessity be a rather gross estimation, but if these same estimations are used with various population groups, data can be provided that will allow comparison among groups. (See Table II.) Riboflavin intake recorded in sixteen countries ranges from an average intake of

1.79 mg/day in the United States to 0.60 mg/day in India. [5,42]

The 1965 Food Consumption Survey conducted by USDA[43] used the 24-hr recall method in which the homemaker estimated food eaten the previous day by individual household members. One might well argue about the accuracy of the figures but can hardly feel any real concern over riboflavin intake in this country if the figures are even a rough reflection of riboflavin nutriture among the whole population. No population group fell below 79% of the riboflavin level recommended in the NRC Allowances, 1968. Only when the intake of a nutrient fails to reach 66 2/3% of the Recommended Dietary Allowances is the intake considered "low." The only groups not meeting or even surpassing the level of the 1968 allowances were females, aged 20-75 years and over, whose intake ranged from 99 to 79% of the recommended level, and males, aged over 75 years, whose intake averaged 82% of the Recommended Dietary Allowances.

Data collected in the Ten-State Nutrition Survey[41] failed to support evidence from the USDA Food Consumption Survey that none of the population groups had a "low" intake of riboflavin (Table III). The

TABLE II. Intake Levels of Riboflavin of Population Groups in Various Regions, from Dietary Survey Data

	Milligrams riboflavin per day per		
Region	Capita	1000 kcal	Remarks
United States			USDA Food Intake Survey,
Range	1.18-2.56	0.75-1.79	1965
Average	1.79	0.90	
Europe			Data from 47 population
Range	0.9-2.1	—	groups
Majority	1.0-1.8	0.35-0.73	
Latin America			Data from 49 population
Range	0.3-1.8	—	groups
Majority	0.4-1.0	0.20-0.61	
Asia and Far East			Data from 91 population
Range	0.3-1.2	—	groups
Majority	0.3-0.7	0.13-0.40	
Near East			Data from 76 population
Range	0.3-1.8	—	groups
Majority	0.4-1.2	0.15-0.78	
Africa			Data from 52 population
Range	0.2-1.4	—	groups
Majority	0.5-0.7	0.25-0.65	

[a]After Table I. "FAO Requirements of Vitamin A, Thiamin, Riboflavin, and Niacin— Report of a Joint FAO/WHO Expert Group," FAO Nutrition Meetings Report Series No. 41, World Health Organization Technical Report Series No. 362, Rome, Italy.[5]

TABLE III. *Low and Deficient Levels of Riboflavin as Identified by Urinary Riboflavin and Divided According to Age and Ethnic Groups*

Age groups	Number	Deficiency %	Deficiency + low %
<6	1,744	4.3	19.9
6-9	2,503	1.9	14.2
10-16	5,081	2.5	17.1
17-49	6,326	0.8	9.6
50-59	1,404	1.0	7.9
60 yr and over	2,726	1.0	8.0

Ethnic groups	Number	Deficiency, %	Deficiency + low %
White	10,318	1.2	7.8
Black	6,123	3.2	21.9
Spanish American	3,778	0.7	11.6
Oriental	278	1.6	6.8
American Indian	102	1.9	9.8

Urinary Riboflavin Deficient and Low Standards
(μg/g creatinine)

Years	Deficiency	Low	Acceptable
1-3	<150	150-499	≥500
4-6	<100	100-299	≥300
7-9	<85	85-269	≥270
10-15	<70	70-199	≥200
Adult	<29	27-79	≥80

[a] After Tables 11D and 11E, United States Department of Health, Education and Welfare, Public Health Service Center for Disease Control, 1971.

Ten-State Survey differed from the Food Consumption Survey in that not only was a different method of determining adequacy of riboflavin intake used (urinary excretion of riboflavin instead of riboflavin ingestion) but also the population samples were skewed toward those of the lower socioeconomic level. However, many individuals not falling below the poverty line were used in the Ten-State Survey. Among the number sampled who fell above the poverty line, 1.1% showed deficient levels of riboflavin excretion (9.0%, Deficient and Low) as compared with 2.9% deficient (17.8%, Deficient and Low) in the sample falling below the poverty line. Females generally had lower excretions of riboflavin than did the males, a fact that supports the lower intake of riboflavin by women as reported in the USDA Food Consumption Survey.[42-44]

Of the groups tested, children under 6 years of age of all ethnic groups and the entire black population had the highest percentage of subjects excreting levels of riboflavin considered deficient and low. Among the children under 6 years of age, 4.3% showed deficient levels of riboflavin excretion, while of the blacks of all age groups 2.3% fell within the deficient classification. When, however, the deficient and low percentages were combined, more blacks of all age groups (21.9%) than children of all ethnic groups (19.9%) were found to have riboflavin excretion levels suggestive of an unsatisfactory intake of the vitamin.

Thus, in the United States a reasonable doubt does seem to exist about the adequacy of intake of riboflavin by certain groups of the population. In South and East Asia, and in certain countries of Africa and Latin America, however, no doubt can exist about the inadequacy of intake of riboflavin because clinical manifestations of a deficiency are widespread.[5] Little attention has been devoted to the study and prevention of hyporiboflavinosis because, even when severe, a deficiency of riboflavin rarely incapacitates the individual. In addition, riboflavin deficiency rarely occurs as an isolated entity. Failure of a vitamin deficiency to incapacitate a human physically at a particular point in time tells one nothing, however, about the effect of this deficiency on the human's mental and physical state in general, his productivity, his disposition toward degenerative diseases, or his projected life span. At a time in which the importance of preventive medicine and the role that good nutrition plays in the maintenance of health have at last been realized, the possible long-range consequences of an inadequate intake of any nutrient cannot be regarded lightly.

5. RECOMMENDATIONS FOR IMPROVING NUTRITIONAL INTAKE

In developing countries where actual ariboflavinosis exists, one of the main problems, exclusive of need for individual nutrients, is that energy needs of the population cannot be met by the present level of food production. Greater food production, in general, is required with particular emphasis on the cultivation of crops that contain high levels of protein and riboflavin. Furthermore, correct methods of preservation and storage of foods containing riboflavin should be taught to the population so that all the available vitamin is conserved for consumption.

In the United States, as well as in the developing countries, effective nutrition education for the masses could do much to improve intake of all nutrients including riboflavin. Persons who purchase and prepare the food need to be taught not only how better to spend their food dollars in order to get the most nutrients for the amount spent but also how best to handle and prepare these foods for consumption so that the nutrient content is retained.

Probably the most efficient device for an immediate improvement in the intake of riboflavin in the United States as well as in other parts of the world would be requirement by the various governments that all bread and bread products—flour, meal, rice and other refined cereals—be enriched. Cereals are the primary source of calories in many areas of the world, and in the United States their consumption varies inversely with the income of the population. Therefore, the population below the poverty line which was shown in the Ten-State Nutrition Survey[41] probably to have an inadequate intake of riboflavin would be the group most benefited by an enrichment program. Improvement in riboflavin nutriture of children in Germany through enrichment of bread during World War II was indicated by the study of McCance and Strangeways.[27] Determination of riboflavin nutriture in pregnant Israeli women of the lower social brackets first in 1945 and then in 1958 after mandatory enrichment had been in effect in Israel for 10 years indeed makes a convincing argument for enrichment.[17] In the 1945 survey, 21% of the subjects studied had definite signs of ariboflavinosis, and excretion of riboflavin in urine was 95 mg/100 ml urine as against 350 mg/100 ml in middle-class pregnant women. In contrast to the earlier survey, no certain case of ariboflavinosis could be found in 1958. Furthermore, 77.3% of the women surveyed showed "high" excretion of riboflavin, 22.3% had "acceptable" values, and only 0.4% were found to have "low" excretions of the vitamin.[47]

Methods by which milk could be made readily available to all children under 6 years of age should be investigated in order to assure adequate riboflavin intake in this age group. The contribution of riboflavin by milk to children between ages three and five is approximately 60% of the total vitamin intake (Fig. 3), and the limited nature of food intake in the very young would make milk an even greater contributor of riboflavin in children under three years of age. It is disturbing to note that young children, the group most vulnerable to the effect of inadequate nutrition, is that segment of the population in which a possible deficiency of riboflavin is most suspected.[4]

A more equitable distribution of resources throughout the population groups of the entire world, including the United States, would seem to be the means by which an adequate intake of nutrients could most readily be achieved and the one toward which all socially conscious

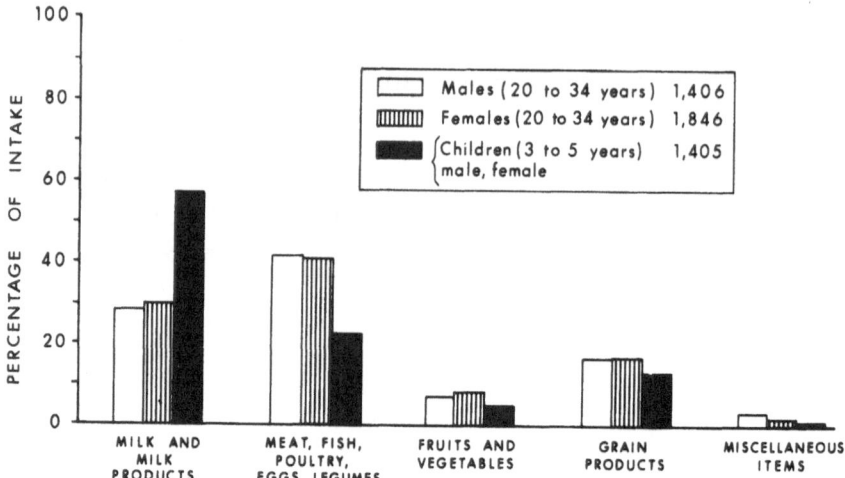

Fig. 3. Percent riboflavin contributed by various food groups in one day. (Adapted from "Food Intake and Nutritive Value of Diets of Men, Women and Children in the United States, Spring 1965. A Preliminary Report." Agricultural Research Service 62-18, United States Department of Agriculture, 1969.[43])

nutritionists should work. An adequate income, however, does not always insure good nutrition. In addition to working for social and economic reforms within the world, nutritionists must also work diligently as a group to improve the connotation of the term "nutrition" and at the same time attempt to prevent development of "food cults." Nutrition through the efforts of nutrition educators must come to denote an exciting science to the young receptive mind so that the youth of the world will grasp the significance of good nutrition and will turn some of their energy toward improving not only their own food intake but also that of the people around them.

6. REFERENCES

1. *Amer. J. Clin. Nutr.* 1967. Letter to the Editor, Riboflavin requirement of animal and man, related to protein requirement or energy turnover **20**:507-510.
2. Bro-Rasmussen, F. 1958. The riboflavin requirement of animals and man and associated metabolic relations, *Nutr. Abstr. and Rev.* **28**:1-23, 369-386.
3. Byerly, T. C. 1960. The effects of agricultural practices on the composition of foods. B. Foods of Animal Origin, *in:* "The Nutritional Evaluation of Food Processing," (R. S. Harris and H. Von Loesecke, eds.), pp. 43-47, John Wiley & Sons, Inc., New York.

4. Dimler, R. J., Altschul, A. M., Planck, R. W., Geddes, W. F., Stewart, R. A., and Liener, I. E. 1960. Effects of commercial processing of cereals on nutrient content, *in:* "The Nutritional Evaluation of Food Processing," (R. S. Harris and H. Von Loesecke, eds.), pp. 197-237, John Wiley & Sons, Inc., New York.

5. FAO Requirements of vitamin A, thiamin, riboflavin and niacin. Report of a joint FAO/WHO expert group. 1967. FAO Nutrition Meetings Report Series No. 41, World Health Organization Technical Report Series No. 362, Rome, Italy.

6. Feaster, J. F., Heid, J. L., Proctor, B. E., Goldblith, S. A., Deatherage, F. E., Hendel, C. E., and Fellers, C. R. 1960. Effects of commercial processing on the composition of fruits and vegetables, *in:* "The Nutritional Evaluation of Food Processing," (R. S. Harris and H. Von Loesecke, eds.), pp. 109-172, John Wiley & Sons, Inc., New York.

7. Fenton, F. 1960. Losses in nutrients during large-scale preparation for direct feeding, *in:* "The Nutritional Evaluation of Food Processing," (R. S. Harris and H. Von Loesecke, eds.), pp. 391-418, John Wiley & Sons, Inc., New York.

8. Food and Drug Administration, Department of Health, Education and Welfare. 1971. Proposed improvement of nutrient levels of enriched foods, *Federal Register* 36:23074, Dec. 3.

9. Food and Nutrition Board. 1943. "Recommended Dietary Allowances," Natl. Research Council Repr. & Circ. Series No. 115, Washington, D.C.

10. Food and Nutrition Board. 1945. "Recommended Dietary Allowances," Natl. Research Council Repr. & Circ. Series No. 122, rev. ed., Washington, D.C.

11. Food and Nutrition Board. 1948. "Recommended Dietary Allowances," Natl. Research Council Repr. & Circ. Series No. 128, rev. ed., Washington, D.C.

12. Food and Nutrition Board. 1953. "Recommended Dietary Allowances," Natl. Acad. Sci.-Natl. Research Council Pub. 302, rev. ed., Washington, D.C.

13. Food and Nutrition Board. 1958. "Recommended Dietary Allowances," Natl. Acad. Sci.-Natl. Research Council Pub. 589, rev. ed., Washington, D.C.

14. Food and Nutrition Board. 1964. "Recommended Dietary Allowances," Natl. Acad. Sci.-Natl. Research Council Pub. 1146, 6th rev. ed., Washington, D.C.

15. Food and Nutrition Board. 1968. "Recommended Dietary Allowances," Natl. Acad. Sci.-Natl. Research Council Pub. 1964, rev. ed., Washington, D.C.

15a. Food and Nutrition Board. 1974. "Recommended Dietary Allowances," Natl. Acad. Sci.—Natl. Research Council Publication, rev. ed., Washington, D.C.

16. Griswold, Ruth M. 1962. "The Experimental Study of Foods," pp. 317-321, Houghton Mifflin Co.,Boston.

17. Guggenheim, K., Brzezinski, A., Ilan, J., and Kallner, B. 1959. Nutritional evaluation of flour enrichment with riboflavin in Israel, *Amer. J. Clin. Nutr.* 7:526-531.

18. Holman, W. I. M. 1954. Biochemical investigations into the B-vitamin metabolism of children having the experimental diets, *in:* "Studies on the nutritive value of bread and on the effect of variations in the extraction rate of flour on the growth of undernourished children," (E. M. Widdowson and R. A. McCance, eds.), Medical Research Council Special Report Series No. 287, Appendix C, Her Majesty's Stationery Office, London.

19. Horwitt, M. K., Harvey, C. C., Wills, C. W., and Lichert, E. 1950. Correlation of urinary excretion of riboflavin with dietary intake and symptoms of ariboflavinosis, *J. Nutr.* 41:247-264.

20. Horwitt, M. K. 1966. Nutritional requirements of man with special reference to riboflavin, *Amer. J. Clin. Nutr.* 18:458-466.

21. Hytten, F. 1964. "Physiology of Human Pregnancy," Blackwell Scientific Publications, Oxford, England.

22. Jukes, T. H. 1971. Fact and fancy in nutrition and food science, *J. Amer. Diet Assoc.* **59**:203-211.

23. Keyes, A., Brozek, J., Henschel, A., Mickelsen O., and Taylor, H. L. 1950. "The Biology of Human Starvation," Vol. 1, University of Minnesota Press, Minneapolis.

24. Kleiber, M. 1932. Body size and metabolism, *Hilgardia* **6**:315-353.

25. Krehl, W. A., and Hodges, R. E. 1965. The interpretation of nutrition survey data, *Amer. J. Clin. Nutr.* **17**:191-199.

26. Lewis, J., Bunker, M. L., and Essien, R. 1972. A pilot study of the reliability of creatinine excretion of children as an index for comparison of urinary metabolites. *Federation Proc.* (Abstr.) **31**: (2):704.

27. McCance, R. A., and Strangeways, W. M. B. 1954. Protein metabolism and oxygen consumption during starvation in infants, young adults and old men, *Brit. J. Nutr.* **8**:21-32.

28. Mitchell, H. S., Rynbergen, H. J., Anderson, L., and Dibble, M. V. 1968. "Cooper's Nutrition in Health and Disease," 15th ed., p. 103, J. B. Lippincott Company, Philadelphia.

29. Morgan, A. F. 1960. Losses of nutrients in foods during home preparation, *in:* "The Nutritional Evaluation of Food Processing," (R. S. Harris and H. Von Loesecke, eds.), pp. 442-461, John Wiley & Sons, Inc., New York.

30. Morgan, A. F., Harris, R. S., and Levenberg, R. K. 1960. Losses of nutrients in foods during home preparation, *in:* "The Nutritional Evaluation of Food Processing." (R. S. Harris and H. Von Loesecke, eds.), pp. 442-491, John Wiley & Sons, Inc., New York.

31. Noble, I. 1970. Thiamine and riboflavin retention in cooked variety meats, *J. Am. Diet. Assoc.* **56**:225-228.

32. Oldham, H., *Johnston, F., Kleiger, S., and Hedderich-Arismendi, H. 1944. A study of the riboflavin and thiamine requirements of children of preschool age, J. Nutr.* **27**:435-446.

33. Oldham, H. G., Sheft, B. B., and Porter, T. 1950. Thiamine and riboflavin intakes and excretions during pregnancy, *J. Nutr.* **41**:231-245.

34. Pearson, W. N. 1962. Biochemical appraisal of nutritional status in man, *Amer. J. Clin. Nutr.* **11**:462-476.

35. Pearson, W. N. 1967. Blood and urinary vitamin levels as potential indices of body stores, *Amer. J. Clin. Nutr.* **20**:514-527.

36. Schweigert, B. S., and Lushbough, C. H. 1960. The effects of commercial processing on the nutrient composition of meat, poultry, and fish products, *in:* "The Nutritional Evaluation of Food Processing," (R. S. Harris and H. Von Loesecke, eds.), pp. 261-304, John Wiley & Sons, Inc., New York.

37. Sherman, H. C., and Lanford, C. S. 1940. "Essentials of Nutrition," The Macmillan Co., New York.

38. Siemers, G. F., and Block, R. J. 1960. Methods of increasing the nutritive value of foods, *in:* "The Nutritional Evaluation of Food Processing," (R. S. Harris and H. Von Loesecke, eds.), pp. 492-520, John Wiley & Sons, Inc., New York.

39. Snyderman, S. E., Ketran, K. C., Burch, H. B., Lowry, O. H., Bessey, O. A., Grey, L. P., and Holt, L. E., Jr. 1949. The minimum riboflavin requirement of the infant, *J. Nutr.* **39**:219-232.

40. Stearns, G., Adamson, L., McKinley, J. B., Linner, T., and Jeans, P. C. 1958. Excretion of thiamine and riboflavin by children. *Amer. J. Dis. Child.* **95**:185-201.

41. "Ten-State Nutrition Survey 1968-70." 1972. DHEW Publication No. (HSM) 72-8131.

42. United States Department of Agriculture, Agriculture Research Service. 1968. "Food

Consumption of Households in the United States, Spring 1965. Household Food Consumption, January 1965-66,'' Report No. 1, Washington, D.C.

43. United States Department of Agriculture. 1969. "Food Intake and Nutritive Value of Diets of Men, Women and Children in the United States, Spring 1965. A Preliminary Report,'' ARS 62-18, Washington, D.C.

44. United States Department of Agriculture, Economic Research Service. 1967. "Outlook Issue,'' National Food Situation, NFS-122, Washington, D.C.

45. Van Zante, H. J., and Johnson, S. K. 1970. Effect of electronic cookery on thiamine and riboflavin in buffered solutions, *J. Amer. Diet. Assoc.* **56**:133-135.

46. Wanner, R. L. 1960. Effects of commercial processing of milk and milk products on their nutrient content, *in:* "The Nutritional Evaluation of Food Processing,'' (R. S. Harris and H. Von Loesecke, eds.), pp. 173-196, John Wiley & Sons, Inc., New York.

47. Windmueller, H. G., Anderson, A. A., and Mickelson, O. 1964. Elevated riboflavin levels in urine of fasting human subjects, *Amer. J. Clin. Nutr.* **15**:73-76.

RIBOFLAVIN DEFICIENCY

Grace A. Goldsmith

1. RIBOFLAVIN DEFICIENCY IN ANIMALS

Riboflavin deficiency has been studied in many animal species and always results in failure to grow. This fact might be anticipated in view of the importance of flavoprotein enzymes in cellular metabolism. There have been reported a great variety of lesions, including changes in the skin, loss of hair, degenerative changes in the nervous system and liver, impaired reproduction, and congenital malformations in the offspring. Lesions of the cornea of the eye, cataract formation, and reduced formation of hemoglobin have also been reported. The specificity of some of these lesions has been questioned.

Changes in the skin have been observed in the rat, mouse, hamster, dog, pig, and monkey. In the rat[28,35] the fur becomes ragged, the hairs are of uneven length, the skin is scaly, and there is incrustation of red-brown material. Areas of alopecia may be observed. The lips are red and swollen and the filiform papillae of the tongue are abnormal. Other lesions in the rat include inflammation of the conjunctiva, blepharitis, corneal vascularization and opacity,[7] degeneration of nerve tissue,[63,111] a decrease in hemoglobin formation,[94] and cessation of the estrus cycle.[24] A number of features of riboflavin-deficient rats are illustrated in Figs. 1 and 2.

GRACE A. GOLDSMITH—School of Public Health and Tropical Medicine, Tulane University School of Medicine, New Orleans, Louisiana.

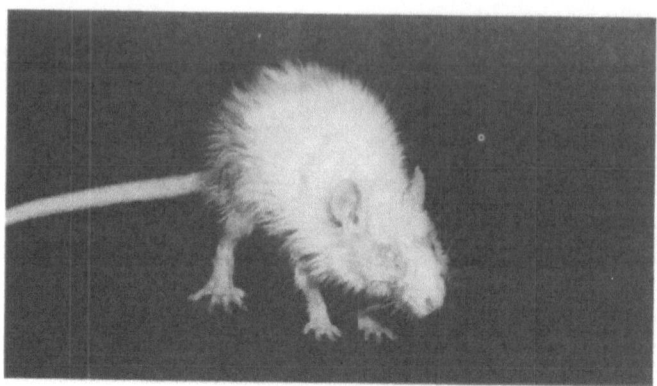

Fig. 1. Animal fed *ad libitum* on a diet deficient in riboflavin for a period of approximately 90 days starting at the time of weaning. (Photograph by E. Hajjar, Francis Delafield Hospital, New York, N.Y.)

Pathologic changes in the skin of rats that are deficient in riboflavin include moderate keratosis and atrophy of the sebaceous glands of the hair follicles.[28] Loss of hair is due to separation of the basal portion of the shaft from the anchoring cells. Lesions in the cornea were described in detail by Bessey and Wolbach.[7] The cornea becomes dull and the blood vessels proliferate extending from the limbus as an anastomosing plexus across the cornea. This plexus is superficial at first but later involves deeper layers. The pathogenesis of these findings is not clear. It has been suggested that the riboflavin in the eye is destroyed by light and vascularization is a compensatory phenomenon. Another hypothesis is that the lacrimal and meibomian glands, which are high in riboflavin, are affected first and that the cornea is involved secondarily through a diminution in the riboflavin content of these secretions. Neither hypothesis has been substantiated.[80]

Maternal riboflavin deficiency in the rat may result in abortion or in severe congenital malformations.[108] The skeleton is primarily affected, prominent findings being shortness of the mandible, cleft palate, shortness of the extremeties or tail, and syndactylism. Abnormalities may involve the teeth,[25] brain, and esophagus in mice.[53] In these studies injections of riboflavin were given to pregnant rats deficient in riboflavin.

Congenital anomalies due to maternal deficiency of riboflavin are not restricted to the skeletal system. Hydrocephalus, lesions of the eye, malformations of the heart, and hydronephrosis have been observed.[41,65] Fetal mortality is high in offspring of deficient animals. In animals that survive, body weights are lower than those of normal animals of the

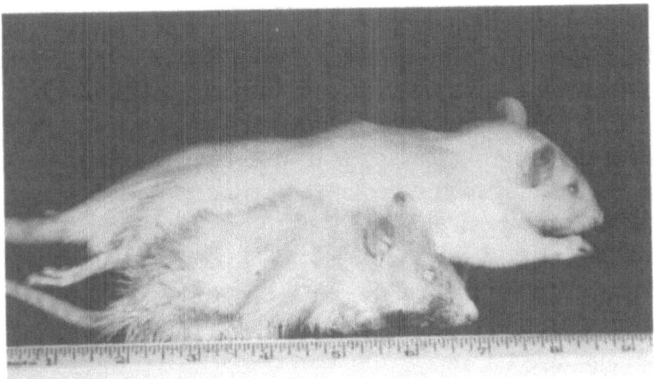

Fig. 2. Severely riboflavin-deficient adult male Holtzman rat shown with its littermate fed *ad libitum* a normal diet during the 90-day experimental period. (Photograph by E. Hajjar, Francis Delafield Hospital, New York, N.Y.)

same age. Biochemical studies of fetuses that developed during maternal riboflavin deficiency show markedly reduced hepatic concentrations of flavin mononucleotide (FMN), flavin adenine dinucleotide (FAD), and riboflavin.[70] It has been postulated that diminished concentrations of FAD, which result in diminished activity of electron transport systems during a critical period of gestation, may explain the pathogenesis of congenital malformations. The subject of congenital malformations due to riboflavin deficiency is discussed in greater detail in Chapter 9.

Riboflavin-deficient rats consume 15–20% more calories than are required by control animals to maintain the same weight.[64] This decrease in efficiency of food utilization may be due to incomplete oxidation of nutrients. Burch et al.[15] suggested that the decrease in flavin enzyme activities in riboflavin deficiency might affect the efficiency of oxidative phosphorylation. Available data did not indicate the precise enzymatic defects responsible for the decreased oxidative rate and lowered efficiency of phosphorylation.

In swine, riboflavin deficiency is characterized by retarded growth, dermatitis, diarrhea, incoordination, nerve degeneration, corneal opacities, and cataract formation.[111] Deficiency in cats results in fatty livers, hypoplasia of testes, cataract formation, and minor changes in the skin.[33]

In dogs, findings in deficiency include weight loss, weakness, and ataxia. As deficiency becomes more severe, there is inability to walk or to stand and spasticity of the extremities develops. Brachycardia, exaggerated sinus arrhythmia, and slow, deep respiration are noted. Coma then appears and the animal dies within 12 hr or sooner. This dramatic collapse is a late manifestation of deficiency and is preceded by dermatitis involving the chest, abdomen, and inner surfaces of the thighs and axillae. In males, the scrotum is characteristically involved.[89,98] Anemia has been reported, but this may have been due to deficiency of folic acid or some other factor. Riboflavin has been shown to be essential for hemoglobin regeneration in dogs that were fed synthetic diets and were subjected to bleeding over a prolonged period.[44]

Pathologic changes in the tissues of dogs that were riboflavin deficient have included fatty degeneration of the liver and, to a lesser extent, of the kidney[88]; atrophy of the bone marrow with an increase in fat content; nodular hemorrhagic areas in the lungs; and degeneration of the brain, spinal cord, and peripheral nerves.[88,89]

In young calves, findings of riboflavin deficiency include redness of the buccal mucosa, lesions at the corners of the mouth and edges of the lip, excessive salivation and lacrimation, and loss of hair.[109]

In chicks, mild riboflavin deficiency of long standing results in curled-toe paralysis, whereas severe deficiency leads to an acute paralysis and dystonia similar to that found in dogs.[82] The eggs of riboflavin-deficient chicks fail to hatch and the developing embryo shows numerous abnormalities.[23,27]

In the monkey, riboflavin deficiency results in loss of weight, a seborrheic scaling type of dermatitis, loss of hair, and incoordination of the limbs.[66] There is a reduction in hemoglobin and in leukocytes in the blood. The levels of riboflavin and its derivatives in plasma decrease markedly. Measurement of flavin adenine dinucleotide appears to be a useful indicator of deficiency. Histologic changes occur primarily in the endocrine system. The thyroid and adrenal glands show no evidence of secretory activity. The function of the gonads appears to be depressed, the liver shows an accumulation of fat, and the peripheral nerves are demyelinated.

The role of riboflavin deficiency in the production of anemia in animals has been uncertain. Anemia was reported in early studies of riboflavin deficiency in rats, mice, dogs, foxes, and swine.[68] In some of these species, subsequent studies suggested that lack of folic acid or vitamin B_{12} might have been responsible for the anemia observed.[33,105] Anemia has not been encountered in cats severely deficient in riboflavin,[33] or in guinea pigs maintained on a diet free of riboflavin for as long as 13 weeks.[45] However, baboons fed a diet free of riboflavin for 2-4 months had hemoglobin levels averaging 6.4 g/100 ml.[29] In contrast, the Cebus monkey, when fed a ration very low in riboflavin, showed no signs of anemia until just before death. This anemia appeared to be due to accompanying anorexia. The anemia in riboflavin-deficient monkeys reported earlier may have been due to folic acid deficiency.[68] Hematological aspects of riboflavin deficiency are discussed in Chapter 8.

In mice with riboflavin deficiency, the intraperitoneal injection of virulent pneumococci leads to more rapid death than does comparable injection in normal animals.[112] In riboflavin-deficient animals, the ability of the liver to inactivate estradiol is decreased.[92]

Riboflavin may have a role in experimental carcinogenesis. In riboflavin-deficient mice, growth of mammary cancer is retarded[75] and regression of lymphosarcoma has been observed.[97] Tumor formation induced by feeding butter-yellow, p-dimethylaminoazobenzine, is increased in animals on a diet low in riboflavin.[69] In one of the few studies related to tumor growth in man, administration of a deficient diet and a riboflavin analogue showed no clear-cut evidence of deficiency nor signs of tumor regression.[60] (See also Chapters 8 and 11.)

Little information is available relative to the manner in which riboflavin deficiency produces the pathologic changes that have been observed. Severely deficient animals may show sudden collapse which is probably due to failure of important enzyme systems.

2. METABOLIC EFFECTS OF RIBOFLAVIN DEFICIENCY

Riboflavin is converted in the body to two coenzymes, flavin mononucleotide (FMN) and flavin adenine dinucleotide (FAD).[26,62] Phosphorylation of riboflavin to flavin mononucleotide (riboflavin-5'-phosphate, or FMN) occurs in the intestinal mucosa.[52] It is not known whether this reaction is necessary for absorption of the vitamin. In riboflavin deficiency, the tissue concentrations of FMN and FAD decrease. In the liver, the activity of hepatic flavokinase also decreases by 50% or more.[85] This enzyme catalyzes conversion of riboflavin to FMN. Accordingly, in deficiency, there may be a decrease in enzymatic synthesis of FMN. The decrease in flavokinase activity may be due to instability of the enzyme in the absence of its substrate, riboflavin. The diminished activity of hepatic flavokinase and the reduced tissue concentrations of FMN do not appear to be related to a decrease in food intake in riboflavin-deficient animals.[85]

Concentrations of FMN are decreased proportionately more than concentrations of FAD, perhaps due to an increase in the activity of FAD pyrophosphorylase in riboflavin deficiency.[84] This is the hepatic enzyme that converts FMN to FAD. Rivlin has postulated that increased activity of hepatic FAD pyrophosphorylase may represent an adaptive mechanism for conserving FAD at the expense of FMN.[84] Many more enzymes require FAD than FMN as a coenzyme. Thus, this mechanism may permit riboflavin to be used for its most essential functions when the supply of the vitamin is limited.

The pattern of liver flavoprotein enzymes is influenced greatly by riboflavin deficiency. Activities of the FMN and FAD requiring enzymes are depressed in deficient animals. Certain enzymes are more sensitive than others to a decrease in the availability of their flavin coenzyme. Burch *et al.*[16] found the following order of sensitivity of hepatic enzymes to riboflavin deficiency in rats: glycolate oxidase, D-amino acid oxidase, glycine oxidase, xanthine oxidase, L-amino acid oxidase, and reduced diphosphopyridine nucleotide dehydrogenase. The decrease in glycolate oxidase and amino acid oxidase paralleled the reduction of FMN. The decrease in xanthine oxidase paralleled the reduction of FAD.

Rivlin[84] has shown that in hypothyroidism hepatic concentrations of FMN and FAD are reduced to about two-thirds of normal and the level of riboflavin to about one-third of normal. The decreased FMN and FAD levels may be attributed in large measure to reduced flavokinase activity. The hepatic profile of flavoprotein enzymes is remarkably similar in hypothyroidism and riboflavin deficiency. The most important site of thyroid hormone control of riboflavin metabolism appears to be the enzyme flavokinase that catalyzes the conversion of riboflavin to FMN. The activity of this enzyme is nearly doubled by administration of thyroid hormone. (See also Chapter 12.)

In the erythrocyte, two key flavoprotein enzymes, glutathione reductase and reduced nicotinamide adenine dinucleotide (NADH)-methemoglobin reductase, are affected by the status of riboflavin nutrition. The addition of FAD to *in vitro* assay of hemolyzed red blood cells of riboflavin-deficient rats augments glutathione reductase activity 200–300% as compared to augumentation of only 70% in hemolyzed cells from rats that have received a high riboflavin diet.[34]

In riboflavin-deficient animals, there is an increase in the weight of the liver in relation to body weight.[16] In riboflavin-deficient rats, the enlarged liver contained a markedly increased level of nitrogen per unit of body weight.[43] The content of fat may be increased,[99] and the glycogen content may also be increased.[19] The latter effect is associated with increased incorporation of alanine-1-^{14}C into glycogen, and increased activity of alanine transaminase.[17]

In rats deprived of riboflavin in which there was impairment of growth, hepatomegaly, and depletion of FAD and catalase in the liver, increased concentrations of glutamic-aspartic and glutamic-alanine transaminase were found in the liver.[72] With dietary depletion and repletion of protein, the transaminase levels followed changes in liver size. Since protein concentration in the liver was not affected, the level of transaminase was directly associated with the degree of anabolism. Earlier findings suggested some stimulation of the adrenal cortex in riboflavin deficiency, which may have a role in the control of glutamic-alanine transaminase in the liver.

In riboflavin-deficient rats, the incorporation of labeled serine into the liver microsomal fraction was less than in normal rats. Injection of riboflavin in deficient animals increased incorporation indicating a possible role of riboflavin in protein biosynthesis.[78]

A study of hepatic enzyme activity in riboflavin-depleted rats showed an increase followed by a decrease of succinate dehydrogenase activity, a progressive decrease in xanthine oxidase activity, and a progressive increase in the activity of alanine aminotransferase. No change in DNA was observed, but the RNA content of liver decreased progressively. The incorporation of amino acid into protein was studied *in vitro* in pH 5 enzyme microsomal fractions of rat liver. Reduced incorporation was observed which was partially overcome by the subcutaneous injection of riboflavin.[79]

The effect of heat on the stability of monoamine oxidase of rat liver mitochondria was decreased in riboflavin-deficient animals as compared to those supplemented with the vitamins.[76] In riboflavin-deficient rats, no changes in monoamine oxidase activity or in endogenous norepinephrine content were found in the brain.[61] In the heart, there was significantly increased norepinephrine content in association with a slight decrease in monoamine oxidase activity. If total heart weight was used as a reference point, the increase in norepinephrine content disappeared and the decrease in monoamine oxidase activity became significant. In the liver, there was a significant decrease in monoamine oxidase activity.

In riboflavin-deficient mice, the hepatic architecture is markedly changed. Electron microscopy shows that the mitochondria become very much enlarged and exhibit increases in the number and length of cristae.[103] The structure begins to return toward normal within a few hours after riboflavin administration. Whether the changes in morphology of the mitochondria are associated with diminution in function remains controversial. Several investigators have shown diminished efficiency of oxidative phosphorylation,[15,64] but this has not been observed by others.[10,31]

Hepatic concentrations of ribonucleic acid (RNA) and deoxyribonucleic acid (DNA) are essentially normal early in riboflavin deficiency but are depressed in later stages.[19] Concentrations of protein[71] and of pyridine nucleotides[15] in liver tend to be essentially normal.

Riboflavin deficiency affects amino acid metabolism. Tryptophan has been the amino acid studied most widely. An increased amount of xanthurenic acid is formed from tryptophan, and deficient rats excrete excessive amounts of anthranilic acid, another tryptophan metabolite, in the urine.[67] Some of the effects of riboflavin deficiency on tryptophan metabolism may be due to the diminished availability of pyridoxal phosphate. Riboflavin is needed for the conversion of pyridoxine phosphate to pyridoxal phosphate,[107] which in turn is required as a coenzyme in several steps in the degradation of tryptophan.

In weanling rats given diets containing casein, gluten, or gluten plus lysine, supplemented with either 100 μg or 10 μg riboflavin, values for FAD and total riboflavin in liver were found to be considerably less in animals fed gluten than in those fed casein. Free riboflavin and FMN in the liver of rats receiving gluten plus 10 μg riboflavin were greater than in animals fed casein or gluten plus lysine. Data indicated a significant interaction between dietary riboflavin and protein. Variations in riboflavin coenzymes in tissues suggested that supplementation of wheat gluten with lysine did not completely meet the demands of the tissues for essential amino acids.[56]

Riboflavin deficiency has an influence on free amino acid levels of tissue, particularly liver.[18] In pair-fed rats that received a 16% protein diet for 45 days, riboflavin deficiency increased free amino acid nitrogen concentration in liver, muscle, and plasma. The decreased oxidation of amino acids, which may result in an increase of the free amino acid pool, may enhance hepatic gluconeogenesis. It was postulated that in addition to accumulation of free amino acids in liver due to decreased oxidation, mobilization of amino acids from breakdown of peripheral tissue proteins occurred.

A decrease of energy or protein intake in chicks decreased riboflavin requirement under restricted feeding regimens.[20] In severe riboflavin deficiency, efficiency of utilization of both energy and protein was decreased significantly under *ad libitum* conditions of feeding. Neither energy nor protein utilization was affected by riboflavin deficiency when both energy and protein were restricted to 70% of that consumed by chicks fed *ad libitum*.

A number of abnormalities of lipid metabolism are found in riboflavin deficiency. The livers of animals have a marked increase in triglyceride content.[99] Dehydrogenation of fatty acids is reduced and, accordingly, the concentrations of linoleic, linolenic, and arachidonic acids in serum and liver are decreased.[71] These effects occur only in advanced deficiency states.

Tissues of riboflavin-deficient rats were found to have higher amounts of trienoic acid and a significantly higher trienoic to tetraenoic acid ratio than tissues of control rats fed either *ad libitum* or pair-fed with riboflavin-deficient animals.[11] The ratio of trienoic to tetraenoic fatty acids observed in the lipids of liver and heart of riboflavin-deficient rats were similar to that found in rats with essential fatty acid deficiency.

In a study of linoleate utilization in rats depleted of riboflavin and essential fatty acids, supplementation with riboflavin and linoleate (as safflower oil) produced no greater increase in liver phospholipid arachidonate than did supplementation with safflower oil alone.[110] Accordingly, riboflavin appeared to have no effect on arachidonate level.

The polyunsaturated fatty acid composition of liver lipids was studied in rats fed a diet deficient in riboflavin, essential fatty acids, or both.[12] In all three groups of animals, there was an increase in the ratio of trienoic to tetraenoic fatty acids in the liver. Increase in riboflavin intake in each of these groups of animals was not effective in correcting the biochemical lesion of essential fatty acid deficiency.

Albino rats fed a high cholesterol diet for 12 weeks showed appreciable depletion of riboflavin and choline in the liver and in blood.[6] Administration of massive doses of riboflavin and choline prevented the depletion of these vitamins from the tissues and exerted a cholesterol-lowering effect in the liver and blood. It was suggested that the high cholesterol diet might increase the requirement of riboflavin.

Riboflavin deficiency was found to have an effect on the metabolism of oxypurines in chicks.[21] In chicks that were fed a riboflavin-deficient diet for 3 weeks and exhibited depressed growth and a high incidence of curled-toe paralysis, the precursors of uric acid—hypoxanthine or xanthine—accumulated in the liver and kidney. These observations showed that dietary riboflavin, which is incorporated into xanthine dehydrogenase, is essential for oxypurine metabolism. The uric acid concentration in plasma of deficient chicks was low, suggesting a disturbance of uric acid synthesis in the liver and kidney.

Riboflavin deficiency made the Wistar rat susceptible to the formation of stress-induced gastric ulcers.[54] The stress procedure was innocuous for the well-nourished rat. The administration of riboflavin protected the rat from these lesions. General inanition played only a minor role in the susceptibility.

Chronic ethanol ingestion in the rat was found to prevent the fatty liver observed in riboflavin deficiency and to diminish the fall in succinic dehydrogenase activity induced by riboflavin deficiency.[32]

An interesting observation is that in growing organisms the requirement for riboflavin to saturate the tissues approximates 700 μg/1000 cal.[68] This requirement appears to be uniform for species ranging from mice to calves and horses. Animal experiments have suggested that excess carbohydrate reduces riboflavin requirement and, conversely, excess fat increases the need for this vitamin. Bro-Rasmussen[14] states that these findings apply only to animals such as dogs and poultry where the intestinal flora has little effect on riboflavin requirement. For other animals, for example, the rat and the cat, intestinal synthesis of riboflavin may be markedly influenced by the composition of the diet. Synthesis, in turn, may influence the animal's requirement for riboflavin.

3. RIBOFLAVIN DEFICIENCY IN MAN

Riboflavin deficiency in man is due to an inadequate dietary intake of the vitamin or to some conditioning factor that increases requirement or impairs absorption or utilization. Intake of riboflavin must be low for many months before symptoms become evident. Signs of deficiency are more common during periods of physiologic or pathologic stress. They may appear when growth is rapid in childhood or during pregnancy and lactation.[42] Deficiency may occur as a result of trauma, including burns and surgical procedures, and has been observed frequently in a number of chronic debilitating diseases such as long continued fevers, e.g., rheumatic fever, tuberculosis, and subacute bacterial endocarditis; chronic congestive heart failure; hyperthyroidism; and malignancy.[39] Malabsorption may occur in chronic diarrheal disorders or after operations on the gastrointestinal tract. In cirrhosis of the liver, riboflavin deficiency may occur possibly due, in part, to poor utilization of the vitamin.

A relationship has been observed between the retention of riboflavin and the retention of protein. When protein is broken down, negative nitrogen balance occurs and there may be an increase in excretion of riboflavin in the urine.[37,83,93] This fact has been reported in acute starvation, uncontrolled diabetes mellitus, and post trauma. However, considerable evidence suggests that there is no constant relationship between urinary riboflavin and nitrogen excretion.[68] A breakdown of riboflavin coenzymes has been found in man when in shock.[77]

Riboflavin deficiency is seen frequently in association with pellagra and for many years the lesions of riboflavin deficiency were considered to be part of the pellagra syndrome. Deficiency has been observed, often, in hospitalized patients[40] and has been encountered in nutrition surveys both in this country and in other parts of the world.[3,40,49,81,104]

3.1. Clinical Aspects of Riboflavin Deficiency

3.1.1. Experimental Human Deficiency

Riboflavin deficiency was not recognized as a clinical entity until it was induced experimentally in human subjects by Sebrell and Butler in 1938.[90,91] The diet, which furnished 0.55 mg riboflavin daily, was similar to one used by Goldberger and Tanner in studies of pellagra in 1925.[36] Deficiency developed between day 94 and day 130 in 13 of 18 subjects. Clinical findings consisted of lesions of the lips and of angles of the mouth and a seborrheic type of dermatitis. The lips became red and denuded along the line of closure. Maceration and fissures developed at the angles of the mouth. The dermatitis involved the nasolabial folds, the alae nasi, the vestibule of the nose, and occasionally the ears and skin around the eyelids, especially the inner and outer canthi. The lesions disappeared following the administration of riboflavin.

These clinical findings were similar to those reported by Stannus in association with pellagra in Nyasaland in 1912.[96] Similar findings have been reported from various parts of the world: Ceylon,[5] Jamaica,[87] West Africa,[73,74] Singapore,[57] South India,[34] and Malaya.[57] Most observers believed that the lesions were on the basis of a dietary deficiency since they could be cured by administration of the vitamin B complex. Goldberger and Tanner[36] reported comparable findings in the United States.

Experimental deficiency was induced in 1948 by Horwitt and his associates.[48] Male subjects were given diets that supplied 0.55 mg riboflavin per day. Signs of deficiency appeared in less than 6 months. Findings included angular stomatitis, seborrheic dermatitis involving the scrotum, and, in a few subjects, diminution in the ability to perceive flicker. Horwitt suggested that the type of lesion encountered may be dependent on trauma, irritation, infection, or other injury to which tissues are subjected, because riboflavin is needed for normal tissue repair.

Since these early experimental studies, clinical and therapeutic investigations have suggested that a number of other signs and symptoms may result from lack of riboflavin. Sydenstricker and associates[101] and Spies *et al.*[95] reported ocular signs and symptoms that were cured by administration of riboflavin. Jolliffe and co-workers[51] described a magenta color of the tongue that was thought to be characteristic of deficiency of this vitamin. While ocular pathology and glossitis are seen in patients with riboflavin deficiency, they are not constant findings. Specificity of the eye lesions is a subject of controversy. Current evidence indicates that, while eye changes may occur in riboflavin deficiency, comparable abnormalities may be found in a number of other conditions including infection, trauma, and deficiency of dietary substances other than riboflavin.

Experimental production of riboflavin deficiency with analogues of riboflavin has clarified some of the clinical features of the deficiency state. Lane *et al.*[59] found that sore throat and angular stomatitis were usually the first findings to appear. Subsequently, they noted glossitis, seborrheic dermatitis of the face, and dermatitis over the trunk and extremities, followed by anemia and neuropathy. The anemia was normocytic and normochromic and was associated with diminished reticulocytosis and red-cell hypoplasia of the bone marrow. [1,58] Incorporation of radioactive iron into erythrocytes was decreased. [50] (See Chapter 8.)

Anemia in riboflavin deficiency may be related to disturbances in folic acid metabolism. Hepatic and serum levels of folic acid decrease,[13,46,70] and conversion of folic acid[30] to ^5N-methyltetrahydrofolic acid is impaired. [46] The abnormalities of folic acid metabolism are probably due to diminished activities of flavoprotein enzymes that are required for utilization of folic acid. [70]

3.1.2. Endemic Riboflavin Deficiency

Early symptoms of ariboflavinosis are soreness and burning of the lips, mouth, and tongue, with exaggeration of discomfort on eating highly seasoned foods. Visual symptoms have been described, also, including photophobia, lacrimation, burning and itching of the eyes, visual fatigue, and dimness of vision not related to errors of refraction. [100]

The objective signs of riboflavin deficiency include cheilosis, angular stomatitis, seborrheic dermatitis, glossitis, and superficial vascularization of the cornea (Figs. 3-7). [51,95,101,102] Lesions of the lips may begin with redness and denudation along the line of closure, or the first abnormality may be pallor and maceration at the angles of the mouth. The lips may become dry and chapped, with shallow ulcerations or crusting. As lesions of the angles of the mouth progress, fissures may extend out from the buccal mucous membrane for a centimeter or more. These fissures may be covered with yellow crusts. After healing occurs, scars may remain at the angles of the mouth and the lips may become atrophic. The lesions at the angles of the mouth have been designated angular stomatitis, or perleche in the older literature (Fig. 6). The lesions of the lips are termed cheilosis (Fig. 5).

All of the changes described above were considered to be specific evidence of riboflavin deficiency at one time, but it has been shown

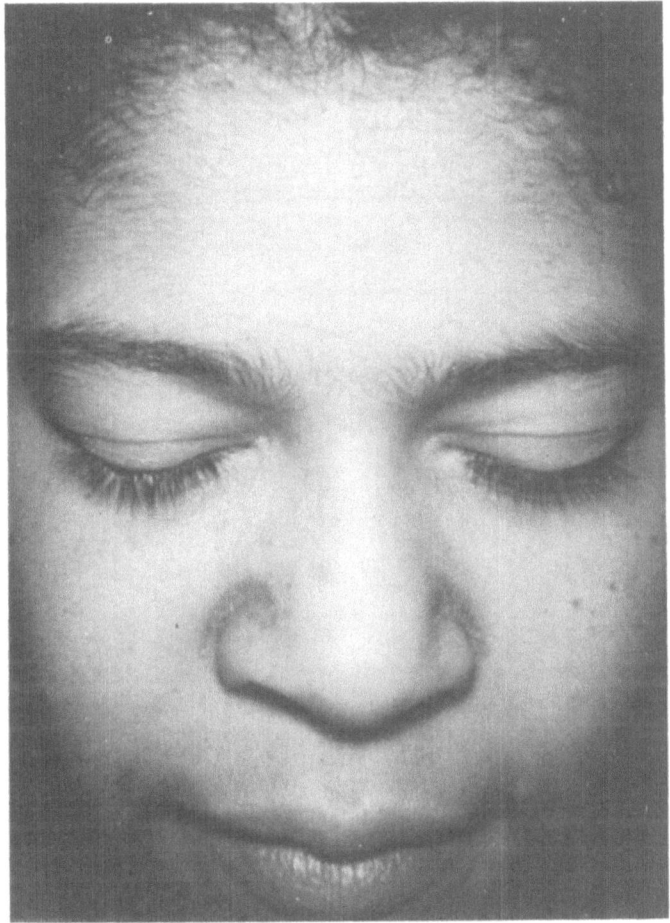

Fig. 3. Seborrheic dermatitis due to riboflavin deficiency.

subsequently that similar lesions may be the result of a deficiency of niacin[38] or iron, or that they follow the administration of the pyridoxine antagonist deoxypyridoxine. Occasionally, changes at the angles of the mouth are observed in persons with malocclusion or are the result of poorly fitting dentures. Cheilosis may develop due to wind, cold, or trauma or may be the result of allergy.

The seborrheic dermatitis of riboflavin deficiency is found in the nasolabial and nasomalar folds (Fig. 3), the alae nasi, the vestibule of the nose, or around the outer and inner canthi of the eyes and on the ears. It is characterized by a red, scaly, greasy appearance. Hard

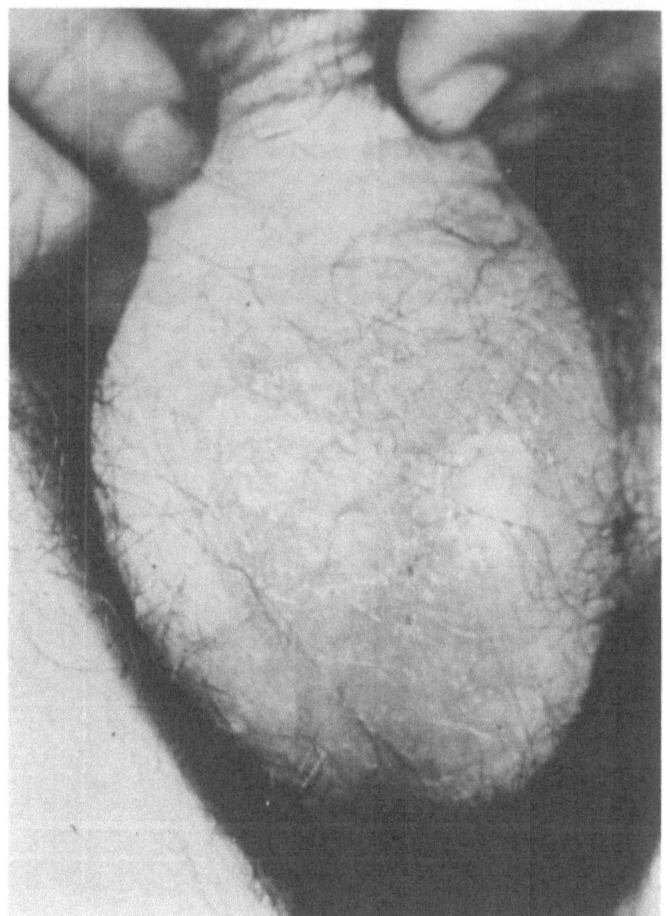

Fig. 4. Scrotal dermatitis due to riboflavin deficiency. (Courtesy of M. K. Horwitt.)

sebaceous plugs or fine filiform comidones may be seen over the bridge of the nose, on the malar prominences, and on the chin. Dermatitis may involve the scrotum and vulva. Characteristically, there is redness, scaling, and desquamation of the superficial skin, which in some instances becomes raw and weeps (Fig. 4).[48] Lesions may extend to adjacent areas of the thigh.

In riboflavin deficiency, the tongue may become purplish red or magenta in color.[51] The papillae may be swollen, flattened, or mushroom-shaped, resulting in a pebbled appearance, or they may become

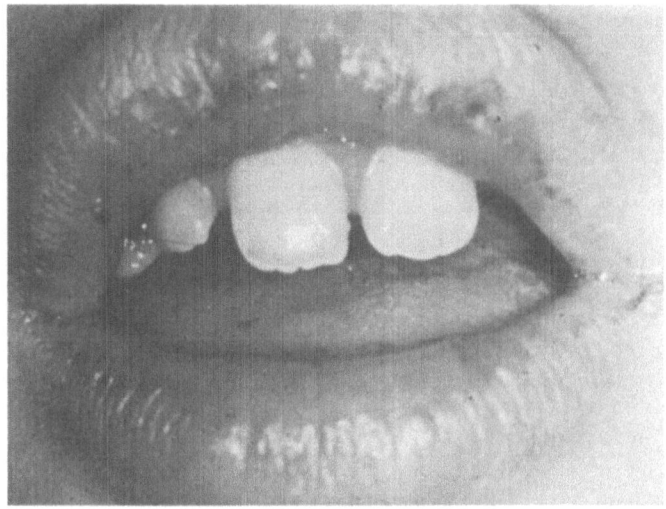

Fig. 5. Cheilosis and angular stomatitis of riboflavin deficiency.

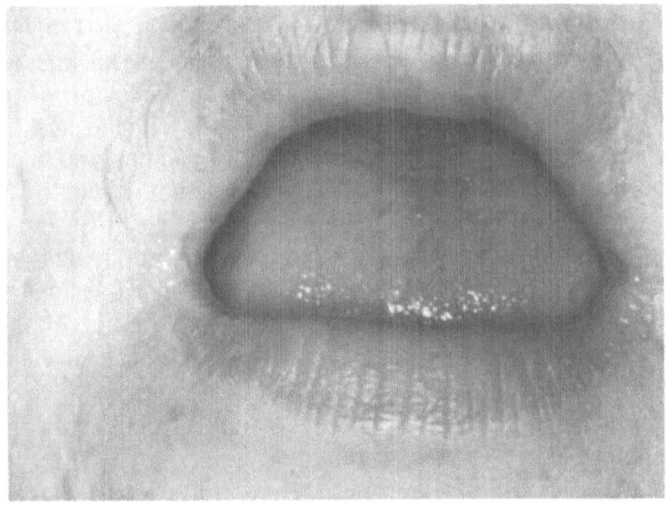

Fig. 6. Angular stomatitis of riboflavin deficiency.

atrophic (Fig. 7). At times, the tongue is deeply fissured. It is often impossible, by observation alone, to differentiate the appearance of the tongue in riboflavin deficiency from that due to deficiency of several other B vitamins, namely, niacin, folic acid, or vitamin B_{12}.

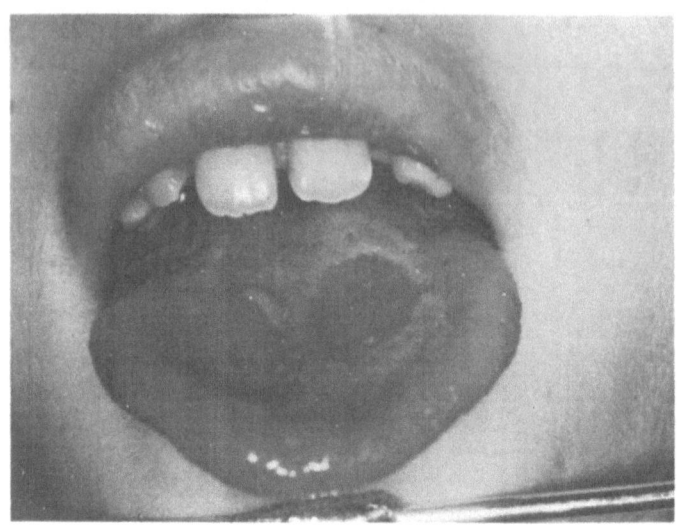

Fig. 7. Glossitis due to riboflavin deficiency.

The eye lesions consist of injection and proliferation of the limbic plexus surrounding the cornea and can be seen at first only with a slit lamp or hand lens.[101] Subsequently, circumcorneal injection may be visible without magnification. Capillaries of the limbic plexus proliferate and extend into the superficial layers of the cornea, anastomosing to form tiers of loops. Superficial punctate opacities and ulcerations of the cornea may develop. These can be demonstrated by staining the eye with fluorescein. The conjunctiva may become diffusely inflamed and the eyelids red, swollen, and matted together with a sticky exudate. Photophobia may be intense. Improvement of ocular lesions has not occurred in all instances following administration of riboflavin. In several studies, no correlation was observed between corneal vascularization and dietary intake of riboflavin. Evidence suggests, however, that riboflavin deficiency can cause vascularization of the cornea, in which instance response to treatment is rapid.[101]

In children with ariboflavinosis, retarded intellectual development and electroencephalographic changes have been reported.[2]

3.2. Diagnosis of Riboflavin Deficiency

A diagnosis of riboflavin deficiency can be made only by correlating dietary, clinical, and laboratory findings, since there are no pathognomonic signs of this disorder. The presence of several of the characteristic clinical features and a history of a dietary intake of less than 0.6 mg daily over a prolonged period strongly suggest deficiency. Biochemical tests can be of considerable assistance in corroborating the diagnosis.

When the diet includes less than 0.6 mg of riboflavin per day, 24-hr urine excretion is usually below 50 μg.[48] Excretion can be measured in relation to the output of creatinine in random specimens of urine. An excretion of less than 27 μg riboflavin/g creatinine has been suggested as indicative of deficiency, while an excretion of 27-79 μg is considered low.[106] Administration of a 1.0-mg test dose of riboflavin subcutaneously with measurement of excretion in the urine for 4 hr thereafter is useful in estimation of tissue stores of the vitamin. In experimental riboflavin deficiency, excretion in 4 hr was 19 μg after 4-8 months on the restricted diet.[47,48] In persons receiving 0.7-1.1 μg riboflavin daily, the 4-hr excretion varied from 56 to 81 μg. In subjects receiving 1.6 mg riboflavin daily, the average excretion was 235 μg. (See also Chapter 2.)

Consolazio *et al.*[22] suggested that the urinary excretion of riboflavin appears to be dependent upon many factors including the daily intake of the vitamin and also of protein, and the subsequent level of nitrogen balance and protein catabolism. An elevated excretion of riboflavin is indicative of adequate reserves, or catabolism of body protein for use as energy, or both.

The tetracylines affect nitrogen and riboflavin metabolism and bring about negative nitrogen balance and increased riboflavin excretion in the urine.[55] The mechanisms responsible for these effects can only be hypothesized. Tetracycline antibiotics have been shown to inhibit oxidative phosphorylation in the mitochondria of animal tissues.

Measurement of concentrations of free riboflavin, flavin mononucleotide, and flavin adenine dinucleotide in plasma or of riboflavin content of white blood cells or erythrocytes are not of much assistance in the diagnosis of deficiency in man. In some subjects but not all, free riboflavin and FMN decrease in plasma in riboflavin deficiency. No change has been reported in the riboflavin content of white blood cells or in FAD in plasma, but the tests have not been explored adequately. Red cell concentrations of riboflavin decrease when dietary intake is restricted, and levels of less than 14μg/100 ml may be indicative of potential deficiency.[8]

Recently, activity of the enzyme erythrocyte glutathione reductase and the magnitude of increase in activity of the enzyme after ingestion of riboflavin have been shown to correlate with the dietary intake of the vitamin.[9] Augmentation of enzyme activity by riboflavin is greatest in patients whose intake has been least adequate. This test appears to be a useful method of evaluating the status of riboflavin nutrition[86] and should be investigated further.

3.3. Prevention and Treatment of Riboflavin Deficiency

Riboflavin deficiency has not occurred in adult subjects who have received 0.8–0.9 mg of the vitamin daily. However, larger amounts of riboflavin than this are needed for saturation of body stores. The best food sources of riboflavin are milk, liver, meat, eggs, and some of the yellow and leafy green vegetables. Cereal and bread contain very little of this vitamin, but the enrichment of flour, bread, and certain cereals with riboflavin has contributed significantly to the dietary supply.

In the treatment of riboflavin deficiency, the vitamin should be administered in amounts of 5 mg, two or three times daily. Oral administration is satisfactory except in an occasional patient where there are abnormalities of absorption. In persons who receive parenteral feeding, riboflavin should always be included in the formula. Lesions of riboflavin deficiency heal rapidly, requiring only a few days to a few weeks for a return to normal.

Riboflavin deficiency is a common condition in many parts of the world, but the disease appears to cause rather minor problems. This is surprising since severe abnormalities and sudden collapse are encountered in animals. In view of the importance of riboflavin in cellular metabolism, it might have been anticipated that severe deficiency in man would result in death, but this has not been reported. It may be speculated either that riboflavin is conserved well by the body or that diets dangerously low in this vitamin are not encountered. The true prevalence of the deficiency state and its effects upon health require further study.

4. REFERENCES

1. Alfrey, C. P., Jr., and Lane, M. 1970. The effect of riboflavin deficiency on erythropoiesis, *Seminars Hemat.* 7:49–54.
2. Arakawa, T., Mizuno, T., Chiba, F., Sakai, K., Watanabe, S., and Tamura, T. 1968. Frequency analysis of electroencephalograms and latency of photically induced, average evoked responses in children with ariboflavinosis, *Tohoku J. Exptl. Med.* 94:327–335.

3. Aykroyd, W. R., Jolliffe, N., Lowry, O. H., Moore, P. E., Sebrell, W. H., Shank, R. E., Tisdall, F. F., Wilder, R. M., and Zamecnik, P. E. 1949. Medical resurvey of nutrition in Newfoundland 1948. *Canad. Med. Assn. J.* **60**:329-352.

4. Aykroyd, W. R., and Krishnan, B. G. 1936. Stomatitis due to vitamin B_2 deficiency, *Indian J. Med. Res.* **24**:411-417.

5. Bahr, P. H. 1915. "A report on researches on sprue in Ceylon, 1912-1914," p. 165, Cambridge University Press, Cambridge, England.

6. Banerjee, B., and Chakrabarti, C. H. 1970. Effect of high cholesterol diet on tissue levels of riboflavin and choline, *J. Vitaminol.* **16**:235-236.

7. Bessey, O. A., and Wolbach, S. B. 1939. Vascularization of the cornea of the rat in riboflavin deficiency, with a note on corneal vascularization in vitamin A deficiency, *J. Exptl. Med.* **69**:1-12.

8. Bessey, O. A., Horwitt, M. K., and Love, R. H. 1956. Dietary deprivation of riboflavin and blood riboflavin levels in man, *J. Nutr.* **58**:367-383.

9. Beutler, E. 1969. Effect of flavin compounds on glutathione reductase activity: *in vivo* and *in vitro* studies, *J. Clin. Invest.* **48**:1957-1966.

10. Beyer, R. E., Lamberg, S. L., and Neyman, M. A. 1961. The effect of riboflavin deficiency and galactoflavin feeding on oxidative phosphorylation and related reactions in rat liver mitochondria, *Canad. J. Biochem.* **39**:73-88.

11. Bhat, K. S., and Belavady, B. 1967. Polyunsaturated fatty acid levels in liver and heart of riboflavin deficient rats, *Indian J. Biochem.* **4**:38-40.

12. Bhat, K. S., and Belavady, B. 1970. Effects of riboflavin deficiency and realimentation on essential fatty acid nutritional status of rats, *Indian J. Biochem.* **7**:178-180.

13. Bovina, C., Landi, L., Pasquali, P., and Marchetti, M. 1969. Biosynthesis of folate coenzymes in riboflavin-deficient rats, *J. Nutr.* **99**:320-324.

14. Bro-Rasmussen, F. 1958. The riboflavin requirement of animals and man and associated metabolic relations. Part II: Relation of requirement to the metabolism of protein energy, *Nutr. Abst. Rev.* **28**:369-386.

15. Burch, H. B., Hunter, F. E., Jr., Combs, A. M., and Schutz, B. A. 1960. Oxidative enzymes and phosphorylation in hepatic mitochondria from riboflavin-deficient rats, *J. Biol. Chem.* **235**:1540-1544.

16. Burch, H. B., Lowry, O. H., Padilla, A. M., and Combs, A. M. 1956. Effects of riboflavin deficiency and realimentation on flavin enzymes of tissues, *J. Biol. Chem.* **223**:29-45.

17. Chatterjee, A. K., and Ghosh, B. B. 1967. Effect of riboflavin deficiency on *in vivo* incorporation of C_{14} labelled alanine into liver glycogen, *Experientia* **23**:633-634.

18. Chatterjee, A. K., and Ghosh, B. B. 1968. Effect of riboflavin deficiency on free amino acid nitrogen concentrations of liver, muscle and plasma, *Experientia* **24**:786-787.

19. Chatterjee, A. K., Roy, A. K., and Ghosh, B. B. 1969. Effect of riboflavin deficiency on nucleic acid metabolism of liver in the rat, *Brit. J. Nutr.* **23**:657-663.

20. Chou, S. T., Sell, J. L., and Kondra, P. A. 1971. Interrelationships between riboflavin and dietary energy and protein utilization in growing chicks, *Brit. J. Nutr.* **26**:323-333.

21. Chou, S. T. Effect of riboflavin deficiency on the metabolism of oxypurines in chicks. 1971. *Canad. J. Physiol. Pharmacol.* **49**:1059-1062.

22. Consolazio, C. F., Johnson, H. L., Krzywicki, H. J., Daws, T. A., and Barnhart, R. A. 1971. Thiamin, riboflavin and pyridoxine excretion during acute starvation and calorie restriction, *Amer. J. Clin. Nutr.* **24**:1060-1067.

23. Cowan, J. N., Boucher, R. V., and Buss, E. G. 1961. Physiological characteristics associated with mutant gene in chicken that causes deficiency of riboflavin 4. The effect of estrogen, *Poultry Science* **40**:1390.

24. Coward, K. H., and Morgan, B. C. E. 1941. The determination of vitamin B by means of its influence on the vaginal contents of the rat, *Biochem. J.* **35**:974.
25. Deuschle, F. M., Takacs, E., and Warkany, J. 1961. Postnatal dentofacial changes induced in rats by prenatal riboflavin deficiency, *J. Dental Res.* **40**:366-377.
26. Dixon, M., and Webb, E. C. 1964. "Enzymes," 2d ed., pp. 405-410, Academic Press, New York.
27. Engel, R. W., Phillips, P. H., and Halpin, J. G. 1940. The effect of a riboflavin deficiency in the hen upon embryonic development of the chick, *Poultry Science* **19**:135.
28. Follis, R. H., 1948. "The Pathology of Nutritional Diseases," Part IV, p. 159, Charles C Thomas, Springfield, Ill.
29. Foy, H., Kondi, A., and Mbaya, V. 1964. Effect of riboflavin deficiency on bone marrow function and protein metabolism in baboons, Preliminary Report, *Brit. J. Nutr.* **18**:307-318.
30. Foy, H., and Mbaya, V. 1966. Serum vitamin B_{12} and folate levels in normal and riboflavin-deficient baboons (papio anubis), *Brit. J. Haemat.* **12**:239-245.
31. Frei, J., and Ryser, H. 1956. Relations entre oxydation phosphorylante et structure des mitochondries hepatiques de rats carences en vitamintes B et B_2, *Experientia* **12**:105-107.
32. French, S. W. 1966. Effect of chronic ethanol ingestion on liver enzyme changes induced by thiamine, riboflavin, pyridoxine, or choline deficiency, *J. Nutr.* **88**:291-302.
33. Gershoff, S. N., Andrus, S. B., and Hegsted, D. M. 1959. The effect of the carbohydrate and fat content of the diet upon the riboflavin requirement of the cat, *J. Nutr.* **68**:75-88.
34. Glatzle, D., Weber, F., and Wiss, O. 1968. Enzymatic test for the detection of a riboflavin deficiency, NADPH-dependent glutathione reductase of red blood cells and its activation by FAD *in vitro, Experientia* **24**:1122.
35. Goldberger, J., and Lillie, R. D. 1926. A note on an experimental pellagralike condition in the Albino Rat, *U.S. Pub. Health Rept.* **41**:1025.
36. Goldberger, J., and Tanner, W. F. 1925. A study of pellagra-prevention action of dried beans, casein, dried milk, and brewers yeast, with a consideration of the essential preventive factors involved, *U.S. Pub. Health Rept.* **40**:54-80.
37. Goldsmith, G. A. 1964. The B vitamins: thiamine, riboflavin, niacin. Nutrition: A Comprehensive Treatise, *in* "Vitamins, Nutrient Requirements, and Food Selection" (G. H. Beaton and E. W. McHenry, eds.), Vol. 2, pp. 153-154, Academic Press, New York.
38. Goldsmith, G. A. 1956. Experimental niacin deficiency in man, *J. Amer. Diet. Assoc.* **32**:312.
39. Goldsmith, G. A. 1943. Incidence and recognition of riboflavin and niacin deficiency in medical diseases, *Southern Med. J.* **36**:108-116 (February).
40. Goldsmith, G. A. 1945. Nutrition studies in the New Orleans area, *Fed. Proc.* **4**:263-268 (September).
41. Grainger, R. B., O'Dell, B. L., and Hogan, A. G. 1954. Congenital malformations as related to deficiencies of riboflavin and vitamin B_{12} source of protein, calcium to phosphorus ratio and skeletal phosphorus metabolism, *J. Nutr.* **54**:33-48.
42. Guggenheim, K., Brzezinski, A., Ilan, J., and Kallner, B. 1959. Nutritional evaluation of flour enrichment with riboflavin in Israel. *Amer. J. Clin. Nutr.* **7**:526-531.
43. Guggenheim, K., and Diamant, E. J. 1959. Body composition of rats in B-vitamin deficiencies, *Brit. J. Nutr.* **13**:61-67.
44. György, P., Robscheit-Robbins, F. S., and Whipple, G. H. 1938. Lactoflavin

(riboflavin) increases hemoglobin production in the anemia dog, *Amer. J. Physiol.* 122:154.

45. Hara, H. 1960. Pathologic study on riboflavin deficiency in guinea pigs, *J. Vitaminol. (Kyoto)* 6:24-42.

46. Honda, Y. 1968. Folate derivatives in the liver of riboflavin-deficient rats, *Tohoku J. Exptl. Med.* 95:79-86.

47. Horwitt, M. K., Harvey, C. C., Hills, O. W., and Liebert, E. 1950. Correlation of urinary excretion of riboflavin with dietary intake and symptoms of ariboflavinosis, *J. Nutr.* 41:247-264.

48. Horwitt, M. K., Liebert, E., Kreider, O., and Wittman, P. 1948. Investigations of human requirements for B-complex vitamins, *Bull. Natl. Res. Council*, No. 116.

49. Hou, H. C. 1949. Nutritional diseases in China, *Nutrition Rev.* 7:193-195.

50. Jamdar, S. C., Udupa, K. R., and Chatterji, A. 1968. Study of hematopoiesis in riboflavin deficient rats with ^{59}Fe as tracer, *J. Vitamin (Osaka)* 14:219-222.

51. Jolliffe, N., Fein, H. D., and Rosenblum, L. A. 1939. Riboflavin deficiency in man, *New Eng. J. Med.* 221:921-926.

52. Jusko, W. J., and Levy, G. 1967. Absorption, metabolism and excretion of riboflavin-5'-phosphate in man, *J. Pharm. Sci.* 56:58-62.

53. Kalter, H. 1959. Congenital malformations induced by riboflavin deficiency in strains of inbred mice, *Pediatrics* 23:222-230.

54. Kim, Y. S., and Lambooy, J. P. 1967. Riboflavin deficiency and gastric ulcer production in the rat: a procedure for the study of susceptibility to stress-induced gastric ulcers, *J. Nutr.* 91:183-188.

55. Kunin, C. M., and Finland, M. 1961. Clinical pharmacology of the tetracycline antibiotics, *Clin. Pharmacol. Ther.* 2:51-69.

56. Lakhanpal, R. K., Harrill, I., and Bowman, F. 1969. Effect of protein and riboflavin on plasma amino acids and hepatic riboflavin-coenzymes, *J. Nutr.* 99:497-501.

57. Landor, J. V., and Pallister, R. A. 1935. Avitaminosis B2, *Trans. Roy. Soc. Trop. Med. Hyg.*, 29:121-134.

58. Lane, M., and Alfrey, C. P., Jr. 1965. The anemia of human riboflavin deficiency, *Blood* 25:432-442.

59. Lane, M., Alfrey, C. P., Jr., Mengel, C. E., Doherty, M. A., and Doherty, J. 1964. The rapid induction of human riboflavin deficiency with galactoflavin, *J. Clin. Invest.* 43:357-373.

60. Lane, M., Fahey, J. L., Sullivan, R. D., and Zubrod, C. G. 1958. The comparative pharmacology in man and the rat of the riboflavin analogue 6,7-dimethyl-9-(2'-acetoxy-ethyl)-isoalloxazine, U-2112, *J. Pharmacol. Exptl. Ther.* 122:315-326.

61. Leodolter, S., and Genner, M. 1971. Monoamine oxidase activity and norepinephrine content of organs from rats fed on a vitamin B_2-deficient diet, *Arch. intern. de Pharmacodynamie et de Therapie.* 190:393-401.

62. Lipmann, F. 1969. The biochemical function of B vitamins, *Perspect. Biol. Med.* 13:1-9.

63. Lippincott, S. W., and Morris, H. P. 1941. Morphologic changes associated with pathothenic acid deficiency in the mouse, *J. Natl. Cancer Inst.* 2:39-46.

64. Luse, S. A., Burch, H. B., and Hunter, F. E., Jr. 1962. Ultrastructural and enzymatic changes in the liver of the riboflavin deficient rat, *Intern. Cong. Electron Microscopy*, Vol. 5, Academic Press, New York.

65. Mackler, B. 1969. Studies of the molecular basis of congenital malformations, *Pediatrics* 43:915-926.

66. Mann, G., Watson, P. L., McNally, A., and Goddard, J. 1952. Primate Nutrition.

II. Riboflavin deficiency in the cebus monkey and its diagnosis, *J. Nutr.* **47**:225-241.

67. Mason, M. 1953. The metabolism of tryptophan in riboflavin-deficient rats, *J. Biol. Chem.* **201**:513-518.

68. Mickelson, O. 1967. Present knowledge of riboflavin, *in* "Present Knowledge in Nutrition," 3rd ed, pp. 61-65, The Nutrition Foundation, Inc., New York.

69. Miller, J. A., Miner, D. L., Rusch, H. P., and Baumann, C. A. 1941. Diet and hepatic tumor formation, *Cancer Research* **1**:699-708.

70. Miller, Z. A., Poncet, I., and Takacs, E. 1962. Biochemical studies on experimental congenital malformations: flavin nucleotides and folic acid in fetuses and livers from normal and riboflavin-deficient rats, *J. Biol. Chem.* **237**:968-973.

71. Mookerjea, S., and Hawkins, W. W. 1960. Some anabolic aspects of protein metabolism in riboflavin deficiency in the rat, *Brit. J. Nutr.* **14**:231-238.

72. Mookerjea, S., and Jamdar, S. C. 1962. Liver transaminase activity in riboflavin-deficient rats, *Canad. J. Biochem. Physiol.* **40**:1065-1070.

73. Moore, D. F. 1930. Partial loss of central acuity of vision for reading and for distance in school children and its possible association with food deficiency, *West African Med. J.* **4**:46-48.

74. Moore, D. F. 1939. Retrobulbar neuritis c̄ pellagra in Nigeria, *J. Trop. Med. Hyg.* **42**:109-114.

75. Morris, H. P., and Robertson, W. V. B. 1943. Growth rate and number of spontaneous mammary carcinomas and riboflavin concentration of liver, muscle, and tumor of C3H mice as influenced by dietary riboflavin, *J. Natl. Cancer Inst.* **3**:479-489.

76. Moussa B., Youdim, H., and Sourkes, T. L. 1965. The effect of heat inhibitors and riboflavin deficiency on monoamine oxidase, *Canad. J. Biochem.* **43**:1305-1318.

77. *Nutrition Reviews.* 1945. "Vitamins in the therapy of shock and anoxia" **3**:89-91, Nutrition Foundation, Inc., New York.

78. Pandit, V. I., and Chakrabarti, C. H. 1970. Effect of vitamin B_1 and B_2 avitaminosis on certain hepatic enzyme activities and protein biosynthesis in rats, *Enzymologia* **39**:111-119.

79. Pandit, V. I., and Chakrabarti, C. H. 1970. *In vitro* incorporation of ^{14}C serine into proteins of crude liver microsomal fraction of riboflavin deficient rats, *Indian J. Exptl. Biol.* **8**:89-91.

80. Parsons, H. T. 1944. Further studies on human requirements for riboflavin, *Fed. Proc.* **3**:162.

81., Pett, L. B., and Hanley, F. W. 1947. A nutrition survey among school children in British Columbia and Saskatchewan, *Canad. Med. Assoc. J.* **56**:187-192.

82. Phillips, P. H., and Engel, R. W. 1938. Neuromalacia, its occurrence and histopathology in the chick on low riboflavin diets, *Poultry Science* **17**:444.

83. Pollack, H., and Bookman, J. J. 1951. Riboflavin excretion as a function of protein metabolism in the normal, catabolic and diabetic human being, *J. Lab. Clin. Med.* **38**:561-573.

84. Rivlin, R. S. 1970. Riboflavin metabolism, *New Eng. J. Med.* **283**:463-472.

85. Rivlin, R. S., Menendez, C., and Langdon, R. G. 1968. Biochemical similarities between hypothyroidism and riboflavin deficiency, *Endocrinology* **83**:461-469.

86. Sauberlich, H. E., Judd, J. H., Jr., Nichoalds, G. E., Broquist, H. P., and Darby, W. J. 1972. Application of the erythrocyte glutathione reductase assay in evaluating riboflavin nutritional status in a high school student population, *Amer. J. Clin. Nutr.* **25**:756-762.

87. Scott, H. H. 1918. An investigation into an acute outbreak of "central neuritis," *Ann. Trop. Med. Parasitol.* **12**:109-196.

88. Sebrell, W. H. 1929. Fatty degeneration of the liver and kidneys in the dog apparently associated with diet, *U.S. Publ. Health Rept.* **44**:2697-2701.
89. Sebrell, W. H., and Onstott, R. H. 1938. Riboflavin deficiency in dogs, *Public Health Rept.* **53**:83.
90. Sebrell, W. H., and Butler, R. E. 1938. Riboflavin deficiency in man; a preliminary note, *U.S. Public Health Rept.* **53**:2282-2284.
91. Sebrell, W. H., and Butler, R. E. 1939. Riboflavin deficiency in man (ariboflavinosis), *U.S. Public Health Rept.* **54**:2121-2131.
92. Singher, H. O., Kensler, C. J., Taylor, H. C., Jr., Rhoads, C. P., and Unna, K. 1944. The effect of vitamin deficiency on estradiol inactivation by liver, *J. Biol. Chem.* **154**:79-86.
93. Smith, J. M., Lu, S. D. C., Hare, A., Dick, E., and Daniels, M. 1959. The effect of nitrogen intake upon the urinary riboflavin excretion of young male adults, *J. Nutr.* **69**:85-94.
94. Spector, H., Maass, A. R., Michaud, L., Elvehjem, C. A., and Hart, E. B. 1943. The role of riboflavin in blood regeneration. *J. Biol. Chem.* **150**:75-87.
95. Spies, T. D., Bean, W. B., and Ashe, W. F. 1939. Recent advances in the treatment of pellagra and associated deficiencies, *Ann. Intern. Med.* **12**:1830-1844.
96. Stannus, H. S. 1912. Pellagra in Nyasaland, *Trans. Roy. Soc. Trop. Med. Hyg.* **5**:112-119.
97. Stoerk, H. C., and Emerson, G. A. 1949. Complete regression of lymphosarcoma implants following temporary induction of riboflavin deficiency in mice, *Proc. Soc. Exptl. Biol. Med.* **70**:703-704.
98. Street, H. R., Cowgill, G. R., and Zimmerman, H. M. 1941. Further observations of riboflavin deficiency in the dog, *J. Nutr.* **22**:7-24.
99. Sugioka, G., Porta, E. A., Corey, P. N., and Hartroft, W. S. 1969. The liver of rats fed riboflavin-deficient diets at two levels of protein, *Amer. J. Pathol.* **54**:1-19.
100. Sydenstricker, V. P. 1941. Clinical manifestations of ariboflavinosis, *Amer. J. Public Health* **31**:344-350.
101. Sydenstricker, V. P., Sebrell, W. H., Cleckley, H. M., and Kruse, H. D. 1940. The ocular manifestations of ariboflavinosis; a progress note. *J. Amer. Med. Assoc.* **114**:2437-2445.
102. Sydenstricker, V. P., Geeslin, L. E., Templeton, C. M., and Weaver, J. W. 1939. Riboflavin deficiency in human subjects, *J. Amer. Med. Assoc.* **113**:1697-1700.
103. Tandler, B., Erlandson, R. A., and Wynder, E. L. 1968. Riboflavin and mouse hepatic cell structure and function. 1. Ultrastructural alterations in simple deficiency, *Amer. J. Pathol.* **52**:69-95.
104. Ten-State Nutrition Survey 1968-70. 1972. DHEW Publication No. (HSM) 72-8131, Department of Health, Education and Welfare, Washington, D.C.
105. Terrill, S. W., Ammerman, C. B., Walker, D. E., Edwards, R. M., Norton, H. W., and Becker, D. E. 1955. Riboflavin studies with pigs, *J. Animal Sci.* **14**:593.
106. U.S. Interdepartmental Committee on Nutrition for National Defense. 1963. Manual for "Nutrition Surveys," 2d ed., Superintendent of Documents, U.S. Government Printing Office, Washington, D.C.
107. Wada, H., and Snell, E. E. The enzymatic oxidation of pyridoxine and pyridoxamine phosphates. 1961. *J. Biol. Chem.* **236**:2089-2095.
108. Warkany, J., and Schraffenberger, E. 1944. Congenital malformations enduced in rats by maternal nutritional deficiency. VI. The preventive factor, *J. Nutr.* **27**:477.
109. Wiese, A. C., Johnson, B. C., Mitchell, H. H., and Nevens, W. B. 1947. Riboflavin deficiency in the dairy calf, *J. Nutr.* **33**:263.

110. Williams, M. A., McIntosh, D. J., Hincenbergs, I. U., and Tamai, K. T. 1967. Comparative effects of pyridoxine, riboflavin and thiamine on linoleate utilization in rats, *Biochem. Biophys. Acta.* **137**:388–390.
111. Wintrobe, M. M., Buschke, W., Follis, R. H., and Humphreys, S. 1944. Riboflavin deficiency in swine, *Bull. Johns Hopkins Hosp.* **75**:102.
112. Wooley, J. G., and Sebrell, W. H. 1942. Nutritional deficiency and infection, *Public Health Rept.* **57**:149.

8

EXPERIMENTAL DIETARY AND ANTAGONIST-INDUCED HUMAN RIBOFLAVIN DEFICIENCY

Montague Lane, Frank E. Smith, and Clarence P. Alfrey, Jr.

1. INTRODUCTION

By the mid-1930s many clinical symptoms and signs attributable to riboflavin deficiency were described in pellagrins and in other dietary deficiencies. [7-9,31,46,58,62,73,82] The specificity of lesions due to ariboflavinosis, however, was uncertain because of the multiplicity of nutrient deficiencies in endemic malnutrition and the unavailability of pure riboflavin for studying selectively the effects of supplementation of the vitamin. With regard to deficiencies of the B group of vitamins, Sydenstricker[77] stated, "these substances commonly occur together

MONTAGUE LANE, FRANK E. SMITH, AND CLARENCE P. ALFREY, JR.—Sadie Darsky Laboratory for Clinical Cancer Research, Division of Clinical Oncology, Department of Pharmacology and the Department of Medicine, Baylor College of Medicine, Houston, Texas. Some of the studies reported in this chapter were supported by the United States Public Health Service Grants CA 08017 and CA 10893.

in their natural sources and have closely related functions in essential metabolic processes so that any circumstance that causes inadequate intake, poor utilization, or rapid depletion of one of these vitamins is almost certain to affect the whole group.'' Consequently, when synthetic riboflavin became available various investigations of experimental clinical riboflavin deficiency were undertaken to determine which symptoms, signs, and laboratory findings were due to dietary deprivation of the vitamin and could be reversed by it specifically.

When analogues of riboflavin were synthesized, some were found to possess riboflavin antagonist properties. Several of these have been studied as potential anticancer agents in human subjects. It has been possible with the use of an antagonist to induce isolated clinical deficiency of riboflavin rapidly and to characterize its manifestations, several of which had not previously been attributed to deficiency of the vitamin. The features of dietary riboflavin deficiency are reviewed here for the purpose of comparing them to antagonist-induced deficiency in man.

2. DIETARY INDUCTION OF DEFICIENCY

2.1. Experimental Diets

The diets that have been used to study the role of riboflavin in clinical nutrition reflect the evolution of knowledge concerning the roles of various nutrients, particularly vitamins, the isolation and availability of pure vitamin preparations, and the development of analytical methods for the vitamins. Thus, the first diet used to study the effect of administered synthetic riboflavin[64] was quite similar to that used by Goldberger and Tanner[31] to induce pellagra. It consisted of corn meal, cowpeas, lard, casein, flour, white bread, calcium carbonate, tomato juice, cod liver oil, syrup, and syrup of iodide of iron. Sebrell and Butler supplemented the basic diet after 86 days with 30 mg ascorbic acid and 3.3 mg thiamin chloride. They stated that the diet was ''somewhat low in nicotinic acid and contains very little riboflavin.'' They also studied the differential effects of 100 mg/day of nicotinic acid and 0.025 mg riboflavin/kg body weight on the observed lesions. Subsequently, other workers[45,70-72,77,78] reported studies of the effects of riboflavin on patients with varying nutritional histories maintained on pellagra-producing diets. When analytical techniques for riboflavin and other vitamins were developed, diets were devised that consisted of more palatable foods and the content of several of the B vitamins, including riboflavin, was known in relationship to calories, protein, fat, and carbohydrate. In addition, these diets were usually supplemented with various quantities of some or all of the following: vitamins A and D, ascorbic acid, thiamin hydrochloride, calcium pantothenate, pyridoxine, nicotinamide, folic acid, biotin, di- or tri-calcium phosphate, and ferrous sulfate. Thus, efforts were made to provide palatable diets that were limited only in riboflavin content, and different levels of riboflavin intake were investigated to establish the minimum human requirements for this vitamin.

2.2. Clinical Manifestations of Deficiency

2.2.1. Skin and Mucous Membrane Lesions

Sebrell and Butler[64,65] initially ascribed to the experimental deficiency of riboflavin a clinical syndrome consisting of cheilosis (pallor of the mucosa of the lip in the angles of the mouth followed by maceration and the development of superficial transverse fissures with little inflammatory reaction which were moist and covered with a honey-colored crust; reddening of the lips along the line of closure with thinning and denudation of the mucosa); and a scaly, slightly greasy desquamation on a mildly erythematous base on the nasolabial folds, on the alae nasi, in the vestibule of the nose, and on the ears and eyelids. The syndrome developed in 94–130 days. These lesions were similar to those described in endemic B complex deficiency states by others. The lesion at the corner of the mouth is now usually referred to as angular stomatitis, and the lip lesion, which may proceed to fissuring, is called cheilosis. In a later paper, Kruse et al.[45] described a glossitis in which the papillae were flattened or mushroom-shaped and the tongue was purplish-red or magenta. These observations were made on patients diagnosed as having clinical evidence of ariboflavinosis who were then placed on a riboflavin-deficient diet, rather than on normal subjects given an experimental diet. There followed in the literature reports that similar lesions in patients with nutritional deficiency states responded[70,71,78] or failed to respond[55,56] to riboflavin therapy. The diet employed by Sebrell and Butler provided 0.5 mg riboflavin/day. Careful studies by Williams et al.,[83] in which subjects previously in good nutritional states were restricted to 0.7 mg riboflavin daily (0.35 mg/1000 cal) for 288 days; by Keys et al.,[42] whose subjects received 0.75 mg/day (0.31 mg/1000 cal) for 5 months; and by Horwitt et al.,[36] whose subjects received 0.75-0.85 mg riboflavin/day for 12-18 months indicated that at these levels of riboflavin intake there were no signs of clinical riboflavin deficiency.

In a study that utilized a diet providing 0.5 mg riboflavin in 2200 cal, Horwitt et al.[37,38] reported that one of fifteen subjects developed cheilosis, three developed angular stomatitis, and two of these patients also demonstrated seborrheic dermatitis similar to that described by Sebrell and Butler. Scrotal dermatitis, previously described in pellagra, was found to be an important sign of experimental riboflavin deficiency. This consisted of erythema, scaling, desquamation, and weeping of the scrotal skin that spared the median raphé and was noted in 12 of 15 subjects. Glossitis was not observed in any subject. The aforementioned findings occurred in 9-17 months, and subjects responded promptly to riboflavin therapy. These workers also found that erythema of the scrotum, without scaling, occurred in a large percentage of hospitalized patients who were adequately nourished but incontinent. Some of the other lesions observed in the riboflavin-restricted patients appeared to depend on preceding local irritation, infections, and other traumas. They suggested, therefore, that riboflavin may be required for normal tissue repair and that the clinical expression of signs of riboflavin deficiency might be a function not only of the degree of the deficiency but of local tissue trauma.

In another study of eight patients, with a diet that provided an equivalent amount of riboflavin (0.55 mg/day), less protein (41 g/day) and niacin (5.8 mg/day), but a B_{12} supplement (0.001 mg/day), Horwitt et al.[40] recorded that the following findings appeared in 27-36 weeks: erythema of buccal and palatal mucosa and "beefy" redness of the tongue with little or no papillary atrophy in four subjects, angular stomatitis in six subjects, scrotal dermatitis in five subjects, and conjunctivitis and seborrheic dermatitis in two subjects. The conjunctivitis appeared in one subject during the first week of supplementation with riboflavin and there was a simultaneous worsening of the seborrheic dermatitis, angular stomatitis, cheilosis, and scrotal dermatitis. The lesions cleared with continued riboflavin supplementation during the next four weeks. These studies have established that angular stomatitis, cheilosis, erythema of the buccal and palatal mucosa and tongue, seborrheic dermatitis, scrotal dermatitis, and possibly conjunctivitis are manifestations of riboflavin deficiency.

2.2.2. Ocular Manifestations

In pellagrins eye lesions that responded to riboflavin therapy were first described by Spies et al.[70,71] These lesions were characterized by burning of the eyes, lacrimation, bulbar and palpebral conjunctivitis, and mydriasis. Sydenstricker et al.[77] noted that conjunctivitis and photophobia in pellagrins responded to riboflavin. Kruse et al.[45] reported ocular signs and lesions in nine patients known to be receiving insufficient riboflavin, five of whom clearly had deficiency diseases. Symptoms included itching and burning of the eyes, mild to severe photophobia, dim vision in poor light, and partial blindness. On slit-lamp examination, in addition to conjunctivitis, corneal changes were noted that included opacities, superficial and deeper invasion of the cornea by capillaries that arose from the anterior ciliary vessels, and interstitial infiltration of the cornea with exudate. The lesions healed with riboflavin therapy. These authors concluded that the principal ocular lesion of ariboflavinosis is keratitis and that it is accompanied by circumcorneal vascular injection and by conjunctivitis of varying severity.

Other reports suggested that these findings lacked specificity,[56,70] but proliferation of the limbic plexus was found to be common in aviators who were subject to severe glare and eyestrain and who were also deficient in riboflavin.[80] Not a single study of experimental dietary riboflavin deficiency has documented the occurrence of corneal vascularization on slit-lamp examination. In one study an increase in flicker fusion threshold was found in some patients,[37] and in another study by this same group of investigators two patients developed conjunctivitis. The previously mentioned hypothesis of Horwitt and his co-workers that lesions in riboflavin deficiency may appear in relation to tissue trauma has been suggested by them as a possible explanation for whether or not corneal vascularization develops.[34]

2.2.3. Central Nervous System Changes

Electroencephalographic abnormalities have been noted in 8- and 9-year-old boys with endemic ariboflavinosis.[5] However, in addition to having low blood riboflavin levels, these children had low levels of serum folate. It is interesting that the two children with serum folate levels in the normal range had normal theta and alpha energies on analysis of EEG integrated voltage at frequency bands and normal latency of photically induced average responses. These studies do not clearly implicate riboflavin deficiency as the basis for the observed abnormalities in the other children and suggest, in fact, that folate deficiency may have accounted for the results observed.

2.2.4. Urinary Excretion of Riboflavin

Early studies described the urinary excretion of riboflavin by human beings.[21,27,32,33,43,61] Later studies had various objectives including (1) determination of the relationship between intake and excretion; (2) establishment of the daily riboflavin requirement; and (3) diagnosis of riboflavin deficiency. Several conclusions may be drawn from the available literature. The urinary excretion of riboflavin, in general, is proportional to the dietary intake, that is, low levels of intake are associated with low urinary excretion and increased excretion with an increased intake. [26,66,72,83] Riboflavin is conserved when its intake is restricted, whatever the status of previous stores. Thus, the administration of a riboflavin restricted diet to an adequately nourished individual results in a prompt reduction in urinary excretion. [16]

Subjects maintained on levels of riboflavin intake that eventually produce signs of riboflavin deficiency excrete progressively smaller amounts of the vitamin in the urine with continuation of the restricted intake over many months. While signs of riboflavin deficiency occur only in subjects with very low urinary excretion of riboflavin, the finding of low urinary riboflavin excretion is in itself not diagnostic, since it may reflect only a brief period of severe reduction in intake of riboflavin. [39] When large doses of riboflavin are administered to adequately nourished individuals, the majority of the riboflavin can be recovered in the urine. However, when riboflavin intake has been restricted for some time and supplemental riboflavin is administered, only a small proportion appears in the urine initially. [42] As supplementation continues, there is a progressive rise in urinary excretion as body stores of the vitamin are replenished. When the oral supplement of riboflavin is increased, a greater amount is unaccounted for by urinary excretion, suggesting that it is destroyed or not absorbed. [66] Finally, estimates of daily riboflavin requirements based on basal urinary excretion and the excretion of test doses indicate that for the average individual a daily intake above 1.1 mg but somewhat less than 1.6 mg is sufficient to preserve tissue stores. [39]

2.2.5. Blood Levels

A fluorimetric method[17] was utilized by Bessey et al.[11] to study the effects of prolonged dietary restriction of riboflavin (0.5–0.55

mg/day). The studies indicated that measurements of plasma flavin components were less reliable than in erythrocytes. The first significant fall in erythrocyte flavin levels occurred after 45 days on the deficient diet; levels continued to fall progressively thereafter. At 9 months the levels of patients on the deficient diet were 10-13.1 μg/100 ml red blood cells compared to 20.2-27.6 μg/100 ml for patients on intakes of 2.4-3.55 mg/day. Measurement of erythrocyte flavin appears to be an accurate means of assessing chronic dietary deprivation of riboflavin.

2.2.6. Red Blood Cell Enzymes

The activities of glutathione reductase (GR) and NADH-methemoglobin reductase, two flavin enzymes in erythrocytes, can be stimulated by the addition of FAD. In the case of GR, this stimulation of the enzyme is not affected appreciably by dialysis or dilution, but the stimulation of NADH-methemoglobin reductase activity is removed by dilution.[12] FAD appears to be the prosthetic group of GR.[18,41,63] It has been shown that the activity of erythrocyte GR is stimulated by FAD to a much greater extent in riboflavin-deficient rats than in rats with an adequate riboflavin intake.[30]

Of considerable interest are studies relating GR activity and riboflavin nutritional status in humans. Bamji[10] reported that in patients with clinical ariboflavinosis GR activity and red blood cell flavin were lower than in healthy subjects and that FAD activity of GR *in vitro* was more marked for the deficient subjects. When healthy subjects were placed on different levels of riboflavin-deficient diets, GR activity fell in proportion to the degree of riboflavin restriction and stabilized in a few days at a particular riboflavin intake. Beutler[13-14] also found that baseline GR activity correlated with daily riboflavin intake and that there was a weaker correlation between riboflavin intake and GR activity after FAD stimulation. FAD produced some stimulation of erythrocyte hemolysate GR activity from all subjects, which usually was greater in those with low initial activity. The administration of 5 mg riboflavin for 8 days increased the basal GR activity of patients previously on 0.67-3.7 mg riboflavin/day indicating that even with adequate intake of riboflavin erythrocyte GR is not fully saturated. The level of erythrocyte FAD was increased by riboflavin administration. Subsequently, Mandula and Beutler[57] have found that FAD and FMN can be synthesized from riboflavin by intact red cells and that incubation of red cells with riboflavin can result in increased activity of GR. The foregoing suggests that measurements of erythrocyte GR activity reflect dietary intake of riboflavin and that significant reduction of erythrocyte flavin indicates depletion of tissue stores.

3. ANTAGONIST-INDUCED DEFICIENCY

Many analogs of riboflavin have been synthesized. A number of these antagonize one of more functions of the vitamin in various biological systems (see Chapter 10). It is established that riboflavin deficiency induced by dietary restriction or some antagonists can inhibit the growth of transplanted tumors in rodents. [4,19,20,35,59,75] The relationship of riboflavin to cancer is discussed in Chapter 11. This approach to the treatment of human neoplasia seemed worthy of exploration and has been the subject of investigations in our laboratories for the past 18 years. As discussed earlier in this chapter, experience by others with riboflavin-restricted diets indicated that many months of restriction were required for the evolution of clinical signs of deficiency and that such signs did not occur in all subjects. We considered riboflavin restriction alone to be an impractical approach to the treatment of cancer patients, and the use of an antagonist appeared to be essential for a therapeutic endeavor. These studies have enabled us to induce isolated clinical riboflavin deficiency rapidly, to describe its clinical signs and symptoms and some of its laboratory expressions, to compare these with those of dietary deficiency, and to study some of its effects on malignant disease.

3.1. Clinical Pharmacology of Antagonists

The riboflavin antagonists that have antitumor activity in rodents have certain properties in common, with some exceptions. Like the vitamin, they are yellow, exhibit fluoresence in ultraviolet light, and are poorly soluble in water. In general, they inhibit the growth of *Lactobacillus casei* and of young rodents, they are weak antagonists whose inhibitory effects require a high ratio of antagonist to riboflavin, and their effects are reversible with riboflavin. Detailed pharmacological studies have been performed with only a few of these antagonists.

3.1.1. 6,7-Dimethyl-9-(2'-acetoxyethyl)-isoalloxazine (U-2112)

The analog we initially selected for study, 6,7-dimethyl-9-(2'-acetoxyethyl)-isoalloxazine, was chosen because (a) analogues previously available had failed to induce signs of riboflavin deficiency or antitumor effects in man[74]; (b) this agent had a relatively favorable inhibitory ratio, that is, 100:1 in bacteria and 50–100:1 in rats; and (c) it produced complete regression of several types of established transplanted rat tumors.[24] Nine patients with various forms of cancer were placed on a diet containing less than 2 mg riboflavin daily and received doses of U-2112 from 0.75 to 6 g/day for 20-84 days. There were no signs of riboflavin deficiency nor were antitumor effects noted in these patients. In an effort to understand this failure, studies of the clinical pharmacology of the drug were undertaken.[48] U-2112 was absorbed following oral administration to human subjects. Peak flavin levels occurred in the plasma approximately 2 hr after ingestion and decreased to pretreatment levels in 24 hr. The plasma peak level increased with dose, but large dosage increments produced relatively small increases in plasma flavin concentration at doses above 50 mg. A 500-mg single dose resulted in a peak plasma flavin concentration of approximately 45 µg/100 ml plasma. Recovery of flavin in the urine within 48 hr ranged from 20% of a 50-mg oral dose to 2.7-5.1% of a 6.0-g oral dose.

A similar pattern of decreasing percent recovery as dose is increased, but with a greater total amount of flavin in urine, was obtained with riboflavin administered orally; at each dose level the percent recovery was higher for U-2112 than for riboflavin. When U-2112 was administered intravenously, 95-99% was recovered as total flavin in the urine in 24 hr. As determined by the rapidity of return of 24-hr urine flavin levels to pretreatment values, there appeared to be no significant accumulation of the drug in the body.

The most significant aspect of the clinical pharmacology of this drug was its metabolic fate. Approximately 1% of the urine flavin was unchanged U-2112; 48% was its hydrolysis product, 6,7-dimethyl-9-(2'-hydroxyethyl)-isoalloxazine, (U-2113); and the remainder consisted of three flavins that lacked antiriboflavin or riboflavin-like activity. The hydroxyethyl compound is only one-tenth as inhibitory of the growth of *L. casei* compared to the acetoxyethyl derivitive. In rats, on the other hand, approximately 11% of the urine flavin was unchanged U-2112. Since the plasma levels and urine flavin recovery at similar doses were comparable in rats and in human subjects, yet rats became riboflavin deficient, we suggested that the species difference in drug metabolism might be one possible explanation for the lack of activity of the drug in man.

3.1.2. Sodium-6,7-dimethyl-9-(2'-hemisuccinoxyethyl)-isoalloxazine (U-6538)

This compound was synthesized by Petering to provide a highly soluble riboflavin antagonist that could be administered parenterally. Its pharmacological properties were studied in bacteria, rodents, and humans.[49] The drug inhibited the growth of *L. casei* at a ratio of U-6538 to riboflavin of 1666:1. However, if the drug was added to the bioassay medium after it had been autoclaved and cooled, bacterial growth was not inhibited. Inhibitory effects were observed only if U-6538 was added to bioassay medium that subsequently was autoclaved, cooled, and inoculated with bacteria. Chromatograms of this material demonstrated that the drug had been partially hydrolyzed to 5,7-dimethyl-9-(2'-hydroxyethyl)-isoalloxazine (U-2113), which accounted for the inhibition of bacterial growth. Intact U-6538 was devoid of activity as a riboflavin antagonist for *L. casei.* U-6538 injected into weanling rats inhibited their growth and also produced regression of the Murphy–Sturm lymphosarcoma in Sprague–Dawley rats. After intramuscular injection or intravenous infusion of the drug into human subjects, plasma flavin levels peaked at 30–60 min and were directly proportional to the administered dose. Patients with plasma flavin levels of 10 μg/ml usually experienced flank pain, oliguria, and crystalluria. Urinary excretion of a single low dose was 90–100% in 24 hr, but with doses above 600 mg recovery in urine at 24 hr fell as low as 67%. The crystals in the urine were shown to be the metabolite 6,7-dimethyl-9-(2'-hydroxyethyl)-isoalloxazine (U-2113). The patients studied did not develop signs that could be definitely ascribed to riboflavin deficiency. The amount of U-6538 that could be administered was limited because of its hydrolysis to the relatively insoluble U-2113 and resultant crystalluria. It was calculated that the total active riboflavin antagonist received by patients treated with U-6538 parenterally was similar to that of patients treated orally with U-2112. Since the latter drug was ineffective clinically, further studies with U-6538 did not appear warranted.

3.1.3. 10-*d*-Dulcityl-7,8-dimethyl-isoalloxazine (galactoflavin)

This drug was selected for study on the basis of its activity as an antitumor agent in mice.[75] Its pharmacology has been studied by Lane and Brindley.[52] At a ratio of galactoflavin to riboflavin of 323:1, the growth of *L. casei* was half-minimum and complete growth inhibition was observed at a ratio 625:1. In rats, 1.2–2.5% of a single oral dose of 50 mg/kg was recovered in the urine and plasma levels of 9–25 μg/100 ml occurred in 30–60 min. Chromatography of plasma and urine revealed a single fluorescent component with the same mobility as galactoflavin in various solvent systems. In human subjects treated with single oral doses of 1–3 g galactoflavin, peak plasma levels ranged from 21 to 94 μg/100 ml and levels of 13–52 μg/100 ml were detected at 4 hr. There was a moderate degree of patient-to-patient variation with respect to urine flavin recovery, but each individual excreted a fairly constant quantity of flavin in the urine for each dose. Urine flavin recovery as percent of administered dose was greater at low than at high doses. The individual patient excreted approximately the same amount of flavin in the urine with total daily doses above 1.5 g/day. Continous treatment with doses of 0.5-1 g every 8 hr resulted in daily total urine flavin of 86-145 mg. Chromatography of plasma and urine revealed a single major flavin component with the mobility of galactoflavin in several solvent systems. In these studies five patients were treated with galactoflavin from 22 to 68 days and received total doses of 66-165 g. Two patients developed sore mouth and throat, cheilosis, and angular stomatitis, but in only one case did the findings abate after discontinuation of galactoflavin and substitution of a regular diet. Another patient developed reticulocytopenia and anemia and responded with reticulocytosis and a rise in hemoglobin concentration after the drug was discontinued and a regular diet was substituted. Plasma flavin concentrations and urine flavin recoveries were generally higher in humans than in rats treated with doses of galactoflavin that were comparable based upon body weight. Significant metabolic transformation of galactoflavin was not detected in either species. In view of the similarities in the pharmacology of galactoflavin in both species, the antitumor activity of the drug in rodents and the suggestive signs of riboflavin deficiency observed in this clinical pharmacological trial, galactoflavin was selected for further study as an antitumor agent in man.

3.2. Galactoflavin-Induced Riboflavin Deficiency

3.2.1. Method of Induction

Our approach to the induction of riboflavin deficiency with galactoflavin[51] took into account several considerations. Since the drug was a weak reversible antagonist, it seemed desirable to restrict riboflavin intake severely. The diet had to be adequate in terms of calories, carbohydrate, protein, fat, and essential nutrients other than riboflavin. The pharmacological studies indicated that urinary galactoflavin excretion occurred at total daily doses of 1.5-3 g/day and did not increase at higher doses. This dose range was therefore employed. Since cancer patients were to be the subject of these investigations, it was important to select individuals whose nutritional status was unimpaired and who had not experienced significant weight loss. These stipulations were required to minimize the possible effects of prior malnutrition and neoplastic disease on the manifestations of riboflavin deficiency. The specificity of lesions attributable to riboflavin deficiency had to be documented by their reversal with riboflavin while galactoflavin and the restricted diet were still being administered. Finally, patients with measureable tumors were selected so that antitumor activity could be evaluated.

3.2.1A. DIET. Initially, the basic diet was prepared according to the following formula: dextrose 280 g; safflower oil emulsion 100 g; calcium caseinate 120 g; 2% methyl cellulose 100 ml; sodium chloride 6 g; potassium chloride 6 g. Sufficient water was added to bring the total volume to 1500 ml. L-cystine was administered in gelatin capsules, 0.25 g each, in the proportion of 0.75 g/1400 cal of diet, to compensate for the L-cystine deficiency of casein. The diet formula contained 1400 cal and 300 μg of riboflavin/100 ml. This formula was supplemented by a vitamin and mineral mixture that was provided in three gelatin capsules, one of which was given morning, noon, and evening. The daily supplement consisted of vitamin A, 5000 U; vitamin D, 1000 U; thiamin hydrochloride, 3 mg; nicotinamide, 15 mg; pyridoxine hydrochloride, 2 mg; folic acid, 5 mg; cyanocobalomin, 1 μg; calcium pantothenate, 5 mg; cobaltous chloride·$6H_2O$, 2 mg; ascorbic acid, 75 mg; d-α-tocopheryl acid succinate, 5 mg; ferrous sulfate, 22 mg; cupric sulfate·5 H_2O, 4 mg; potassium iodide, 0.2 mg; manganous sulfate·5 H_2O, 1.5 mg; sodium molybdate·2 H_2O, 0.5 mg; zinc sulfate·7 H_2O, 5.3 mg; magnesium sulfate·7 H_2O, 61 mg. After four patients were studied, the diet formula was modified to reduce the content of riboflavin. This diet is shown in Table I. The formula was prepared each morning, refrigerated, and mixed in a blender before each serving. We have found this formula to be well tolerated and have continued to use it. Patients generally receive six servings a day. Sufficient formula is given to provide the same number of calories patients are estimated to eat on a regular diet in the hospital. The quantity of diet is modified if a patient complains of hunger or being "too full," or if body weight is not maintained. It has been our experience that

TABLE I. Formula for Riboflavin-Deficient Diet

Dextrose	280 g	N/1 sodium bicarbonate	71 ml
Safflower oil emulsion	100 g	NaCl	2 g
"Vitamin-free" casein	100 g	KCL	2 g
Methyl cellulose, 2%	100 ml	H_2O q.s.	1500 ml

Supplement—L-cystine, 0.75 g/1000 ml.
1000 ml—provides 1400 cal and 33 μg riboflavin.

within two or three days the patients become accustomed to the formula. The monotony of the liquid diet is interrupted by occasional serving of stewed fruits. Patients with teeth are given small servings of carrots and celery to maintain the integrity of dental structures. No more than three cups of coffee, prepared from powdered coffee (15 μg riboflavin per cup), are allowed each day.

3.2.1B. GALACTOFLAVIN REGIMEN. The drug is administered 0.5 hr prior to each feeding of formula. The majority of patients now receive 0.25 g six times a day, although some have been treated with 0.5-g doses. There is no evidence that the higher dose has accelerated the development of clinical signs of deficiency, and this dose has been associated with slight nausea in some patients.

3.2.1C. SELECTION OF PATIENTS. Twenty-four white and black men and women from 27 to 72 years of age with different types of cancer have been studied. Many of these patients were considered nutritionally normal in terms of dietary history, maintainence of usual body weight, physical examination, and various laboratory parameters prior to study. Twenty-three of the patients were treated with galactoflavin for at least 6 weeks.

3.2.2. Clinical Manifestations

Initial reports from our laboratory[50-52] documented the following expressions of galactoflavin-induced riboflavin deficiency: sore throat, cheilosis, angular stomatitis, glossitis, seborrheic dermatitis, and anemia. These changes were all reversed upon administration of riboflavin. In subsequent studies of 16 patients, these findings have received confirmation. We have also observed other hematological changes. A peripheral neuropathy has been shown to accompany prolonged treatment with galactoflavin. Riboflavin deficiency has been shown to inhibit the growth of some human neoplasms and to produce hematological improvement in polycythemia rubra vera.

3.2.2A. CHEILOSIS AND ANGULAR STOMATITIS. One or both of these findings occurred within 1.5 to 7 weeks in 19 of 23 patients treated for 6 weeks or longer. Occasionally both lesions began simultaneously, but often one preceded the other. Angular stomatitis occurred alone in four patients and cheilosis alone in two patients. Usually angular stomatitis was bilateral and the lesions varied in severity. Lesions that were several millimeters deep were often covered by a honey-colored crust or crusted blood. These lesions would split open and bleed during eating or yawning and were painful. Cheilosis also caused slight to moderate discomfort when the fissures were deep, but the lips rarely bled. Surface epithelium was denuded and the lips appeared dry and shiny, especially at the mucocutaneous border. Applications of petrolatum would relieve most of the lip discomfort but did not cause the lesions to heal. Healing occurred within 10 days after riboflavin administration.

3.2.2B. ORAL MUCOSAL CHANGES. Within 2-5 weeks about one-half of the patients complained of dryness and soreness of the throat upon awakening that tended to subside during the day. Hyperemia and edema of the posterior pharynx, fauces, uvula, and even the buccal mucosa were observed in these patients. Some patients also were distressed by soreness of the mouth throughout the day. Smears and cultures of the mouth revealed normal flora in most instances. A few patients had white plaques that proved to be *Candida albicans.* These responded to treatment with mycostatin suspension rinses and gargles. Changes in the oral mucosa were reversed within 1 week of riboflavin therapy.

3.2.2C. GLOSSITIS. Glossitis occurred in 18 of 23 patients in 3-6 weeks. Typically, this began with flattening and then disappearance of the filiform papillae first from the tip and edges and then from the dorsum of the tongue. The fungiform papillae enlarged and became mushroom-shaped, some assuming a "cystic" appearance. In the most advanced cases, the tongue was slightly edematous and completely smooth except where hypertrophied fungiform papillae pebbled the surface. The color of the tongue was usually magenta or beefy red, but in severely anemic patients it was pale pink (Fig. 1). Some patients complained of numbness, tingling, burning, or soreness of the tongue. Occasionally, there was diminution in the ability to distinguish taste sensations. In every instance, symptoms subsided, taste returned, and the appearance of the tongue was restored to normal within 14 days upon reversal of the deficiency state with riboflavin.

3.2.2D. DERMATITIS. Seborrheic dermatitis, characterized by drying of the epidermis and heaping up of scale, occurred in approximately half of the patients in 2-7 weeks. This usually developed on the nose, nasolabial folds, cheeks, and postauricular skin. These areas had a somewhat greasy appearance. Sometimes the involved skin was slightly reddened. Scrotal dermatitis was observed in one-third of the male subjects. The skin of the anterior surface of the scrotum became erythematous and there was scaling and desquamation of superficial epithelium with weeping and maceration of the skin in the most severe

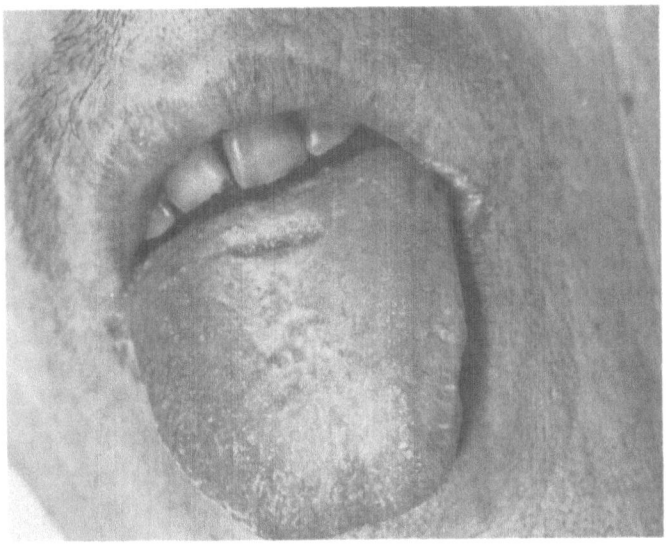

Fig. 1. Glossitis and angular stomatitis during galactoflavin-induced riboflavin deficiency. Note absence of filiform papillae and hypertrophied fungiform papillae. (From Lane et al.[51] Courtesy of Rockefeller University Press, New York.)

cases. The lesions occasionally spread to the groin and medial aspect of the thighs and were fairly well demarcated from uninvolved adjacent skin. In a few patients, the lesions were accompanied by symptoms of burning and itching that were relieved by 1% hydrocortisone ointment and local measures designed to keep the involved areas clean and dry. The appearance of the skin returned to normal only after administration of riboflavin. Generalized dryness of the skin, with small, flaky scales, especially over the trunk and extremities, was noted in one-fourth of the patients. These lesions did not subside in all patients after riboflavin therapy.

3.2.2E. Hematological Findings. Peripheral Blood. The most consistent expressions of galactoflavin-induced riboflavin deficiency were reticulocytopenia and anemia, which occurred in every patient.[53] Initially, each patient had a normal or elevated percentage of reticulocytes and within 2-8 weeks a decrease in reticulocytes was observed. In all but four patients the reticulocytes were absent from the blood in 3-9 weeks. The degree of anemia that developed was directly related to the duration of maintained recticulocytopenia. In several patients who were anemic prior to study, the development of reticulocytopenia was soon followed by severe degrees of symptomatic anemia for which blood transfusion was required. Prior to administration of riboflavin decreases in hemoglobin concentration of 3-9.7 g/100 ml in periods from 37 to 108 days occurred in a group of eight patients who were not transfused. The administration of riboflavin in doses of 5-10 mg/day resulted in an increase in reticulocytes in 2-5 days with a median of 4 days. In several patients small doses of riboflavin were evaluated to determine the minimum requirement for reticulocyte response. This was established as a total daily oral intake of 0.5 mg riboflavin in patients continuing to receive 1.5-3 g/day of galactoflavin. With daily administration of 0.5-1.0 mg of riboflavin orally reticulocyte increases began on the fifth day and did not exceed 2%. Large doses (5-10 mg/day) of riboflavin orally or of riboflavin-5'-monophosphate sodium intramuscularly (5-15 mg/day) produced greater peak reticulocyte levels for comparable degrees of anemia. In cases of severe anemia (hematocrit 7-18 vol%), peak reticulocyte values ranged from 10 to 29% and occurred in 3 to 8 days.

In all cases in which the red blood cells were morphologically normal prior to study, examination of films of the peripheral blood at the height of anemia demonstrated the red cells to be normocytic and normochromic. Red blood cell indices were normal. Patients with abnormal red cells (usually hypochromic and microcytic) prior to study showed only the same abnormalities at the height of the anemia.

The 24-hr urinary erythropoietin content has been determined by Alexanian in two patients with polycythemia vera prior to study and at the height of deficiency; and, in two other patients, at the height of deficiency. Erythropoietin was found to increase appropriately in the patients with polycythemia vera as the hematocrit decreased and

TABLE II. Urine Erythropoietin Content[a] in Riboflavin Deficiency

Patient	Diagnosis	Predeficiency		Deficiency	
		Hct., %	Erythropoietin level, standard B units/day	Hct., %	Erythropoietin level, standard B units/day
M.W.	Lymphosarcoma	30	—	26	41
B.F.	Hodgkin's disease	39	—	25	70
F.W.	Polycythemia vera	53	0.7	43	1.4
R.T.	Polycythemia vera	58	0.4	42	1.5

[a]Method of R. Alexanian, W. K. Vaughn, and M. W. Ruchelman, J. Lab. Clin. Med. 70:777-785 (1967).

TABLE III. *Effects of Galactoflavin-Induced Riboflavin Deficiency on Peripheral Leukocyte and Platelet Counts in Patients with Lymphosarcoma and Hodgkin's Disease Who Had Splenomegaly*

Patient	Diagnosis	Period	WBC/ cu mm	Platelets/ cu mm
J. B.	Lymphosarcoma	Prestudy	4,700	58,000
		Deficiency	1,800	10,000
		Reversal	6,000	144,000
C. C.	Lymphosarcoma	Prestudy	5,100	164,000
		Deficiency	1,900	62,000
		Reversal	4,200	162,000
M. W.	Lymphosarcoma	Prestudy	5,800	156,000
		Deficiency	24,000	56,000
		Reversal	21,000	138,000
C. S.	Hodgkin's disease	Prestudy	2,800	132,000
		Deficiency	850	204,000
		Reversal	9,700	532,000
B. F.	Hodgkin's disease	Prestudy	5,600	171,000
		Deficiency	1,500	100,000
		Reversal	7,700	290,000

to be markedly increased in the anemic patients (Table II). Erythropoietin production does not appear to be inhibited by riboflavin deficiency.

In the initial group of eight patients previously reported, one patient with colon cancer had a drop in peripheral leukocyte count from 6750 cells/cu mm to 3300/cu mm at the height of the deficiency, and a rise in leukocyte count to 5850/cu mm after treatment with riboflavin. The platelets decreased from 160,000/cu mm to 100,000/cu mm in a patient with lung cancer. None of the other patients had significant changes in peripheral leukocyte or platelet counts. It did not appear that riboflavin deficiency had a major effect on leukocytes or platelets. However, subsequent studies in patients with lymphosarcoma and Hodgkin's disease (Table III) and polycythemia vera clearly demonstrated that under certain circumstances riboflavin deficiency can produce significant leukopenia and thrombocytopenia. Two of the patients had moderate leukopenia and one also had thrombocytopenia prior to study. All but one patient (M. W., see Table III) developed leukopenia, and that patient's peripheral white cells consisted of 80% lymphoblasts. In the other patients, the leukocytes and platelets in the peripheral blood appeared to be normal. Only one patient (C.S.) did not show a decrease in platelets. In each instance of leukopenia or thrombocytopenia, riboflavin administration resulted in an increase of the depressed blood elements. The presence of splenomegaly—a clinical feature in each of these

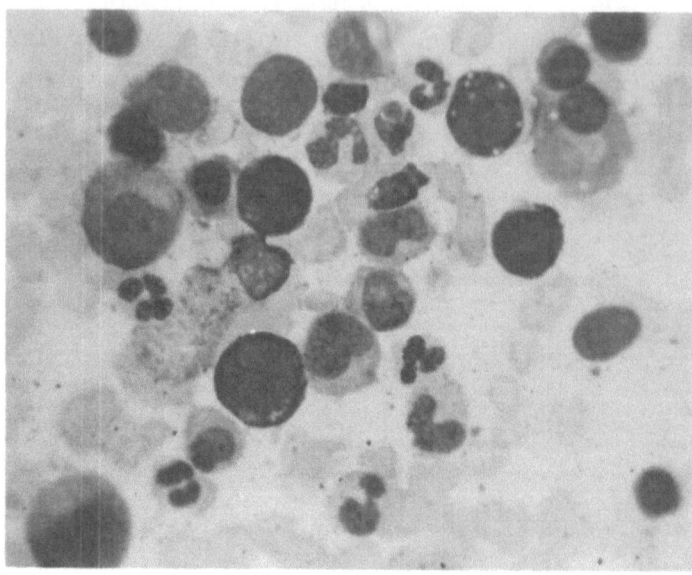

Fig. 2. A bone marrow specimen obtained from a patient 12 days after initiation of riboflavin deficiency. Note the vacuolization of the pronormoblasts. (From Lane and Alfrey.[53] Courtesy of Henry M. Stratton, Inc., New York.)

patients—suggests that the spleen may have played a contributory role in the development of leukopenia or thrombocytopenia. It is possible that prior to induction of riboflavin deficiency there was increased removal of leukocytes and platelets by the enlarged spleen, but this was compensated for by increased production of cells in the marrow. Riboflavin deficiency might have a minimal inhibitory effect on leukocyte and platelet production that would not be reflected in the appearance of the bone marrow or in the peripheral blood counts in patients without splenomegaly. However, in the presence of splenic sequestration, a small inhibition of marrow production might conceivably result in overt leukopenia and thrombocytopenia. While this explanation may not be completely satisfying, the development of leukopenia and thrombocytopenia in some patients made riboflavin deficient, and the increase in leukocytes and platelets with riboflavin therapy while galactoflavin administration was continued, implies that the vitamin has a role in the maintenance of leukocytes and platelets. Effects of riboflavin deficiency on white blood cells and platelets may not be evident even when red cell production has ceased, unless other disease conditions, such as splenomegaly, coexist.

Bone Marrow. During the induction of riboflavin deficiency the bone marrow undergoes a series of characteristic changes. Within the first 2 weeks after initiation of galactoflavin therapy and the deficient diet, there is an increase in the percentage of pronormoblasts. Cytoplasmic and nuclear vacuoles are found in many of these cells (Fig. 2). The erythrocyte series undergoes progressive hypoplasia. The M:E ratio in a group of six patients who had serial bone marrow examinations increased from a mean of 4, prior to treatment, to 19 at the end of deficiency. The percentage of orthochromic and polychromatophilic normoblasts is markedly decreased in the deficient patient (Table IV). In some instances, no erythroid precursors could be found in marrow aspirates and clot sections obtained at the height of deficiency. The absence of megaloblastic changes would indicate that if riboflavin deficiency has some effects in man on the metabolism of either folate or vitamin B_{12}, these are insufficient to influence erythropoiesis or are masked by the administration of these vitamins to patients. The cells of the myeloid series and megakaryocytes appeared normal in all patients, including those who developed leukopenia and thrombocytopenia, and myelopoiesis

TABLE IV. Effects of Riboflavin Deficiency on Marrow Erythroid Precursor Cells

Patient	Period	Pronormo-blasts, %	Basophilic normo-blasts, %	Ortho-chromic and polychro-matophilic normo-blasts, %	All other cells, %	M. E. ratio
V. T.	Prestudy	0.3	1.3	26.4	72.0	1.9
	Deficiency	1.0	2.4	7.9	88.7	7.8
	Reversal	0.9	1.6	15.4	82.1	4.6
C. R.	Prestudy	0.9	2.4	14.8	81.9	4.5
	Deficiency	1.3	1.5	5.2	92.0	11.5
R. C.	Prestudy	0.5	14.9	17.9	66.7	2.0
	Deficiency	1.6	11.9	9.6	76.9	3.3
G. H.	Prestudy	1.8	9.2	23.8	65.2	1.9
	Deficiency	0.5	1.8	0.3	97.4	38.5
J. M.	Prestudy	0.8	0.3	7.3	91.6	10.9
	Deficiency	1.2	0.0	1.0	97.8	44.5
W. J.	Prestudy	0.8	5.3	20.5	73.4	2.8
	Deficiency	2.2	4.2	5.7	87.9	7.3
	Reversal	1.4	3.8	34.0	60.8	1.6

From Lane and Alfrey.[53] Courtesy of Henry M. Stratton, Inc., New York.

was orderly. The bone marrow responded promptly to riboflavin administration with a decrease in M:E ratio, due to repopulation principally with late nucleated erythroid cells. The pattern of erythroid hyperplasia persisted for several weeks.

Iron Metabolism. The plasma iron concentration has been determined in the majority of patients prior to study, during deficiency, and following reversal with riboflavin. Increases in plasma iron concentrations occurred in every case and ranged from 34 to 264 μg/100 ml. Reversal of the deficiency with riboflavin resulted in a rapid decrease in plasma iron concentration to levels as low as 8 μg/ml. There was an inverse relationship between erythroid activity in the marrow and the plasma iron concentration.

Parallel changes were reflected in studies of the plasma iron disappearance. The $t_{1/2}$ of injected radioiron ranged from 34 to 92 min prior to study. At the height of deficiency the $t_{1/2}$ ranged from 90 to 410 min, and following reversal of deficiency from 19 to 60 min.

The plasma turnover rate, which is the number of milligrams of iron entering and leaving the plasma per unit time, is directly related to the plasma iron concentration and inversely related to the plasma iron $t_{1/2}$. In these patients, the plasma turnover rate prior to and following induction of riboflavin deficiency was unchanged, since the increase in plasma iron concentration was paralleled by an increase in plasma iron disappearance time. The incorporation of radioiron by red blood cells was markedly reduced during the deficiency state, ranging from 0 to 7% 1 week after injection of radioiron. The low incorporation occurred at the time of severe reticulocytopenia and in association with a high plasma iron concentration and a prolonged plasma iron disappearance time. These findings are characteristic of erythroid hypoplasia. Since incorporation of iron into red cells was negligible and the plasma iron turnover rate was unchanged, the turnover of storage iron was increased.

Within 7-11 days after initiation of reversal of the deficiency with riboflavin, a second injection of radioiron was administered to several patients. In each instance, the plasma iron disappearance was very rapid (19-58 min), the plasma iron concentration was low (8-52 μg/100 ml), and uptake of injected radioiron by red cells was complete in 7 days. These results indicated recovery of red cell production, with rapid removal of iron from the plasma iron pool.

The distribution of radioiron uptake by the tissues 24 hr after its injection was determined by linear scanning.[1] Radioiron is removed principally by sites of erythropoiesis in normal subjects, and the linear scan reveals considerable uptake over the chest, abdomen, and pelvis. By contrast, in the riboflavin-deficient patient with red cell hypoplasia

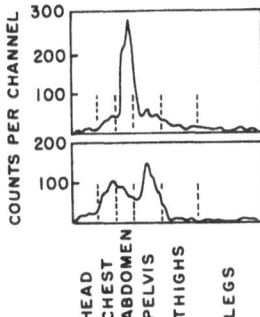

Fig. 3. The distribution of radioiron along the head-toe axis 24 hr after intravenous injection. Scan above is of a riboflavin deficient patient and that below of a normal individual. (From Alfrey and Lane.[1] Courtesy of Henry M. Stratton, Inc., New York.)

most of the exchange between plasma and tissue iron occurs in the liver. The linear scan in these patients showed that most of the injected radioactivity was incorporated in the organs of the upper abdomen (Fig. 3). This pattern of iron distribution was observed in patients with other causes of erythroid hypoplasia.[3] Even after reversal of riboflavin deficiency and restoration of erythropoiesis, the radioiron was removed from the liver very slowly (0.4%/day or less), indicating the stability of the hepatic storage pool.[2]

3.2.2F. NEUROLOGICAL FINDINGS. Peripheral neuropathy has been documented as a feature of galactoflavin-induced riboflavin deficiency in four patients. These patients received the riboflavin deficient diet for at least 90 days and a total dosage of at least 175 g galactoflavin. In one patient, symptoms began shortly after reversal of the deficiency with riboflavin. The neuropathy has a stocking-glove distribution. Initially, patients complained of hyperesthesia and then of coldness, numbness, and pain in the hands and feet. These symptoms fluctuated from day-to-day both in quality and intensity, were aggravated by exposure to heat or cold, occasionally subsided completely for several days, but then persisted. Objective evidences of neurological dysfunction usually developed weeks to months after the onset of these symptoms. Sensory modalities were affected primarily, including first diminished perception of light touch, then of pain, temperature, vibration, and finally of position. Muscle tenderness was noted in two patients. Subsequently, the deep tendon reflexes became hypoactive to absent. Two patients walked with an ataxic gait as a result of sensory losses, since motor modalities were affected only minimally. The lower extremities were afflicted more severely than the upper extremities. Tests of peripheral nerve conduction eventually reflected slowing of sensory conduction and increased latency. However, these changes did not become manifest despite repeated tests until the patients had well developed symptomatology and physical findings, so that conduction studies could not be used to detect early evidences of neuropathy. The cerebrospinal fluid pressure was normal, and examination of the fluid was unremarkable in all but one case. That patient had a febrile illness approximately 1 week before the development of objective signs of neuropathy, and the spinal fluid protein concentration gradually increased from 80 mg% at that time to 270 mg% over the next 3 months and was normal 5 months later. There was no pleocytosis. This patient's neuropathy was more severe than in the other cases and may have actually been due to a Guillain-Barré syndrome. Recovery from the neuropathy has been slow. Complete recovery occurred in less than 9 months in two patients. Two patients died 1 month and 13 months after onset of neuropathy, and both had some persistant neurological deficits. The patient whose spinal fluid was abnormal was capable of walking unassisted, but her gait was broad based, and she still had hypoactive reflexes and some ataxia of the lower extremities 4 years after the initial symptomatology. The administration of large oral and parenteral doses of riboflavin, other vitamins of the B-complex and prednisone did not appear to hasten neurological improvement in these patients. Since our recognition of this neuropathy, we have limited the daily dose of galactoflavin to 1.5 g, the total dose of 75 g, and the treatment period to 8 weeks.

3.2.2G. METABOLIC EFFECTS. Body Weight. Although some patients lost weight during the study, it appeared to be related to inability to maintain an adequate intake of formula as a result of progression of neoplastic disease. Patients who had a constant intake of formula and whose neoplastic disease did not appear to progress maintained body weight throughout several months of riboflavin deficiency (Fig. 4).

Urinary Riboflavin. When patients were placed on the deficient formula, the 24-hr urine riboflavin fell immediately, as expected. Those patients on the diet providing 33 μg/1400 cal had levels below 0.05 mg/day. Galactoflavin administration resulted in a prompt increase in riboflavin excretion to peak levels of 2-3 mg/day. Over a period of weeks, the increased excretion of riboflavin persisted but progressively diminished in amount until the vitamin could no longer be detected. Only a small percentage of riboflavin administered orally or parenterally to deficient subjects receiving galactoflavin appeared in the urine during the first few days of reversal. These observations indicate that galactofla-

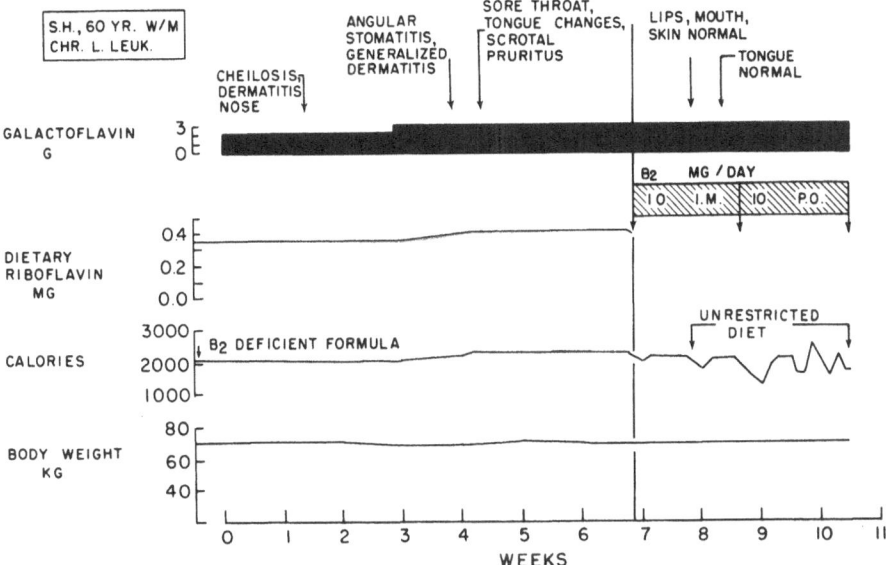

Fig. 4. Course of development and reversal of riboflavin deficiency. Note constancy of body weight. (From Lane et al. [51] Courtesy of Rockefeller University Press, New York.)

vin did not produce the initial increase in the urinary excretion of riboflavin by enhancing renal clearance of the vitamin, but that it probably displaced riboflavin from the tissues. As the tissue stores were replenished, increasing percentages of the administered riboflavin were excreted (Fig. 5).

The increased excretion of riboflavin with galactoflavin therapy and the finding of lower levels of riboflavin, FMN, and FAD, as well as the presence of galactoflavin in the livers of rats that were on normal diets or riboflavin-deficient diets with and without supplemental galactoflavin [51,52] indicate that the antagonist displaced riboflavin from the tissues. The antagonist was not converted into metabolites. In these experiments, galactoflavin increased the depletion of tissue riboflavin and produced a much greater reduction in tissue flavin nucleotides than did dietary deprivation alone. Prosky et al. [60] have also reported that galactoflavin metabolites could not be recovered in the tissues but found no evidence that galactoflavin replaced riboflavin in the tissues. This difference in result may be due to the fact that these authors fed 2 g galactoflavin/kg of diet to 250-g rats, while Prosky et al. fed 200 mg/kg to weanling rats. In their experiments, galactoflavin represented 0.1–0.2% liver flavin. Our studies showed that riboflavin constituted 1.1% of liver flavin of animals on the deficient diet but only 0.6% of

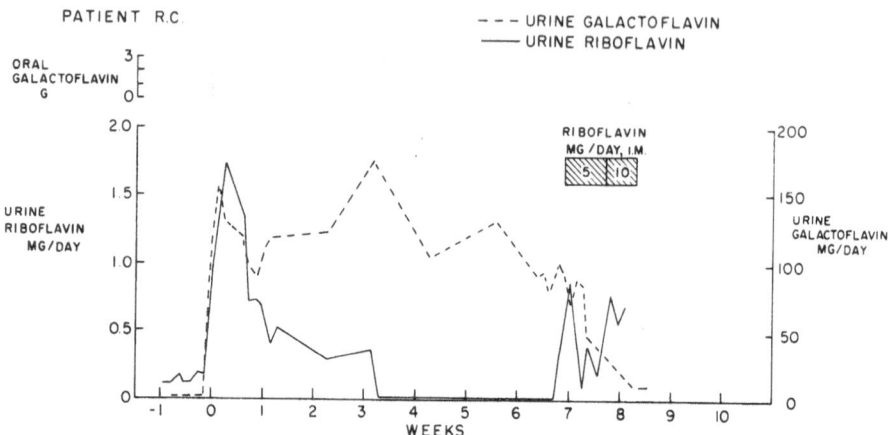

Fig. 5. Riboflavin and galactoflavin content of urine of patient. (From Lane et al.[51] Courtesy of Rockefeller University Press, New York.)

the liver flavin of rats treated with galactoflavin, and the galactoflavin content of these livers exceeded that of riboflavin. In our study, liver FAD and FMN were decreased about equally at 21 days, but in weanling rats[25,60] FMN was clearly more depressed than FAD at 4 weeks.

Other Vitamins. The urinary excretion of pantothenic acid and folic acid was not influenced by riboflavin deficiency. No consistent changes were noted in serum vitamin A and vitamin B_{12} concentrations.

Routine Laboratory Tests. There have been no consistent changes that might be related to induced riboflavin deficiency in the serum electrolytes, liver function tests, urea nitrogen, uric acid, or serum protein electrophoretic patterns. Some patients had decreases in serum cholesterol levels which probably were a reflection of the composition of the semisynthetic diet.

3.2.3. Comparison of Experimental Dietary and Antagonist-Induced Deficiencies

There are obvious similarities between experimental dietary and antagonist-induced riboflavin deficiency, and they relate primarily to changes in the mucous membranes and skin. Thus, angular stomatitis, cheilosis, glossitis, erythematous oral mucous membranes, seborrheic dermatitis, and scrotal dermatitis occur with both types of induced deficiency. Corneal changes have not occurred in induced deficiency and apparently occur only in endemic deficiency, perhaps related to multiple nutritional deficits or to ocular trauma.

In antagonist-induced deficiency, clinical signs become evident in a few weeks compared to many months. One of the consistent features of the deficiency is the development of reticulocytopenia, anemia, morphological changes in red cell precursors, erythroid hypoplasia, and changes in ferrokinetics. These changes have not been reported in human experimental dietary deficiency. Anemia has been noted in some experiments with lower species,[22,44,68,69,81,84] but not in others.[6,79] Anemia responsive to riboflavin has been reported in subjects with endemic multiple deficiency states.[28,29]

Neuropathy has been described in riboflavin-deficient animals,[23,67,76] but not in experimental dietary deficiency in humans. It is clearly a feature of antagonist-induced deficiency, and its development is correlated with prolonged deficiency and high doses of galactoflavin.

The speed of development of the deficiency appears to be due to antagonist-induced loss of riboflavin from the body. Reversal of the anemia with riboflavin during continued administration of galactoflavin indicates that the anemia is due to deficiency of riboflavin and is not simply a toxic effect of the analogue. The finding of vacuolated proerythroblasts and increased urinary erythropoietin during the anemia suggests that the primary lesion occurs in erythroid precursors. Its biochemical etiology has not been defined, but it is unlikely that glutathione reductase is involved since other conditions with low GR levels are not characterized by erythroid hypoplasia and vacuolated proerythroblasts. In some patients with splenomegaly, antagonist-induced deficiency was also accompained by leukopenia and thrombocytopenia that responded to riboflavin therapy.

While the slow reversal of the neuropathy is consonant with recovery from nerve injury, it obfuscates determination of the etiology of the injury. Thus, it can not be stated whether riboflavin deficiency or galactoflavin itself is damaging to peripheral nerves. The animal experiments cited previously would suggest that the deficiency itself could account for the neuropathy.

3.2.4. Effects of Galactoflavin-Induced Deficiency in Neoplastic and Myeloproliferative Diseases

An inadequate number of patients in any single disease category have been studied to estimate the value of galactoflavin-induced deficiency as a form of cancer therapy. Reduction of tumor size occurred in one patient with colon cancer. Two of four patients with lymphosarcoma

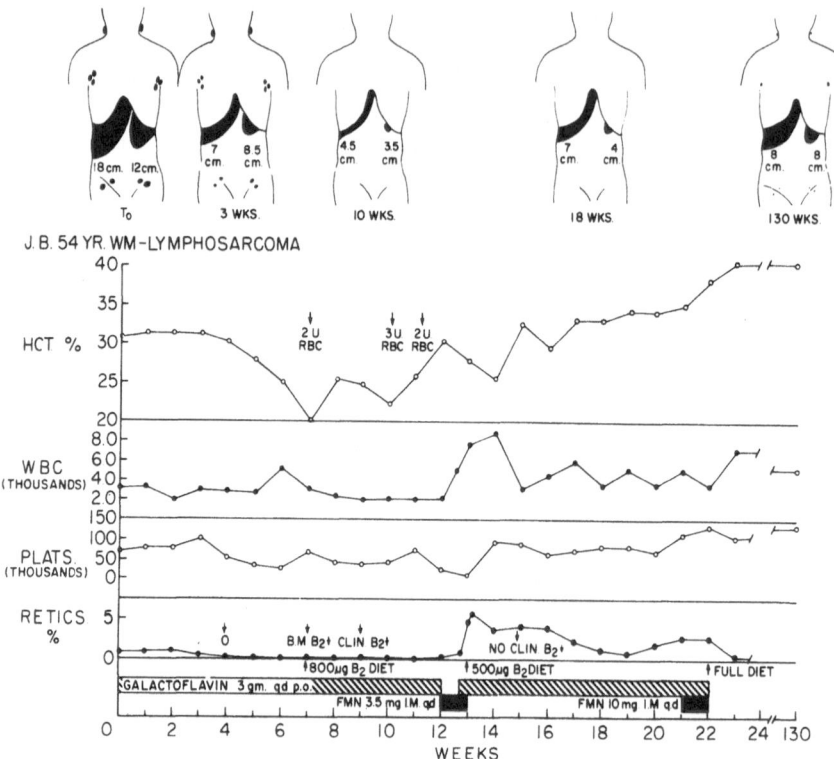

Fig. 6. Clinical course of patient with lymphosarcoma treated with riboflavin-deficient diet and galactoflavin. Patient survived for an additional 18 months in partial remission and succumbed to a myocardial infarction.

had greater than 75% regression of lymphadenopathy and hepatospleno-megaly. These partial remissions lasted 3 months and 4 years, respectively. The clinical course of one of the these patients is depicted in Fig. 6. Two patients with Hodgkin's disease have been treated and one responded. This patient had an almost complete disappearance of evident peripheral and mediastinal lymphadenopathy and of hepatosplenomegaly, when she developed miliary tuberculosis. The riboflavin deficiency program was terminated and she was treated successfully with antituberculosis chemotherapy. There was relapse of Hodgkin's disease in 3 months.

    Provocative observations have been made in patients with polycythemia rubra vera. Five patients were treated and in each case the hematocrit, leukocyte count, and platelet count fell into or below the normal range and there was reduction in liver or spleen size (Table V). Following

TABLE V. Effect of Induced Riboflavin Deficiency on Hematological Parameters of Patients with Polycythemia Vera

Patient	Predeficiency						Deficiency						
	Hct, %	Retics, %	WBC 10^3	Plats 10^3	Liver,[a] cm	Spleen,[b] cm	Hct, %	Retics, %	WBC 10^3	Plats 10^3	Liver,[a] cm	Spleen,[b] cm	Weeks of Treatment
B. W.	62	1.9	17.0	374	6	6	34	<0.1	6.0	180	0	0	12
H. M.	55	1.2	7.7	403	10	22	38	0.1	4.5	365	0	10	4
R. W.	44	1.8	9.0	637	6	4	33	<0.1	4.4	448	5	4	6
F. W.	56	1.0	4.7	295	2	4	42	<0.1	2.8	231	2	1	5
R. T.	58	4.0	29.6	248	11	14	36	<0.1	7.2	41	9	11	6

[a] Distance below right costal margin in mid-clavicular line.
[b] Distance below left costal margin in mid-clavicular line.

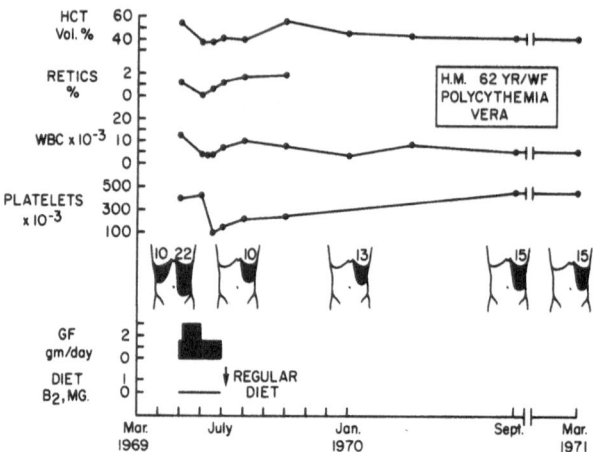

Fig. 7. Clinical course of patient with polycythemia vera treated with riboflavin-deficient diet and galactoflavin. Patient continues to have normal hematocrit, white blood cell, and platelet counts to the present.

reversal of the deficiency, the hematocrit, leukocyte count, and platelet count rose to pretreatment values. The liver and spleen did not increase in size in some patients, or increased in others but not to their size prior to treatment. The first two patients treated then showed a spontaneous fall to normal in peripheral blood elements. This remission lasted 3 yr prior to relapse in one case and is continuing after 3 yr in another. The latter patient had previously relapsed after three courses of radioactive phosphorus and required phlebotomy at 1- to 2-month intervals. This patient's course is depicted in Fig. 7. The other three patients were not observed sufficiently long to determine if similar remission would occur.

4. SUMMARY

The clinical signs and symptoms of dietary deficiency of riboflavin have been characterized through the efforts of many investigators. The overt evidences of deficiency tend to develop very slowly despite severe restriction of the vitamin and do not seem to be of threatening proportions to adults, since they consist primarily of changes in the mucous membranes of the lips and mouth, glossitis, and dermatitis. Consistent or significant ocular abnormalities have not been related to experimental dietary deficiency of the vitamin. Methods have been developed for estimating the adequacy of riboflavin intake and of the stores of riboflavin in the tissues. The minimum daily requirement of riboflavin for maintenance of clinically adequate nutrition has been bracketed within fairly narrow limits. There is undoubtedly much to be learned concerning the metabolic consequences of riboflavin deficiency which is not recognized clinically, but may be manifested at the biochemical level.

The use of a riboflavin antagonist has resulted in rapid development of deficiency with reproduction of the clinical signs of dietary deficiency. It has also been associated with important hematological and neurological effects. Antagonist-induced deficiency has resulted in regression of some human neoplasms, particularly lymphomas, and has produced remission in polycythemia rubra vera. The value of this approach for treatment of cancer patients is uncertain and will require broader clinical trials. It would be desirable to have a more potent riboflavin antagonist for such studies, so that patients could be given a normal diet. However, an antagonist of very high activity, such as a pseudo-irreversible inhibitor, might not be desirable. It is conceivable that a highly potent drug might produce frequent, severe neuropathy, marrow injury, or other unwarranted toxicities.

5. REFERENCES

1. Alfrey, C. P., Jr., and Lane, M. 1970. The effect of riboflavin deficiency on erythropoiesis, Sem. Hemat. 7:49-54.
2. Alfrey, C. P., Jr., Lane, M., and Karjala, R. J. 1966. Modification of ferrokinetics in man by cancer chemotherapeutic agents, Cancer 19:428-432.
3. Alfrey, C. P., Jr., Lynch, E. C., and Hettig, R. A. 1969. Studies of iron kinetics using a linear scanner. I. Distribution of sites of uptake of plasma iron in hematological disorders, J. Lab. Clin. Med. 73:405-417.
4. Aposhian, H. V., and Lambooy, J. P. 1951. Retardation of growth of Walker rat carcinoma 256 by administration of diethyl riboflavin, Proc. Soc. Exptl. Biol. Med. 78:197-199.
5. Arakawa, T., Mizuno, T., Chiba, F., Sakai, K., Watanabe, S., and Tamura, T. 1968. Frequency analysis of electroencephalograms and latency of photically induced average evoked responses in children with ariboflavinosis (preliminary report), Tohoku J. Exptl. Med. 94:327-335.
6. Axelrod, A. E., Lipton, M. A., and Elvehjem, C. A. 1941. Riboflavin deficiency in the dog, Amer. J. Physiol. 133:555-561.
7. Aykroyd, W. R., and Krishnan, B. G. 1936. Stomatitis due to vitamin B_2 deficiency, Indian J. Med. Res. 24:411-417.
8. Aykroyd, W. R., and Krishnan, B. G. 1938. The treatment of stomatitis caused by diet deficiency, Indian J. Med. Res. 25:643-646.
9. Bahr, P. H. 1914. A report on researches in sprue in Ceylon, Cambridge University Press, London.

10. Bamji, M. S. 1969. Glutathione reductase activity in red blood cells and riboflavin nutritional status in humans, *Clin. Chim. Acta* **26**:263-269.

11. Bessey, O. A., Horwitt, M. K., and Love, R. H. 1956. Dietary deprivation of riboflavin and blood riboflavin levels in man, *J. Nutr.* **58**:367-383.

12. Beutler, E. 1969. The effect of flavin coenzymes on the activity of erythrocyte enzymes. *Experentia* **25**:804.

13. Beutler, E. 1969. The correction of glutathione reductase deficiency by riboflavin administration, *J. Clin. Invest.* **48**:7a.

14. Beutler, E. 1969. Glutathione reductase: stimulation in normal subjects by riboflavin supplementation, *Science* **165**:613-615.

15. Beutler, E. 1969. Effect of flavin compounds on glutathione reductase activity: *in vivo* and *in vitro* studies, *J. Clin. Invest.* **48**:1957-1966.

16. Brewer, W., Porter, T., Ingalis, R., and Ohlson, M. A. 1946. The urinary excretion of riboflavin by college women, *J. Nutr.*, **32**:583-596.

17. Burch, H. B., Bessey, O. A., and Lowry, O. H. 1948. Fluorimetric measurements of riboflavin and its natural derivatives in small quantities of blood serum and cells, *J. Bio. Chem.* **175**:457-470.

18. Buzard, J. A., and Kopko, F. 1963. The flavin requirement and some inhibition characteristics of rat tissue glutathione reductase, *J. Biol. Chem.* **238**:464-468.

19. Emerson, G. A., and Tishler, M. 1944. The antiriboflavin effect of isoriboflavin, *Proc. Soc. Exptl. Biol. Med.* **55**:184-185.

20. Emerson, G. A., Wurtz, E., and Johnson, O. H. 1945. The antiriboflavin effect of galactoflavin, *J. Biol. Chem.* **160**:165-167.

21. Emmerie, A. 1936. Determination and excretion of flavins in normal human urine, *Nature* **138**:164.

22. Endicott, K. M., Kornberg, A., and Ott, M. 1947. Hemopoiesis in riboflavin-deficient rats, *Blood* **2**:164-174.

23. Engel, R. W., and Phillips, P. H. 1939. Effect of riboflavin-low diets upon nerves, growth, and reproduction in the rat, *Proc. Soc. Exptl. Biol.* **40**:597-598.

24. Fall, H. H., and Petering, H. G. 1956. Metabolite inhibitors. I. 6,7-dimethyl-9-formyl-methylisoalloxazine, 6,7-dimethyl-9-(2'-hydroxyethyl)-isoalloxazine and derivatives, *J. Am. Chem. Soc.* **78**:370-380.

25. Fass, S., and Rivlin, R. S. 1969. Regulation of riboflavin-metabolizing enzymes in riboflavin deficiency, *Amer. J. Physiol.* **217**:988-991.

26. Feder, V. H., Lewis, G. T., and Alden, H. S. 1944. Studies on the urinary excretion of riboflavin, *J. Nutr.* **27**:347-353.

27. Ferrebee, J. W. 1940. The urinary excretion of riboflavin. Fluorometric methods for its estimation, *J. Clin. Invest.* **19**:251-256.

28. Foy, H., and Kondi, A. 1953. A case of true red-cell aplastic anaemia successfully treated with riboflavin, *J. Pathol. Bacteriol.*, **65**:559-564.

29. Foy, H, and A. Kondi. 1961. Pure red cell aplasia in marasmus and kwashiorkor treated with riboflavine, *Brit. Med. J.*, **1**:937-941.

30. Glatzke, D., Weber, F., and Wiss, O. 1968. Enzymatic test for the detection of riboflavin deficiency. NADPH-dependent glutathione reductase of red blood cells and its activation by FAD *in vitro, Experientia* **24**:1122.

31. Goldberger, J., and Tanner, W. F. 1925. A study of the pellagra-preventive action of dried beans, casein, dried milk, and brewer's yeast, with a consideration of the essential preventive factors involved, U.S. *Pub. Health Rept.*, **40**:54-80.

32. Helmer, O. M. 1935. Vitamin B_1 and B_2 content of human urine, *Proc. Soc. Exptl. Biol. Med.* **32**:1187-1188.

33. Helmer, O. M. 1937. The determination of vitamins B and G in human urine by the rat-growth method, *J. Nutr.* **13**:279-286.

34. Hills, O. W., Liebert, E., Steinberg, D. L., and Horwitt, M. K. 1951. Clinical aspects of dietary depletion of riboflavin. *Arch. Intern. Med.* **87**:682-693.

35. Holly, F. W., Peel, E. W., Mozingo, R., and Folkers, K. 1950. Studies on carcinolytic compounds. I. 6,7-dichloro-9-(1'-D-sorbityl)-isoalloxazine, *J. Am. Chem. Soc.* **72**:5416-5418.

36. Horwitt, M. K., Liebert, E., Kreisler, O., and Wittman, P. 1948. Investigations of human requirements for B-complex vitamins, *Bull. Nat. Res. Council,* No. 116. National Academy of Sciences, Washington, D.C.

37. Horwitt, M. K., Hills, O. W., Harvey, C. C., Liebert, E., and Steinberg, D. L. 1949. Effects of dietary depletion of riboflavin, *J. Nutr.* **39**:357-373.

38. Horwitt, M. K., Sampson, G., Hills, O. W., and Steinberg, D. L. 1949. Dietary management in a study of riboflavin requirements, *J. Amer. Diet. Assoc.* **25**:591-594.

39. Horwitt, M. K., Harvey, C. C., Hills, O. W., and Liebert, E. 1950. Correlation of urinary excretion of riboflavin with dietary intake and symptoms of ariboflavinosis, *J. Nutr.* **41**:247-264.

40. Horwitt, M. K., Harvey, C. C., Rothwell, W. S., Cutler, J. L., and Haffron, D. 1956. Tryptophan-niacin relationships in man, *J. Nutr.* **60**:suppl. 1, 1-43.

41. Icen, A. 1967. Glutathione reductase and human erythrocytes. Purification and properties, *Scand. J. Clin. Lab. Invest. Suppl.* **96**:1-67.

42. Keys, A., Henschel, A. F., Mickelsen, O., Brozek, J. M., and Crawford, J. H. 1944. Physiological and biochemical functions in normal young men on a diet restricted in riboflavin, *J. Nutr.* **27**:165-178.

43. Klein, J. R., and Kohn, H. I. 1940. The synthesis of flavin-adenine dinucleotide from riboflavin by human blood cells *in vitro* and *in vivo, J. Biol. Chem.* **136**:177-189.

44. Kornberg, A., Tabor, H., and Sebrell, W. H. 1945. Blood regeneration in rats deficient in biotin, thiamin or riboflavin, *Amer. J. Physiol.* **145**:54-66.

45. Kruse, H. D., Sydenstricker, V. P., Sebrell, W. H., and Cleckley, H. M. 1940. Ocular manifestations of ariboflavinosis, *U.S. Pub. Health Rept.* **55**:157-169.

46. Landor, J. V., and Pallister, R. A. 1935. Avitaminosis B$_2$. *Trans. Roy. Soc. Trop. Med. Hyg.* **29**:121-134.

47. Lane, M. 1964. Studies on the mechanism of the growth inhibitory action of galactoflavin in rats, *Cancer Res.* **24**:1811-1813.

48. Lane, M., Fahey, J. L., Sullivan, R. D., and Zubrod, C. G. 1958. The comparative pharmacology in man and the rat of the riboflavin analogue, 6,7-dimethyl-9-(2'-acetoxyethyl)-isoalloxazine, U-2112, *J. Pharmacol. Exptl. Therap.* **122**:315-326.

49. Lane, M., Petering, H. G., and Brindley, C. O. 1959. Synthesis, pharmacology, and clinical trial of the riboflavine analogue, sodium-6,7-dimethyl-9-(2'-hemisuccinoxyethyl)-isolloxazine, U-6358, *J. Natl. Cancer Inst.* **22**:346-361.

50. Lane, M., Mengel, C. E., and Doherty, D. J. 1960. Rapid induction of isolated riboflavin deficiency in man, *J. Clin. Invest.* **39**:1004.

51. Lane, M., Alfrey, C. P., Jr., Mengel, C. E., Doherty, M. A., and Doherty, J. 1964. The rapid induction of human riboflavin deficiency with galactoflavin, *J. Clin. Invest.* **43**:357-373.

52. Lane, M., and Brindley, C. O. 1964. Laboratory and clinical studies with the riboflavin antagonist, galactoflavin. *Proc. Soc. Exptl. Biol. Med.* **116**:57-61.

53. Lane, M., and Alfrey, C. P., Jr., 1965. The anemia of human riboflavin deficiency, *Blood* **25**:432-442.

54. Lane, M., and Smith, F. E. 1971. Induced riboflavin deficiency in treatment of patients with lymphomas and polycythemia vera, *Proc. Amer. Assoc. Cancer Res.* **12**:85.
55. Machella, T. E. 1942. Studies of the B vitamins in the human subject. III. The response of cheilosis to vitamin therapy, *Amer. J. Med. Sci.* **203**:114-120.
56. Machella, T. E., and McDonald, P. R. 1943. Studies of the B vitamins in the human subject. VI. Failure of riboflavin therapy in patients with the accepted picture of riboflavin deficiency. *Amer. J. Med. Sci.* **205**:214-222.
57. Mandula, B., and Beutler, E. 1970. Synthesis of riboflavin nucleotides by mature human erythrocytes, *Blood* **36**:491-499.
58. Moore, D. G. F. 1930. Partial loss of central acuity of vision for reading and for distance in school children and its possible association with food deficiency, *West African Med. J.* **4**:46-48.
59. Morris, H. P., and Robertson, W. R. 1943. Growth rate and number of spontaneous mammary carcinomas and riboflavin concentration of liver, muscles, and tumor of C_3H mice as influenced by dietary riboflavin, *J. Natl. Cancer Inst.* **3**:479-489.
60. Prosky, L., Burch, H. B., Bejrablaya, D., Lowry, O. H., and Combs, A. M. 1964. The effects of galactoflavin on riboflavin enzymes and coenzymes, *J. Biol. Chem.* **239**:2691-2695.
61. Roscoe, M. H. 1936. The B vitamins in human urine, *Biochem. J.* **30**:1053-1063.
62. Scott, H. H. 1918. An investigation into an acute outbreak of "central neuritis," *Ann. Trop. Med. Parasit.* **12**:109-196.
63. Scott, E. M., Duncan, I. W., and Ekstrand, V. 1963. Purification and properties of glutathione reductase of human erythrocytes, *J. Biol. Chem.* **238**:3928-3933.
64. Sebrell, W. H., and Butler, R. E. 1938. Riboflavin deficiency in man. A preliminary note, *Pub. Health Rept.* **53**:2282-2284.
65. Sebrell, W. H., and Butler, R. E. 1939. Riboflavin deficiency in man (ariboflavinosis), *Pub. Health. Rept.* **54**:2121-2131.
66. Sebrell, W. H., Butler, R. E., Wooley, J. G., and Isbell, H. 1941. Human riboflavin requirement estimated by urinary excretion of subjects on controlled intake, *Pub. Health Rept.* **56**:510-519.
67. Shaw, J. H., and Phillips, P. H. 1941. The pathology of riboflavin deficiency in the rat, *J. Nutr.* **22**:345-358.
68. Shuckers, C. F., and Day, P. L. 1943. The effects of inanition and riboflavin deficiency upon the blood picture of the rat, *J. Nutr.* **25**:511-520.
69. Spector, H., Maass, A. R., Michaud, L., Elvehjem, C. A., and Hart, E. B. 1943. The role of riboflavin in blood regeneration, *J. Biol. Chem.* **150**:75-87.
70. Spies, T. D., Bean, W. B., and Ashe, W. F. 1939a. Recent advances in the treatment of pellagra and associated deficiencies, *Ann. Int. Med.* **12**:1830-1843.
71. Spies, T. D., Vilter, R. W., and Ashe, W. F. 1939b. Pellagra, beriberi, and riboflavin deficiency in human beings, *J. Amer. Med. Assoc.* **113**:931-937.
72. Spies, T. D., Bean, W. B., Vilter, R. W., and Huff, N. E. 1940. Endemic riboflavin deficiency in infants and children, *Amer. J. Med. Sci.* **200**:697-701.
73. Stannus, H. S. 1912. Pellagra in Nyasaland, *Trans. Soc. Trop. Med. Hyg.* **5**:112-119.
74. Steinfeld, J. L., White, L. P., Petrakis, N. L., and Shimkin, M. B. 1954. Negative effects of some metabolite analogs in human neoplasms, *Cancer Res.* **14**:315-318.
75. Stoerk, H. C., and Emerson, G. A. 1949. Complete regression of lymphosarcoma implants following temporary induction of riboflavin deficiency in mice, *Proc. Soc. Exptl. Biol. Med.* **70**:703-704.
76. Street, H. R., Cowgill, G. R., and Zimmerman, H. M. 1941. Further observations of riboflavin deficiency in the dog, *J. Nutr.* **22**:7-24.

77. Sydenstricker, V. P. 1941. The clinical manifestations of nicotinic acid and riboflavin deficiency (pellagra), *Ann. Int. Med.* **14**:1499-1517.
78. Sydenstricker, V. P., Geeshin, L. E., Templeton, C. M., and Weaver, J. M. 1939. Riboflavin deficiency in human subjects, *J. Amer. Med. Assoc.*, **113**:1697-1670.
79. Terrill, S. W., Ammerman, C. B., Walker, D. E., Edwards, R. M., Norton, H. W., and Becker, D. E. 1955. Riboflavin studies with pigs, *J. Animal Sci.* **14**:593-603.
80. Tisdall, F. F., McCreary, J. F., and Pearce, H. 1943. The effect of riboflavin deficiency on corneal vascularization and symptoms of eye fatigue in R.C.A.F. personnel, *Canad. Med. Assoc. J.* **49**:5-13.
81. Waisman, H. A. 1944. Production of riboflavin deficiency in the monkey, *Proc. Soc. Exptl. Biol. Med.* **55**:69-71.
82. Wheeler, G. A. 1933. The pellagra-preventive value of autoclaved dried yeast, canned flaked haddock, and canned green peas, *Pub. Health Rep.* **48**:67-77.
83. Williams, R. D., Mason, H. L., Cusick, P. L., and Wilder. R. M. 1943. Observations on induced riboflavin deficiency and the riboflavin requirement of man, *J. Nutr.* **25**:361-377.
84. Wintrobe, M. M., Buschke, W., Fallis, R. H., Jr., and Humphreys, S. 1944. Riboflavin deficiency in swine with special reference to the occurrence of cataracts, *Bull. Johns Hopkins Hosp.* **75**:102-114.

RIBOFLAVIN DEFICIENCY AND CONGENITAL MALFORMATIONS

Josef Warkany

1. INTRODUCTION

Experimental riboflavin deficiency has served as a useful tool of teratologic research in mammals. It had been possible for over 100 years to produce congenital malformations in chicks by various environmental disturbances, and for many years a variety of monstrosities had been produced experimentally in amphibia and fishes. Eggs and embryos of animals of lower classes are easily accessible to modification, but mammalian ova that develop in the mother's body are well protected against adverse influences of the outside world. It was generally assumed until 35 years ago that environmental insults to pregnant mammals terminate in death of the embryos—or leave them morphologically intact, resulting in the birth of normal young. It was believed, and often dogmatically stated, that in mammals and in man systemic and internal congenital malformations must be genetically determined and hereditary, since, with the exception of rare amputations by mechanical intrauterine disturbances, no exogenous factors were known that could bring about prenatal deformities in embryos and fetuses. It was thought in particular

JOSEF WARKANY—Children's Hospital Research Foundation and the Department of Pediatrics, College of Medicine, University of Cincinnati, Cincinnati, Ohio. Some of the results presented in this chapter were supported by NIH grants HD00502 and HD05221 and the Charles H. Hood Foundation.

that in mammals symmetrical and serial malformations (that is, defects involving upper and lower extremities) must be hereditary. This belief was expressed not only in the medical literature but also incorporated in the German Law of 1933 for Prevention of Offspring with Heritable Diseases.[59,65] It was known, of course, that heredity could not be proved in all cases and in all syndromes of human congenital malformations, but both sporadic and nonfamilial cases could be explained as new mutations or by various complicated and irregular modes of inheritance. To disprove the axiomatic belief that all systemic and internal malformations are hereditary, experimental evidence of exogenous causation was needed. Such experiments had been done with roentgen rays early in this century, but this work carried little conviction since it was based on a recently invented teratogenic method.

2. EARLY NUTRITION EXPERIMENTS

A more subtle interference with mammalian embryonic development was achieved in swine by withholding certain nutritional factors from the maternal diet.[67] Between 1933 and 1937 Hale[21,22] demonstrated that sows fed a vitamin A-free diet farrowed pigs born "without eyeballs." He proved that the defects of the pigs were not hereditary but were due to the maternal nutritional deprivation in early pregancy. It is understandable that swine because of their size and cost were not useful for large-scale experiments and that it took many years before Hale's work was repeated and expanded.[40]

We used in the 1930s dietary deficiencies in rats to produce rickets and endocrine disorders. By modification of a rachitogenic diet,[53] it was made possible to raise female rats fed such diets and to breed them.[55] When vitamin D was added to the original rachitogenic diet, rats grew and matured slowly, but eventually some of them conceived and delivered young. Among the young there were many—about one third—that had congenital malformations.[56] It was not known at first which nutritional factor was missing in the vitamin D-supplemented Steenbock diet (diet I); in fact it was not certain that the malformations were due to a nutritional deficiency. Much time and effort were spent to prove that they were not caused by some complicated genetic mechanism. But when it was established that supplementation of diet I with dried pig liver afforded complete protection of the young,[55] the nutritional origin of the malformations was considered proved. It was unknown, however, which of the innumerable nutritional factors

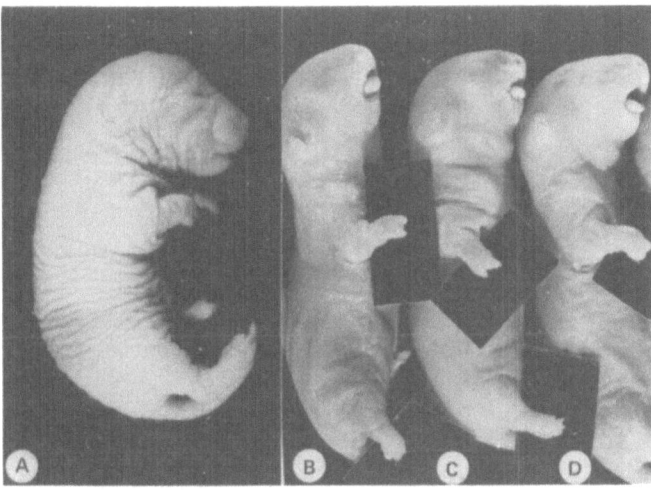

Fig. 1. Newborn rats. A. Control. B-D. Offspring of riboflavin-deficient mothers, showing short mandibles, protruding tongues, malpositioned extremities, and various degrees of syndactylism (approximately × 2).

contained in liver was the preventive one. In spite of this shortcoming, the newly found method could be used for a number of teratologic studies.

It was clear from inspection of the deformed newborns that we were dealing with a syndrome of congenital malformations that involved various parts of the body: the jaws, the palate, and the extremities (Figs. 1 and 2). Limb defects usually were bilateral, and upper as well as lower extremities were abnormal in many specimens. Entire litters were involved and in alternating litters of the same female normal or abnormal young could be produced according to the mother's diet.[57] These observations in themselves already proved that systemic, symmetrical, and serial malformations could be induced in a mammal by adverse environmental conditions. But more information was gained by clearing of the specimens, which permitted visualization of the entire skeleton (Fig. 3),[8] and by histologic sectioning, which revealed details of the tissues. Both methods demonstrated that the nutritional deficiency rendered some organs abnormal, while others were spared; it did not retard growth of all parts but deformed certain structures and left others intact. In this respect, the nutritional deficiency acted like an abnormal gene that produces limited and specific malformations but permits development of the rest of the organism. Needless to say, the dietary inadequacy exerted its injurious influence only on the young carried

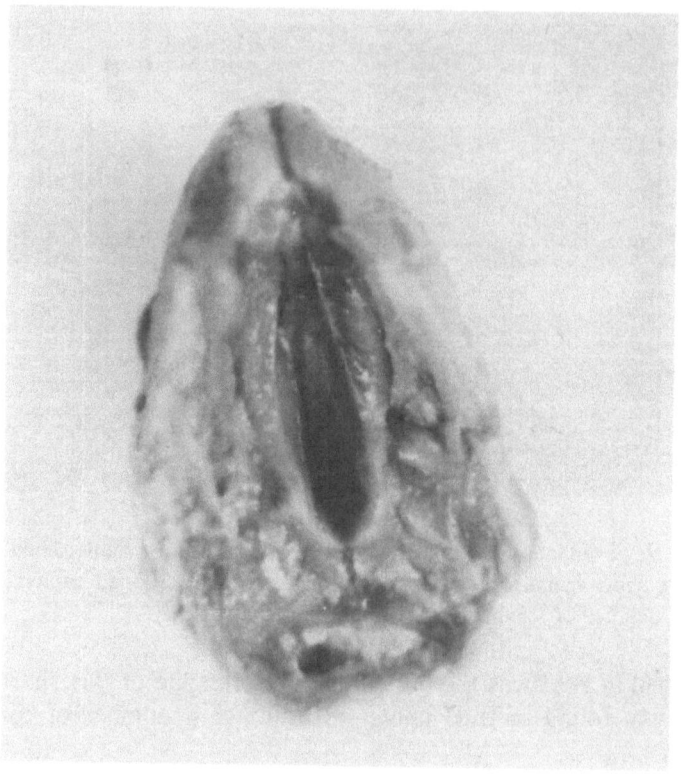

Fig. 2. Cleft palate produced by maternal riboflavin deficiency (× 6).

by the mother during her deficient dietary regime and not on subsequent generations. Occasionally, mildly deformed young could be raised and bred: Their offspring were always normal.

Table I lists the frequency of osseous defects in 100 cleared abnormal specimens. It shows that the tibia was often abnormal, while other bones were affected with decreasing frequency. Several gradients could be recognized. The lower extremities were more vulnerable than the upper; distal bones were more involved than proximal; and preaxial parts were more often abnormal than postaxial, for example, the tibia was sometimes shortened whereas the fibula was not; or the radius was more defective than the ulna (Fig. 3). The pattern of skeletal malformations is so specific that cleared specimens produced by this nutritional method can be easily distinguished from specimens rendered defective by other teratogenic methods.[61] The shortened mandible showed an interesting detail: The

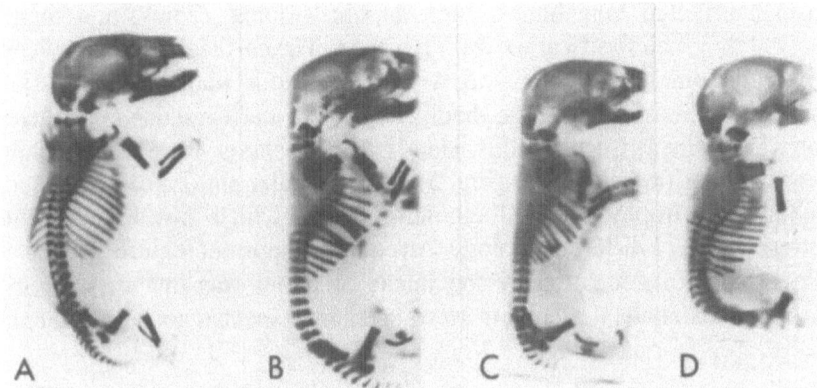

Fig. 3. Cleared specimens of newborn rats. A. Control. B-D. Offspring of riboflavin-deficient mothers. In B short mandible, fused ribs, and a markedly reduced tibia can be seen. In C the tibia is almost completely absent. In D there are no forearm bones and no bones in the lower leg. Note that B has same size as control, whereas D is much smaller.

corpus was markedly reduced while the rami were little affected, indicating like the limb bones a proximodistal gradient. A similar gradient was noted in the costal abnormalities. There was a high incidence of "fused ribs" and the fusions were always in the distal portions of the ribs (near the costochondral junctions) and not near their proximal (vertebral) origin (Fig. 3). The list in the table does not include cleft palate, one of the most interesting malformations produced by diet I. This anomaly is better recognized in intact animals than in cleared specimens (Fig. 2). Cleft palate occurred in 44% of the abnormal specimens[59] and ranked in frequency between those of the ulna and the humerus. Diet I was the first method that permitted experimental production of cleft palate with some regularity.

TABLE I. *Frequency of Osseous Defects in 100 Cleared Abnormal Specimens*

Tibia	93	Ulna	50
Mandible	80	Humerus	34
Ribs	75	Hindfoot	31
Fibula	63	Maxilla	8
Radius	58	Scapula	6
Hand	54	Clavicle	6
Sternum	52	Femur	1

Histologic studies added important information (Fig. 4).[58] Sections through affected long bones, such as tibia, fibula, radius, and ulna, showed that their ossification was disturbed. The cartilaginous ends were relatively long when compared with the osseous diaphyses, and the ossification lines between the diaphysis and the cartilaginous ends were not well defined. Cartilaginous islands and processes were seen within the partly ossified diaphyses (Fig. 5). This irregular pattern can be called a chondrodystrophy but not "achondroplasia," which shows a different pattern and has a different etiology. An equally important feature disclosed by histologic examination of specimens of diet I was that in sections cartilaginous skeletal elements were seen that seemed to be absent in

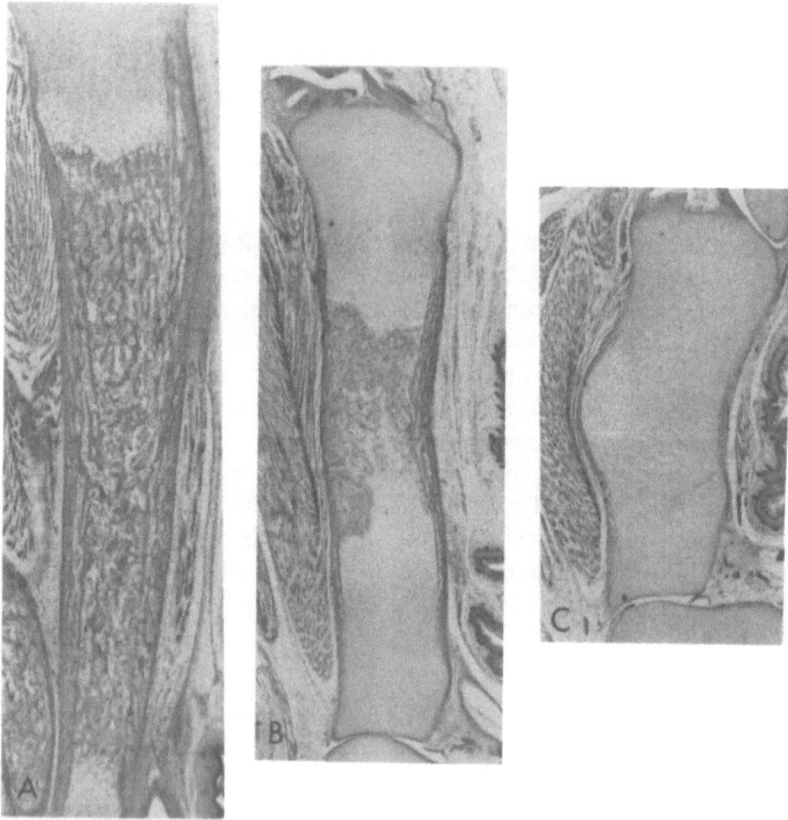

Fig. 4. Longitudinal sections through tibiae of newborn rats. A. Control. B-C. Offspring of riboflavin-deficient mothers showing shortened or absent ossified portions with relatively increased cartilaginous parts (× 18).

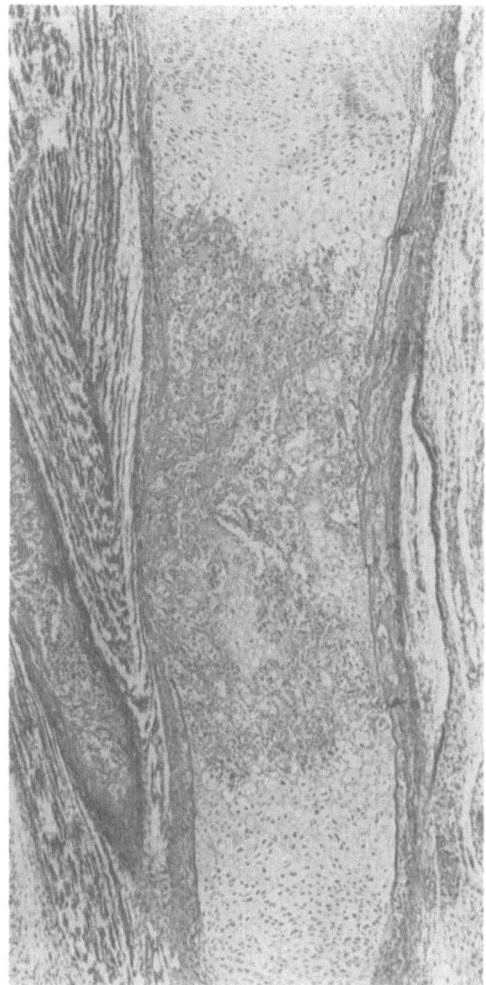

Fig. 5. Section shown in Fig. 4B at higher magnification. In the diaphysis osseous and cartilaginous tissues are intermingled (× 45).

cleared specimens in which only bones were stained specifically (Fig. 6). When syndactylous paws were sectioned, it was frequently seen that the fused digits consisted of broad cartilaginous structures; there was syndactylism already before ossification had taken place (Fig. 7). These histologic findings indicated that the skeletal anomalies produced were not due primarily to failure of ossification but to abnormal development of earlier stages of the skeleton; they were present at least as early as their cartilaginous precursors. Studies of sections of syndactylous paws of embryos sacrificed on the fifteenth day of gestation (Fig. 8) revealed that syndactylism was already present in the membranous stage of the skeleton, that is, before mesenchyme had been converted into cartilage or bone. It was recognized that the nutritional deficiency inhibited the development of certain skeletal structures in their early membranous stages. Since the number of digits becomes recognizable in 14-day rat embryos we thought development of an abnormal number of digits must be determined before day 14 of fetal life, but we could not conclude how long before this time the injury occurred.

Theoretically, the malformations could have been determined at any stage before, in the ovum, soon after fertilization, or at any time during the early gestational periods as late as day 14. The use of alternating

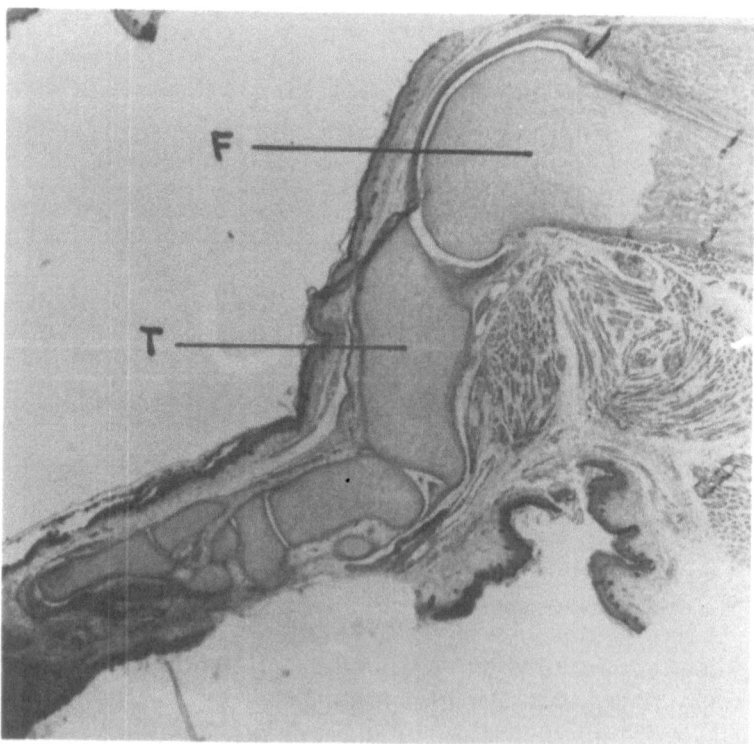

Fig. 6. Longitudinal section through the leg of an abnormal young. While the femoral end (F) is of normal size, the tibia (T) is very small and completely cartilaginous (× 18).

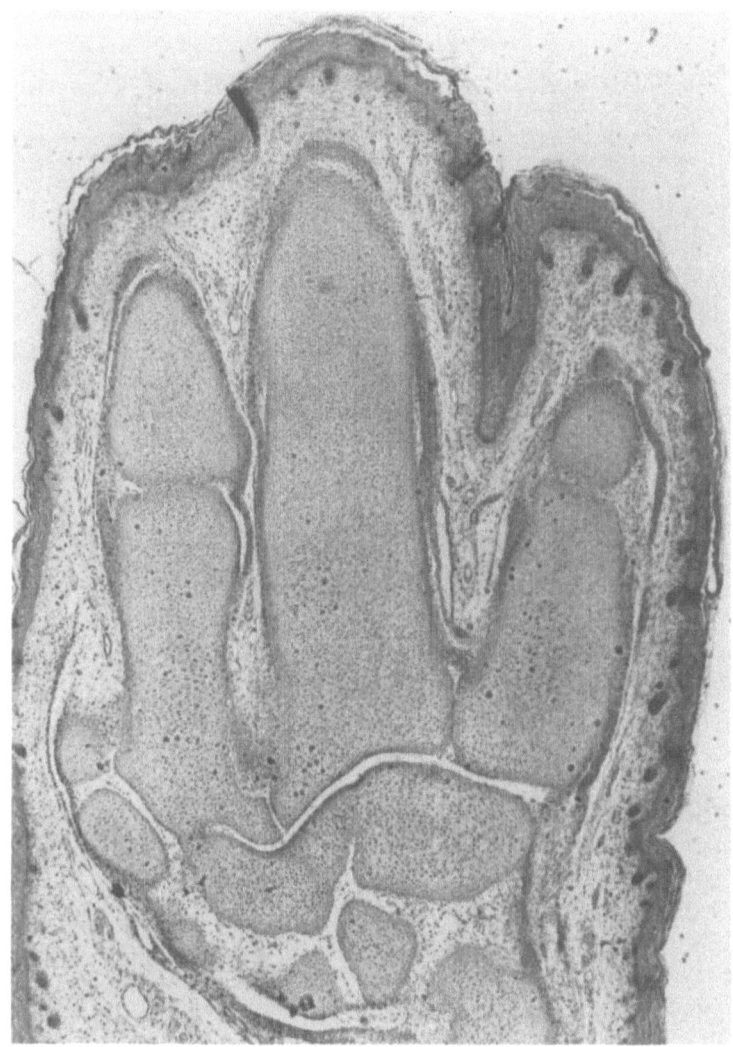

Fig. 7. Section through paw of abnormal newborn young. The broad central digit failed to divide into two digits. Note that the joint between metacarpal and basal phalanx of the syndactylous finger has not developed (× 50).

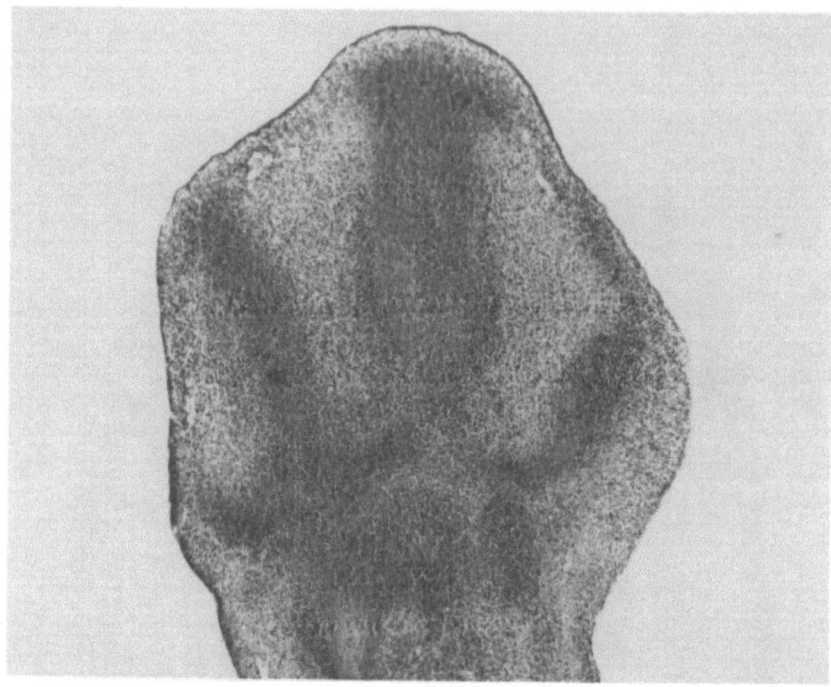

Fig. 8. Section through paw of a day 15 abnormal embryo showing broad and undivided central digit in mesenchymal stage (× 60).

diets offered an approach to this question.[57] It has been mentioned that abnormal offspring could be prevented when a change to the liver-containing diet was made. A series of experiments was instituted in which a change from diet I to the liver-supplemented diet I was made on different days after mating. Thus we hoped to ascertain the day before which the offspring could be protected by adding liver to the mother's diet and the day after which such protection would be impossible: Some rats received the liver supplement one day after mating, another rat on the second day, a third rat on the third day, and so forth, until such experiments with time-limited diets were made for each of the 21 days after conception. The result was that addition of liver up to the thirteenth day protected offspring. After day 14 the addition of liver to diet I did not afford complete protection as some abnormal offspring appeared. It seemed, therefore, that the developmental period between day 13 and day 14 of gestation should be considered as the critical period in which the nutritional factor exerted its influence. The absence or presence of the factor at this limited period determined whether or not malformations appeared.

3. RIBOFLAVIN DEFICIENCY AS A TERATOGENIC METHOD

The above teratologic studies progressed before we knew the nutrient whose lack in diet I was responsible for the malformations. The fact that a liver supplement always prevented the teratogenic effects of diet I was a lead, but this supplement was too complex to give us information about the preventive factor. Many attempts were made to ascertain by trial and error the substance or substances that prevented the malformations. Since diet I was known to be goitrogenic,[46] iodine was given as a supplement, but it failed to prevent the abnormalities. In the same way manganese, casein, wheat germ oil, cod liver oil, alfalfa leaf meal, and others were tested and found to be nonprotective. Because it was known that liver contains vitamins of the B-complex in large amounts, it seemed logical to test those that we could obtain in pure form. It was soon found that a mixture of thiamine, riboflavin, niacin, pyridoxine, and pantothenate prevented the malformations of the pattern of diet I. From then on, it was a matter of ascertaining the preventive B-vitamin or the preventive combinations of the group. Riboflavin proved to be the supplement to diet I that was needed for prevention (Table II).[60] Subsequently the crucial experiments were done with highly purified diets which had become available by that time. In these diets

TABLE II. *The Effect of Vitamin Supplementation of Diet I on the Appearance of Congenital Malformations in Rats*[a]

	Offspring		
Mothers fed diet I supplemented by:	*Total*	*Normal*	*Abnormal*
Riboflavin + thiamine + niacin + pyridoxine + Ca pantothenate	371	371	0
Thiamine + niacin + pyridoxine + Ca pantothenate	51	27	24
Pyridoxine + Ca pantothenate	67	47	20
Thiamine	152	125	27
Niacin	180	161	19
Riboflavin	319	319	0

[a]From Warkany and Schraffenberger.[60]

most of the nutritional factors were of known chemical constitution and the vitamin B complex was represented by crystalline preparations. It was shown that a purified diet that was lacking riboflavin was teratogenic and produced abnormalities identical with those of the pattern of diet I. But, when riboflavin was added to the diet, all young were anatomically normal. It was concluded that these experiments were "in accord with the assumption that a deficiency of riboflavin in the maternal diet is responsible for the abnormalities of the pattern of diet I."[60]

We have abbreviated our discussion of the experiments resulting in the discovery that a diet deficient in riboflavin could cause in rats a syndrome of skeletal congenital malformations. The brief account does not convey the difficulties encountered in the performance of these early experiments. Pregnant animals had to be kept on a borderline deficiency that was damaging the embryos while it kept mothers and fetuses alive. In the beginning, we tried to breed the females repeatedly with and without supplements[57] to prove that the malformations were due to the diet and not to the genetic constitution of the parents; this necessitated day and night "obstetrical care"; without supervision of the deliveries, the young—particularly the abnormals—would have been cannibalized by the mother who suffered from "hidden hunger." Such excessive precautions were necessary at a time when many scientists and physicians doubted that congenital malformations of mammals could be due to adverse environmental conditions during pregnancy. The difficult experimental setup probably was also responsible for the delayed confirmation of our findings. Except for a short confirmatory report,[38] it was not until 1947 that it was demonstrated that malformations of the pattern of diet I could be produced by riboflavin deficiency outside of our laboratory, when Giroud and Boisselot[17] began to make their contributions to this field and Gilman et al.[16] made a confirmatory report. Later Grainger et al.[20] found that addition of riboflavin to the vitamin D-supplemented, Steenbock and Black[53] diet did not completely prevent malformations. But this discrepancy was more apparent than real since the experiments of these authors differed in many respects from those of the earlier investigators. They used a different strain of rats, different basic rations, and different amounts of riboflavin for supplementation.

It was and still is surprising that riboflavin deficiency results in a syndrome that essentially consists of malformations of the skeleton. What does riboflavin have to do with formation of the skeleton and bone? Our histologic observations and experiments of "dating" the beginnings of the developmental deviations[62] led to the conclusion "that the formation of the membranous skeleton which precedes the cartilaginous as well as the osseous skeleton is inhibited by the riboflavin deficiency." Another surprising finding was that some of the deformed animals were of normal size when they were born; that is, differentiation seemed to be more affected by riboflavin deficiency than growth. Since riboflavin had been known to be essential for normal growth of young animals, the observation that it was also essential for differentiation of the membranous skeleton was of considerable interest. It should be emphasized that not all deformed young reached normal size. Many suffered from intrauterine growth retardation like most offspring obtained in various teratologic experiments. But that some young in the presence of riboflavin deficiency could achieve normal size in spite of abnormal differentiation is rather exceptional in teratologic experiments. The relationship of general growth to teratogenesis, neglected in early mammalian studies, has become of increasing interest to pediatricians since the difference of prematurity and intrauterine growth retardation has been rediscovered. [4,64]

4. RIBOFLAVIN ANTIMETABOLITES

The importance of riboflavin for the embryonic development of the rat was further demonstrated by Nelson and co-workers,[37] who introduced galactoflavin, a riboflavin antagonist, as a teratogenic agent. By combination of a riboflavin-deficient diet with a galactoflavin supplement, congenital malformations could be induced in the young of rats more rapidly and in a higher percentage than with the older deficiency method, which required feeding of the riboflavin-deficient diet weeks before mating. If a galactoflavin-containing diet is used, the depletion can be started after mating. The use of galacotoflavin with the maternal riboflavin-deficient diet fed during gestation commonly results in malformations of various soft tissue organs in addition to skeletal malformations, but the osseous and cartilaginous changes produced by galactoflavin closely simulate those obtained by riboflavin deficiency alone.

A riboflavin-deficient diet fed to *mice* before and during pregnancy does not produce congenital malformations. Mice do not reproduce under the dietary conditions teratogenic for rats. But, when pregnant mice of inbred A; DBA; 129; and C57Bl strains were subjected to a riboflavin-deficient, galactoflavin-supplemented diet for 96 hr (beginning 9 or 10 days after conception), the offspring presented a variety of congenital malformations of the skeleton as well as of many soft tissues, including the central nervous system. Offspring of the various strains differed greatly in regard to teratogenic levels of the antimetabolite as well as frequency and severity of specific malformations. [25] Several riboflavin antagonists besides galactoflavin have been used in metabolic and reproductive studies in rats. Although in some of these experiments abnormal offspring have been observed, the young were described as having functional anomalies but not malformations. [27] A specific enzyme inadequacy was induced in infant rats by the use of the riboflavin homologue 7-ethyl-8 methyl flavin. [26] It would be very interesting to test this and other riboflavin homologues in teratologic experiments.

5. COENZYME AND ENZYME STUDIES IN EMBRYONAL TISSUES

The discovery of the role played by riboflavin in developmental processes of mammalian embryos promised elucidation of some problems of cell division and differentiation. It pointed the way to investigation of enzymatic processes on the cellular level, since it was known that riboflavin is incorporated in prosthetic groups of certain enzymes that seemed to direct pathways of embryonic development. [62] During the last decades much has been learned about riboflavin metabolism and about metabolic effects of riboflavin deficiency, [49] but few investigations were directed toward elucidation of cellular processes that result in congenital malformations. One of the coenzymes under consideration is flavin mononucleotide (FMN); and another, flavin adenine dinucleotide (FAD). These two coenzymes form the prosthetic groups of a variety of flavoprotein enzymes. Miller et al. in 1962[35] found a lower flavin content in fetuses from riboflavin-deficient rats than in control fetuses. Experiments performed with embryos of mothers depleted of riboflavin by dietary means are at a disadvantage, since the pure deficiency method does produce malformations in only about one third of the offspring of riboflavin-deficient rats. Thus, embryos collected from such pregnant animals may be a mixture of deformed and normal specimens. This could "dilute" the results of chemical determinations. If, however, the maternal riboflavin-deficient diet is supplemented by the antagonist galactoflavin, the yield of deformed young can be increased to nearly 100%. [37] Shepard et al. [50] found that embryos of mothers treated in this way were already reduced in overall size on days 12 and 13 of gestation; on day 14 it could be recognized that the rate of differentiation of tissues of the treated embryos was delayed and that their tissues contained extensive areas of necrosis in the mesoblast of the extremities and the first branchial arch. Sections of the extremities of the embryos revealed a reduction in the number of cellular mitoses. Embryos and fetuses from day 12 to day 17 subjected to histochemical investigations demonstrated an overall decrease in the reactions for succinic dehydrogenase, whereas malic and lactic dehydrogenases and alkaline and acid phosphatases were not reduced.

The lowered flavin content in fetuses of riboflavin-deficient rats noted by Miller *et al.*[35] suggested to Aksu *et al.*[1] that there may be corresponding deficiencies in the activities of flavin-dependent enzymes such as the terminal electron transport systems (ETP). These investigators who used a riboflavin-deficient, galactoflavin-containing maternal diet demonstrated that the specific activity of the terminal electron transport systems of embryonic tissues was markedly reduced compared to the activity of preparations from control animals during the period of 12–16 days of gestation. These direct determinations agreed with earlier experiments that tentatively assigned the period between day 13 and 14 of gestation as determinative for the skeletal malformations of pure riboflavin deficiency.[57] The early indirect determinations had indicated "that we would not be far off if we were to say that riboflavin deficiency induces the skeletal malformations on the 14th day of gestation."[65]

The studies of Aksu *et al.*,[1] which showed a marked reduction of the activity of the electron transport systems during the critical days of development, demonstrated that the levels of protein in the ETP or R_2 (residual) fractions from treated embryos and fetuses were not decreased, a fact suggesting that normal amounts of enzyme protein or apoenzyme were being produced. As to the role of galactoflavin in these teratologic experiments, it remained to be determined whether the galactoflavin found in fetal tissues was present in a free or bound form. Since galactoflavin did not directly inhibit the activity of the intact electron transport systems in control experiments, it was thought that the antimetabolite could hinder the binding of flavin mononucleotide (FMN) and flavin adenine dinucleotide (FAD) during synthesis of the enzymes, or act by being bound itself to the enzyme in place of the natural flavin coenzyme, thus producing an inactive enzyme or an enzyme of reduced activity. The marked decrease in activity of the electron transport systems, accompanied by a decrease in the rate of formation of high-energy phosphate compounds at critical periods of embryonic development when cellular demands for energy may be greatly increased because of the high rate of cellular multiplication and differentiation, makes understandable the decreased size of embryos by day 12 of gestation and the finding of increased mesenchymal cellular death by day 14. These studies are of special interest since they indicate that fetal tissues are particularly susceptible to the efforts of riboflavin deficiency, whereas the electron transport systems of the placenta and of maternal heart tissue of treated rats are not significantly affected.[50]

The results of Aksu et al.[1] agree well with the hypothesis of Warkany and Schraffenberger, who in 1944[60] attributed the effects of riboflavin to a specific inhibition of proper formation of the embryonic membranous skeleton and not to a general placental insufficiency or a general growth retardation. This hypothesis was further demonstrated by Shepard and Bass,[51] who showed that limb buds of embryos from riboflavin-deficient rats failed to grow in riboflavin-deficient medium whereas the growth of control limb buds was not impaired by exposure to deficient medium. The authors concluded that the major mechanism responsible for production of limb defects is to be sought on a local cell level rather than indirectly by general impairment of the embryo's physiology. In continuation of his work, Mackler[31a] concluded that marked increases in the activities of the terminal electron transport system and mitochondrial ATP'ase take place between days 10 and 14 of gestation in the rat embryo-fetus, and that the rise in enzyme activity is paralleled by a striking change in the number and structure of the mitochondrial cristae as described by electron microscopy. It was suggested that oxidative metabolism may be relatively unimportant to embryonic growth and development until day 11 of gestation in the rat, but that thereafter the electron transport systems and associated phosphorylation processes increase rapidly in activity and in importance to embryogenesis with inhibition of the enzyme systems leading to marked changes in growth and development. Ritter et al.[46a] thought that riboflavin deficiency that may result in diminished flavoprotein concentrations in the electron transport system should be expected to lead to decreased ATP synthesis. But assays of treated embryos 11–14 days old showed only a mild decrease of about 20% below that of controls. This result contrasts with findings in embryos treated with 6-aminonicotinamide which had a much larger ATP reduction. The finding that in riboflavin-deficient animals (of day 14 of gestation) the placental alkaline phosphatase is reduced[43] is of interest, but the relationship of this enzyme deficiency of the placenta to the results of Aksu et al.[1] and Shepard and Bass[51] remains to be elucidated.

It has been shown that the conversion of riboflavin to hepatic FAD is under thyroid control[47] and that both FMN and FAD are reduced in hypothyroidism.[49] It is worth emphasis, therefore, that the goiters of female rats fed the Steenbock and Black diet (supplemented with vitamin D) did not contribute to the origin of the skeletal malformations of the young. If the diet was supplemented with iodine, there were no goiters but malformations occurred in the young; if the diet was supplemented with liver, maternal goiters were present but there were no malformations.[57]

It may be added here that in rats the incidence of malformations produced by hypoglycin was reduce by simultaneous administration of riboflavin,[42] and that in chickens, teratogenic effects of boric acid injections were reduced by riboflavin supplements.[28]

6. INTERPRETATIONS

What is the meaning of the finding that riboflavin deficiency induces congenital malformations in experimental animals? It does not mean that human congenital malformations can be attributed to dietary riboflavin deficiency of the mother. In fact, Brzezinski et al.[5] thought that antenatal riboflavin deficiency of women does not influence the development of the fetus, but in their observations deficiency symptoms made their appearance only during the last trimester of pregnancy,[3] at which time malformations of the type described in animal experiments have long been determined. Inadequate diets in the last two trimesters of gestation may damage the fetus in various respects but cannot cause malformations dating back to organogenesis. Yet the experiments cited were useful because they alerted the medical profession to the possibility that adverse environmental conditions could deform a mammalian embryo during gestation. They helped to accept the idea that rubella and other infectious diseases of a pregnant woman can result in congenital malformations of the child.

At first, however, there were only few observations that showed that in man congenital malformations of the extremities could be attributed to environmental causes.[34,63] But, when between 1959 and 1961, that is, 20 years after our experiments, epidemics of serious limb defects occurred in several areas of the world, the medical community was ready to consider the possibility of exogenous causation. The idea that symmetrical and serial malformations of the extremities *must* be hereditary had been abandoned and a drug, thalidomide, was quickly recognized as the cause of the epidemic.[30,33] When Lenz (in June 1961) heard of a child born with hypoplasia of humeri and femora, aplasia of radii, and tibial polydactyly, he thought at first that the case could best be explained by a dominant new mutation. But when he subsequently learned of many other new observations of reduction malformations of the limbs, he soon considered the possibility of an exogenous causation.[31] The riboflavin deficiency experiments and other teratologic investigations had prepared the ground for quick acceptance of an environmental explanation of the limb defects. It may be mentioned as a curiosity that the thalidomide-induced "phocomelias" had a certain resemblance to the malformation pattern of diet I, in that in both conditions preaxial structures (tibia and radius) were more affected than postaxial bones (fibula and ulna); in fact, the severe limb defects produced by riboflavin deficiency can be considered as "distal phocomelias." But there the similarity ends, and the suspicion of a direct connection of the effects of thalidomide with disturbed riboflavin metabolism[29,52] has not been sustained. Felisati and Nodari[13] failed to protect rabbits from the teratogenic effects of thalidomide by riboflavin, and Bertrand et al.[2] reported that the simultaneous administration of riboflavin and thalidomide to pregnant rats increased the number of resorptions. Dyban and Akimova[10] noted that thalidomide causes death and malformations in rat embryos when the amounts of riboflavin and folic acid in the rations were decreased, and Friedman et al.[15] found that the growth of rats fed a riboflavin-deficient diet was markedly reduced by thalidomide as compared with rats fed a supplemented diet. But there was no evidence that thalidomide functions as a riboflavin antagonist or that the mode of action of thalidomide as a teratogenic agent is elucidated by riboflavin-deficiency experiments.[15]

Other applications of the experiments cited to human teratology are merely speculative and hypothetical. It is possible that the enzyme systems discussed above could be disturbed by causes other than maternal riboflavin deficiency or exposure to galactoflavin, and thus result in congenital malformations, but so far such situations have not been recognized. Yet it may be permissible to end this review with a hopeful note about leads one could possibly get by nutrition experiments of the kind cited above. In a discussion of the relationship of malformations induced by maternal dietary deficiency to malformations of genetic origin, I emphasized[62] that these two kinds of malformations differ completely, both in their origin and in their importance for the species but that they have some points of similarity in their appearance and in their mechanisms of development.

By maternal dietary deficiency congenital malformations can be induced which resemble morphologically malformations of genetic origin. Such malformations have been called phenocopies.[19]

Phenocopies are nonhereditary malformations which simulate malformations induced by mutant genes. For instance, hydrocephaly, cleft palate, ocular colobomas, or reduction malformations of the extremities may be of genetic origin; similar malformations can be produced by various deficiency experiments as nonhereditary phenocopies. Another resemblance between effects of abnormal genes and effects of nutritional deficiencies lies in the formation of syndromes of multiple anomalies. An abnormal gene frequently has a pleiotropic effect, i.e., it causes malformations in various organs, situated in different parts of the body and apparently unrelated to each other in postnatal life. Pleiotropic effects have been described following many experiments using maternal dietary deficiency.[6,18,36,65] A third resemblance is found in the fact that both a genic deficiency and a continuous nutritional deficiency persist throughout pregnancy but act during certain selective phases of the organogenetic period: They have "ambush effects," lying in wait while the embryo develops and attacking when special demands are made by the embryo's metabolism, demands that are not fulfilled because of the genic or nutritional deficiency. This procedure is in contrast to the mechanisms of acute teratogenic agents such as rubella, antimetabolites, thalidomide, and other chemicals that attack the embryo at once at the time of exposure. It has been said[9] that responses that a developing organism can make are directed into a limited number of channels and that environmental disturbances may produce phenocopies by altering some developmental processes in the same way as mutant genes do. If this is correct, knowledge of the abnormal channels opened up by modifying environmental factors may throw some light on the mode of action of some abnormal genes.

Since little is known about the biochemical basis of genes which lead to malformations, a knowledge of the pathways that lead to their phenocopies can be of value since it may permit correction of an inherited disability. This can be illustrated by the case of pallid mutant mice ("pa") that inherit congenital otolith defects and a tendency to abnormal posture and inability to swim. Since it was known that manganese deficiency in chicks,[39] rats,[23,24] and other animals results in disturbances of equilibrium and ataxia, Erway et al.[11] attempted prevention of the genetic abnormalities of "pa" mice by supplements of the maternal diet with manganese. It was found that manganese supplements to the diet of pregnant "pa" mice prevent the otolith defect if fed in high concentrations and at critical times of development. Thus, an inherited defect could be prevented by knowledge of the mechanism that results in similar disturbances in the phenocopies.[12] A comparable situation may exist in avian genetics. A hereditary riboflavin deficiency in chicken eggs has long been known[32] in a strain of Single Comb White Leghorns carrying the recessive riboflavinuria alleles "rdrd," the normal genotype being "RdRd." The embryos of the mutant "rdrd" die at approximately day 13, since birds homozygous for this gene are unable to lay eggs that contain riboflavin sufficient for survival of the embryos. When such eggs were injected with an aqueous solution of riboflavin on the third day of incubation, a number of embryos survived and normal chicks were hatched.[32] This subject is also discussed in Chapter 4. It was shown that the inherited malfunction is due to a deficiency of riboflavin-binding protein in the albumen and yolk of the eggs and in the blood of the laying females.[66] This example illustrates that riboflavin deficiency of embryos need not be due to maternal dietary deficiency but can be caused by a genetic inability to retain riboflavin and to direct it to the embryo when it is needed. Knowledge of the genetically determined metabolic defect can aid in prevention of its deleterious manifestations. Unfortunately, delivery of biochemical supplements to mammalian embryos is more difficult than additions to avian ova.

Attempts have been made to prevent human congenital malformations, particularly cleft palate, by administration of large amounts of vitamins to mothers who had given birth to children with facial clefts. [7,41] Although the results were far from convincing, [14] more subtle approaches could be successful if missing metabolites could be conveyed to embryos at appropriate times. Studies dealing with biochemical effects of riboflavin deficiency on tissues of offspring shortly before [43-45a,54] or soon after birth [48] are of great value since they show developments of biochemical patterns in the perinatal periods. But biochemical changes leading to structural malformations like those described here must be studied much earlier, in organogenic periods when the deviations from the normal begin.

7. SUMMARY

Riboflavin deficiency has been instrumental in promotion of teratologic research and enhancement of our knowledge of etiology and pathogenesis of congenital malformations. But the work done along these lines must be considered a beginning rather than a finished chapter. The fact that withholding of a chemically well-defined nutritional factor can result in enzymatic deficiencies, and that these, in turn, can induce embryonic malformations, has not been used sufficiently in studies of basic causes of congenital malformations. Although great progress has been made in the analysis of inborn errors of metabolism, progress has been slow in the elucidation of the chemical background of inherited and environmentally induced structural malformations of mammals. Nutrition experiments like those discussed in the preceding pages show one way that can lead to clarification of fundamental errors of development that bring about congenital malformations in man and other mammals.

8. REFERENCES

1. Aksu, O., Mackler, B. Shepard, T. H., and Lemire, R. J. 1968. Studies of the development of congenital anomalies in embryos of riboflavin-deficient, galactoflavin fed rats. II. Role of the terminal electron transport systems, *Teratology* 1:93-102.
2. Bertrand, M., Florio, R., Magat, A., and Delatour, P. 1964. Sur la potentialisations des effets embryotoxiques du thalidomide chez la ratte, *C. R. Soc. Biol. (Paris)* **158**:737.
3. Braun, K., Bromberg, Y. M., and Brzezinski, A. 1945. Riboflavin deficiency in pregnancy, *J. Obstet. Gynaecol. Brit. Commonw.* **52**:43.
4. Brent, R. L., and Jensh, R. P. 1967. Intra-uterine growth retardation, *Adv. Teratol.* **2**:139-227.
5. Brzezinski, A., Bromberg, Y. M., and Braun, K. 1947. Riboflavin deficiency in pregnancy. Its relationship to the course of pregnancy and to the condition of the foetus, *J. Obstet. Gynaecol. Brit. Commonw.* **54**:182-186.
6. Cheng, D. W., Bairnson, T. A., Rao, A. N., and Subbammal, S. 1960. Effect of variations of rations on the incidence of teratogeny in vitamin E-deficient rats, *J. Nutr.* **71**:54-60.
7. Conway, H. 1958. Effect of supplemental vitamin therapy on the limitation of incidence of cleft lip and cleft palate in humans, *Plast. Reconstr. Surg.* **22**:450-453.
8. Dawson, A. B. 1926. Note on the staining of the skeleton of cleared specimens with alizarin red S, *Stain Technol.* **1**:123-124.
9. Dunn, L. C. 1939. Heredity and development of early abnormalities in vertebrates, *Harvey Lect.* **35**:135-165.
10. Dyban, A. P., and Akimova, I. M. 1966. The significance of vitamin B complex and genetic factors in reaction to thalidomide in rat embryos, *Arkh. Anat.* **51**:3-17.
11. Erway, L., Hurley, L. S., and Fraser, A. 1966. Neurological defect: manganese in phenocopy and prevention of a genetic abnormality of inner ear, *Science* **152**:1766-1767.
12. Erway, L. C., Fraser, A. S., and Hurley, L. S. 1971. Prevention of congenital otolith defect in pallid mutant mice by manganese supplementation, *Genetics* **67**:97-108.
13. Felisati, D., and Nodari, R. 1963. Effets toxiques et tératogéniques de la thalidomide sur les foetus de lapin, *Schweiz. Med. Wochenschr.* **93**:1559-1562.
14. Fraser, F. C., and Warburton, D. 1964. No association of emotional stress or vitamin supplement during pregnancy to cleft lip or palate in man, *Plast. Reconstr. Surg.* **33**:395-399.
15. Friedman, L., Shue, G. M., and Hove, E. L. 1965. Response of rats to thalidomide as affected by riboflavin or folic acid deficiency, *J. Nutr.* **85**:309-317.
16. Gilman, J. P. W., Berry, F. A., and Hill, D. C. 1952. Some effects of maternal riboflavin deficiency on reproduction in rats, *Canad. J. Med. Sci.* **30**:383-389.
17. Giroud, A., and Boisselot, J. 1947. Répercussions de l'avitaminose B_2 sur l'embryon du rat, *Arch. Fr. Pediatr.* **4**:317-327.

18. Giroud, A. 1970, "The Nutrition of the Embryo," Charles C Thomas Co., Springfield.
19. Goldschmidt, R. B. 1938. "Physiological Genetics," McGraw-Hill Book Co., Inc., New York.
20. Grainger, R. B., O'Dell, B. L., and Hogan, A. G. 1954. Congenital malformations as related to deficiencies of riboflavin and vitamin B_{12}, source of protein, calcium to phosphorus ratio and skeletal phosphorus metabolism, *J. Nutr.* **54**:33-48.
21. Hale, F. 1933. Pigs born without eye balls, *J. Hered.* **24**:105-106.
22. Hale, F. 1937. The relation of maternal vitamin A deficiency to microphthalmia in pigs, *Texas State J. Med.* **33**:228-332.
23. Hill, R. M., Holtkamp, D. E., Buchanan, A. R., and Rutledge, E. K. 1950. Manganese deficiency in rats with relation to ataxia and loss of equilibrium, *J. Nutr.* **41**:359-371.
24. Hurley, L. S., Everson, G. J., and Geiger, J. F. 1958. Manganese deficiency in rats: Congenital nature of ataxia, *J. Nutr.* **66**:309-320.
25. Kalter, H., and Warkany, J. 1957. Congenital malformations in inbred strains of mice induced by riboflavin-deficient, galactoflavin-containing diets, *J. Exp. Zool.* **136**:531-565.
26. Kim, Y. S., and Lambooy, J. P. 1971. Induction of a specific enzyme inadequacy in infant rats by the use of a homologue of riboflavin. *J. Nutr.* **101**:819-830.
27. Lambooy, J. P. 1966. Riboflavin antagonists, *Bibl. Nutr. Diet.* **8**:139-155.
28. Landauer, W., and Clark, E. M. 1964. On the role of riboflavin in the teratogenic activity of boric acid, *J. Exp. Zool.* **156**:307-312.
29. Leck, I. M., and Millar, E. L. M. 1962. Incidence of malformations since the introduction of thalidomide, *Brit. Med. J.* **2**:16-20.
30. Lenz, W. 1961. Diskussionsbemerkung zu dem Vortrag von R. A. Pfeiffer und K. Kosenow: Zur Frage der exogenen Entstehung schwerer Extremitätenmissbildungen, *Tagung der Rheinisch-Westfälischen Kinderärztevereinigung in Düsseldorf* **19**:11.
31. Lenz, W. 1963. Das Thalidomid-Syndrom. *Fortschr. Med.* **81**:148-155.
31a. Mackler, B. 1969. Studies of the molecular basis of congenital malformations, *Pediatrics* **43**:915-926.
31b. Mackler, B. 1970. Studies on mitochondrial energy systems during embryogenesis in the rat, *in*: "Metabolic Pathways in Mammalian Embryos during Organogenesis and Its Modification by Drugs," (R., Bass, F. Beck, H.-J. Merker, D. Neubert, and B. Randhahn, eds.), Freie Universität Berlin.
32. Maw, A. J. G., 1954. Inherited riboflavin deficiency in chicken eggs. *Poult. Sci.* **33**:216-217.
33. McBride, W. G., 1961. Thalidomide and congenital abnormalities. *Lancet* **2**:1358.
34. Meltzer, H. J., 1956. Congenital anomalies due to attempted abortion with 4-aminopteroglutamic acid. *JAMA* **161**:1253.
35. Miller, Z., Poncet, I., and Takacs, E. 1962. Biochemical studies on experimental congenital malformations: Flavin nucleotides and folic acid in fetuses and livers from normal and riboflavin-deficient rats. *J. Biol. Chem.* **237**:968-973.
36. Nelson, M. M., Asling, C. W., and Evans, H. M., 1952. Production of multiple congenital abnormalities in young by maternal pteroylglutamic acid deficiency during gestation. *J. Nutr.* **48**:61-80.
37. Nelson, M. M., Baird, C. D. C., Wright, H. V. and Evans, H. M. 1956. Multiple congenital abnormalities in the rat resulting from riboflavin deficiency induced by the antimetabolite galactoflavin. *J. Nutr.* **58**:125-134.
38. Noback, C. R., and Kupperman, H. S., 1944. Anomalous offspring and growth of Wistar rats maintained on a deficient diet. *Soc. Exp. Biol. Med.* **57**:183-185.
39. Norris, L. C., and Caskey, C. D., 1939. A chronic congenital ataxia and osteodystrophy

in chicks due to manganese deficiency, *J. Nutr.* **17**:407-417.

40. Palludan, B., 1966. *A-Avitaminosis in Swine: A Study of the Importance of Vitamin A for Reproduction.* Munksgaard, Copenhagen.
41. Peer, L. A., Strean, L. P., Walker, J. C., Jr., Bernhard, W. G., and Peck, G. C., 1958. Study of 400 pregnancies with birth of cleft lip-palate infants. Protective effect of folic acid and vitamin B$_6$ therapy, *Plast. Reconstr. Surg.* **22**:422-449.
42. Persaud, T. V. N. 1970. Studies on the mechanism of teratogenic action of hypoglycin, *Teratology* **3**:208 (abstr.).
43. Potier de Courcy, G., and Terroine, T. 1968a. Influence de la carence en riboflavin sur la fonction phosphatasique alcaline des organes maternels et foetaux à différents stades de la gestation, *Ann. Nutr. Alim.* **22**:95-100.
44. Potier de Courcy, G., and Terroine, T. 1968b. Conséquences chez le rat de la carence en riboflavine sur la composition globale de certains tissues maternels et foetaux, *Arch. Sci. Physiol.* **22**:329-355.
45. Potier de Courcy, G., Susbielle, H., and Terroine, T. 1970. Etude du zinc dans l'ariboflavinose tératogène chez le rat, *Arch. Sci. Physiol.* **24**:409-417.
45a. Potier De Cjurcy, G., Desmettre-Miguet, S., Macquart-Moulin, M. R., and Terroine, T. 1974. Evolution enzymatique des tissue foetaux et placantaires de rat en carence teratogene de riboflavine, *J. Embryol. Exp. Morph.* **31**:183-198.
46. Remington, R. E. 1937. Improved growth in rats on iodine deficient diets, *J. Nutr.* **13**:223-233.
46a. Ritter, E. J., Scott, W. J., and Wilson, J. G. 1974. Correlation between teratogenicity and ATP synthesis in embryos from riboflavin deficient and 6-aminonicotinamide treated rats (abstr.), *Teratology* (in press).
47. Rivlin, R. S., and Langdon, R. G. 1966. Regulation of hepatic FAD levels by thyroid hormone. *Adv. Enzyme Regul.* **4**:45-58.
48. Rivlin, R. S. 1969. Perinatal development of enzymes synthesizing FMN and FAD, *Amer. J. Physiol.* **216**:979-982.
49. Rivlin, R. S. 1970. Riboflavin metabolism, *New Eng. J. Med.* **283**:463-472.
50. Shepard, T. H., Lemire, R. J., Aksu, O., and Mackler, B. 1968. Studies of the development of congenital anomalies in embryos of riboflavin-deficient, galactoflavin fed rats, *Teratology* **1**:75-92.
51. Shepard, T., and Bass, G. L. 1970. Organ culture of limb buds from riboflavin-deficient and normal rat embryos in normal and riboflavin-deficient media, *Teratology* **3**:163-167.
52. Skre, H. 1963. Talidomidpolyneuritt. En form for riboflavinavitaminose? *Nord. Med.* **15**:916-918.
53. Steenbock, H., and Black, A. 1925. Fat-soluble vitamins. XXIII. The induction of growth promoting and calcifying properties in fats and their unsaponifiable constituents by exposure to light, *J. Biol. Chem.* **64**:263-298.
54. Terroine, T. 1967. Anomalies biochimiques et avitaminoses tératogènes, *Ann. Biol.* **6**:329-359.
55. Warkany, J., and Nelson R. C. 1941. Skeletal abnormalities in the offspring of rats reared on deficient diets, *Anat. Rec.* **79**:83-100.
56. Warkany, J., and Nelson, R. C. 1942a. Congenital malformations induced in rats by maternal nutritional deficiency, *J. Nutr.* **23**:321-333.
57. Warkany, J., Nelson, R. C., and Schraffenberger, E. 1942b. Congenital malformations induced in rats by maternal nutritional deficiency. II. Use of varied diets and of different strains of rats, *Amer. J. Dis. Child.* **64**:860-866.
58. Warkany, J., and Nelson, R. C. 1942c. Skeletal abnormalities induced in rats by maternal nutritional deficiency, *Arch. Path.* **34**:375-384.

59. Warkany, J., Nelson, R. C., and Schraffenberger, E. 1943. Congenital malformations induced in rats by maternal nutritional deficiency. IV. Cleft palate. *Amer. J. Dis. Child.* **65**:882–894.

60. Warkany, J., and Schraffenberger, E. 1944. Congenital malformations induced in rats by maternal nutritional deficiency. VI. The preventive factor, *J. Nutr.* **27**:477–484.

61. Warkany, J., and Schraffenberger, E. 1947. Congenital malformations induced in rats by roentgen rays, *Amer. J. Roentgen.* **57**:455–463.

62. Warkany, J. 1952–1953. Congenital malformations induced by maternal dietary deficiency. Experiments and their interpretation, *The Harvey Lectures Series* **48**:89–109.

63. Warkany, J., Beaudry, P. H., and Hornstein, S. 1960. Attempted abortion with 4-amino-pteroylglutamic acid (aminopterin). Malformations of the child, *Amer. J. Dis. Child.* **97**:274–281.

64. Warkany, J., Monroe, B. B., and Sutherland, B. S. 1961. Intrauterine growth retardation, *Amer. J. Dis. Child.* **102**:249–279.

65. Warkany, J. 1969. Experimental production of mammalian limb malformations, *in:* "Limb Development and Deformity," (C. A. Swinyard, ed.), pp.140–160, Charles C Thomas, Springfield.

66. Winter, W. P., Buss, E. G., Clagett, C. O., and Boucher, R. V. 1967. The nature of the biochemical lesion in avian renal riboflavinuria. II. The inherited change of a riboflavin-binding protein from blood and eggs, *Comp. Biochem. Physiol.* **22**:897–906.

67. Zilva, S. S., Golding, J., Drummond, J. C., and Coward, K. H. 1921. The relation of the fat-soluble factor to rickets and growth in pigs, *Biochem. J.* **15**:427–437.

BIOLOGICAL ACTIVITIES OF ANALOGS OF RIBOFLAVIN

John P. Lambooy

1. GENERAL BACKGROUND INFORMATION

Life as it exists in its varied forms on earth is dependent on the use of a flavin[1] for cellular metabolic processes. If this essential flavin is isolated from natural sources, there is no exception to the finding that it is a derived form of riboflavin.[2] Thus, the number of ways in which the biological activity of riboflavin might be studied is very large; since the biological activity of an analog[3] of riboflavin might conceivably be studied in any of these many ways, the combination of several analogs with the many systems in which riboflavin functions provides a still larger number of opportunities for exploration within the subject area defined by the title of this chapter.

If such analogs are to be studied as antagonists or antimetabolites of riboflavin, there is no avoiding the need to study, initially, their activities on whole animals or whole microorganisms.

[1] The term flavin is used interchangeably with the term isoalloxazine.
[2] No essential role has yet been described for L-lyxoflavin if it does exist in living tissue, nor has any role been described for nekoflavin.
[3] In this instance, analog is used to include all the flavins that possess structures "analogous" to that of riboflavin.

JOHN P. LAMBOOY—Department of Biochemistry, University of Maryland School of Dentistry.

In this chapter, the subject of biological activity of the analogs will be covered from the point of view of the effects they have on the whole animal or the whole microorganism and then how these effects may be investigated in one way or another at the tissue and cellular level. Not many animals are useful for the study of riboflavin requirements or the action of an antagonist of its use. Because the rat is the best animal for this purpose, emphasis will be placed on results of studies in which it has been used. Also, there are not many. microorganisms that can be used in this way, but fortunately, an excellent, well-characterized and widely used organism is available as *Lactobacillus casei.*[4]

1.1. Biological Activity in the Rat

It is essential for a carefully controlled evaluation of the biological activity of an analog in the rat that the flavin content of the animal and intake by the animal be accurately known. Since the content of the animal can be known only as the result of assay of wholly comparable groups at some equilibrium point, it is necessary to use rats that have been brought to a uniform state of riboflavin deficiency. For this reason, the production of riboflavin deficiency in the rat and some of the associated changes will be discussed in some detail.

Great care must be exercised in the selection of rats to use. The production of the CFN rat (Carworth, Farms, Nelson), a rat derived from the Wistar strain, provided an animal exceptionally well suited for studying riboflavin deficiency and the utilization of riboflavin analogs. These animals have been of immense value in many kinds of nutrition studies, and we have used this strain of animals in all of our research directed toward nutritional evaluation of the analogs.

Although in our earlier studies we used male animals exclusively, the sudden and growing demand for male rats for the enormous drug testing programs initiated by the pharmaceutical companies outstripped the supply of CFN male rats just at the time we became involved in reproduction studies in rats fed diets containing some of our analogs. Quite aside from the special role the females played in reproduction we found them to be superior to males in many aspects of our studies. Their response was more uniform than that of males with regard to the development of riboflavin deficiency, growth response, food con-

---

[4]The best source of the organism is the American Type Culture Collection, 12301 Parklawn Drive, Rockville, Md. 20852. To order specify, *Lactobacillus casei*, ATCC, No. 7469.

sumption, and ease of handling; an additional advantage was that when full grown, being smaller than males, they required less diet. Once we had established our basic facility needs, our animal and diet requirements, and the regimen of care and management, we were not surprised to discover that we could reproduce any of several studies with identical results in separate laboratories in different parts of the country.

1.1.1. Riboflavin Deficiency in the Rat

What constitutes a description of riboflavin deficiency in the rat depends upon the needs and aims of the study as well as many other factors, among which can be mentioned the age, sex, and strain of the rat; the composition of the diet; the care of the cages, food cups, and the drinking water supply; the temperature and humidity of the animal quarters; whether the animals are housed one or more to a cage; and even the number of hours of light and darkness prevailing in the animal room.

If the aim of an investigation is to study the biological activity of an analog of riboflavin to learn if it is vitamin-like, antagonistic, or inert, there are a few characteristics of the deficiency state which, if modified during the administration of the analog, must be evaluated if they are to carry quantitative significance. If such quantitative meaning is to be used for comparative purposes, it is of the great importance that the means by which the deficient state is reached is standardized to the extent necessary to yield reproducible characteristics. When viewed from such a starting point, one might observe if the animals treated with the analog eat more food, gain more weight, live longer, show improvement in appearance, display greater activity, and in other ways appear better off than the deficient controls. If in all or in some of these characteristics the experimental animal is worse off than the deficient control, the analog may be suspected of being an antagonist of riboflavin. It then becomes important to learn if the effects of the analog can be reversed or prevented by the simultaneous administration of riboflavin with the analog and, if so, in what ratio to the analog.

The diet we use, which has been described recently,[18] is fed to the animals from the day of their arrival. The food cup containing somewhat more food than the rat will eat during the feeding period is placed in the cage at the same time each day (usually 3-5 P.M.) and removed the following morning (usually 8-9 A.M.). This routine is followed every day the study is in progress. The animals are weighed to the nearest gram once a week for the first two weeks and then twice a week. When the animal has gained no more than 5 g during a period of 14 consecutive days, it can be considered riboflavin deficient for many purposes. However, when an analog of low biological activity is to be investigated, it may be necessary to use the animals only after they have shown an actual weight loss during the last 7 of the 14 days. Under circumstances where very small quantities of riboflavin are to be used, the preparation of the animals for the study can involve breeding females fed diets containing minimal quantities of riboflavin and using the surviving young as weanlings. These weanlings are then placed on the riboflavin-deficient diet and the above severe criterion applied. [71] The criterion of a gain in weight of no more than 5 g during a 14-day interval will usually result in most of the animals becoming deficient in from 4 to 6 weeks.

Figure 1 illustrates the average riboflavin content and concentration of a group of rats maintained on the same regimen as described above.

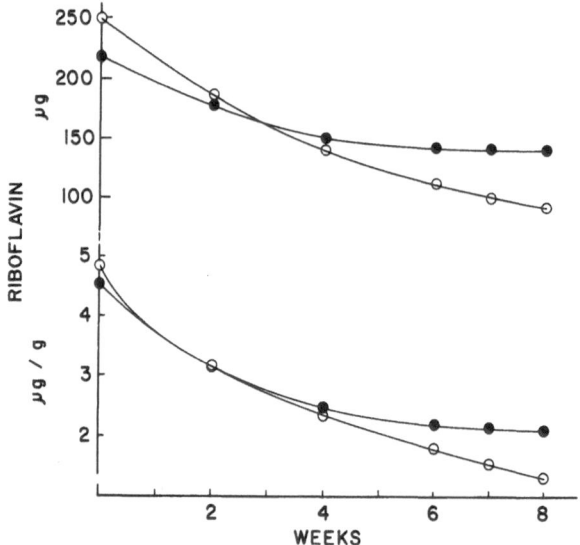

Fig. 1. Change in average content and concentration of riboflavin in groups of rats fed a riboflavin-deficient diet. Solid circles represent total riboflavin determined by the microbiological procedure. Open circles represent ^{14}C-2-riboflavin. Weanling female rats fed ^{14}C-2-riboflavin-containing diet until adulthood, through gestation, and until they had weaned their young. The young were the animals used in these studies. Number of animals at zero time, 16; numbers of animals at other intervals varied from 10 to 12. Standard error of the mean for both assay procedures varied from 3% to 5% of the mean except for the value for the microbiological at week 8 where it was 7%. The assay procedures used were essentially those described by Lambooy *et al.* [77]

The riboflavin expressed in either way reaches essentially a minimum plateau at 4 weeks. The figure shows that the riboflavin in the body at any time is a summation of the residual tissue riboflavin and that which is absorbed from the vitamin synthesized by the microorganisms in the intestinal tract and the very small amount in the diet.[20,77] The figure also shows that the original tissue stores of riboflavin decline at essentially a constant rate. The concentration of riboflavin of approximately 2 μg/g whole animal will be maintained for a few additional weeks and even until the rat dies.

When the deficient rats have maintained their weight unchanged or have lost some weight during the 2-week period, they can be used to show a highly significant response to 1 μg riboflavin per day.[71]

While every effort is made to use weight response as quantitatively the most sensitive indicator of vitamin-like or antagonistic activity, appearance of the animal is also a very important indicator of the animal's response to the biological activity of a flavin. The expected visible response of a riboflavin-deficient rat to riboflavin is (a) greatly increased food intake, (b) gain in weight, and (c) improved appearance. While these changes are inseparably linked when riboflavin is the flavin under study, they have been emphasized because, as will be seen later in this chapter, responses to flavins other than riboflavin, in the presence of adequate flavin and adequate food, may show great variations and may include all three responses listed above or only one or two of them.

A survey of a wide variety of metabolic effects upon many systems as a result of riboflavin deficiency in the rat will be found in Chapter 6. A number of the effects observed are, however, critical to the evaluation of the biological activity of several of the analogs to be discussed and for this reason will be discussed briefly.

The failure of the riboflavin-deficient rat to gain weight is largely due to the reduction in food intake and, to a smaller degree, to reduced utilization of the food that is consumed.[72,81,106] Many studies have shown that riboflavin deficiency, and in some cases the associated diminished food intake, reduces the activity of the riboflavin dependent enzymes of the liver.[12,94] These enzymes, most of which require flavin-adenine dinucleotide (FAD) as coenzyme, are attached to the FAD by easily dissociable bonds. We have directed most of our attention to a study of succinic acid dehydrogenase (SDH) (EC 1.3.99.1) and the electron-transport-linked diphosphopyridine nucleotide dehydrogenase (DPNHD) (EC 1.6.99.3). Both are enzymes required at critical stages in energy production, are mitochondrial enzymes, are involved in the electron transport chain, and utilize FAD as coenzyme. The FAD is covalently bound to SDH and is an integral part of the structure of the mitochondria. The FAD of DPNHD is loosely bound and can be readily separated from the protein by acid extraction.

The specific SDH activity of the liver is severely depressed during riboflavin deficiency,[9,47] but its activity is not reduced in the heart or kidneys.[47,48] The actual changes in SDH in the liver are the result of several factors. Perhaps one of the most unusual findings relative to SDH activity in the liver during riboflavin deficiency is that it may be elevated above what it might have been due to riboflavin deficiency alone, because the reduced food intake is responsible for a very substantial increase.[48] The net result is that the liver of the rat during the development of and the existence of a riboflavin deficiency provides sufficient SDH activity so that it is maintained at essentially a normal level. Thus, in a particular study the SDH of a riboflavin-deficient rat might be 53% of normal if the normal is an animal consuming adequate quantities of food and riboflavin. It might be 40% of normal if the normal is an animal receiving adequate riboflavin but only enough food to keep its weight equal to that of the deficient animal. Finally, the SDH activity might be essentially 100% of normal if one considers as normal the activity for the whole liver in terms of its total activity at the beginning of the deprivation period.[48] The total recovery process following the administration of riboflavin and the rapid increase of food intake is very complicated, but the return of SDH activity per milligram protein is phenomenal and is complete in a period of 8 days. These findings tell us much about the activity of the mitochondria in the liver of the riboflavin-deficient rat.

The above observations were related to the activity of an enzyme that can lose its coenzyme flavin only by biodegradative processes; its specific activity in the liver was found to fall. Another mitochondrial enzyme that it is believed can be readily dissociated and for this reason might appear to be sensitive to the FAD concentrations in the tissue, is DPNHD. However, riboflavin deficiency causes no depression of the activity of this enzyme per milligram of protein in the heart and kidneys, but it does cause a significant although small loss in the liver.[49] That these changes in SDH and DPNHD are not related to riboflavin concentration in the tissues alone is emphasized by the observation that 4 weeks after the rat has become deficient, the riboflavin concentration in the heart, kidneys, and liver is approximately 9, 20, and 9 $\mu g/g$ tissue, respectively.[81] These concentrations are roughly 65%, 95%, and 50% of the corresponding tissues in animals receiving adequate riboflavin. The average whole-body concentration of riboflavin for the deficient rat at the same time is approximately 2 $\mu g/g$. Rats provided riboflavin in quantities of 20 μg/g food, 5 μg/g food, and 12 μg/day have approximate whole-body concentrations of riboflavin of 4.5 μg, 3.9 μg, and 3.1 μg/g fresh tissue, respectively.[71,77,81] When the heart, kidneys, and liver had been removed from the deficient rats described above, the remaining carcass contained 1.3 μg/g tissue.

1.1.2. Biological Activity of Analogs in the Rat

The techniques that are useful for evaluation of an analog of riboflavin in the riboflavin-deficient rat are not unlike those one might use to study the response of such animals to different quantities of riboflavin. [72] The flavin under study must be administered to the rat in critically controlled amounts and sufficiently critical control is not possible if the flavin is mixed in the diet and further, if the quantity of analog mixed in the diet is large, the flavor of the diet is very bitter. If a rat is fed a bitter-flavored but adequate diet, the animal will restrict its food consumption with the net result that the flavin intake and the protein intake will be reduced. Such animals, if adult, lose weight, perhaps not because they consume an unnatural or antagonistic flavin but because the flavin causes them not to consume adequate quantities of food.

The flavins are always given by polyethylene[5] stomach tube in 0.5 ml of the vehicle. The polyethylene tube is used instead of a steel tube[5] because of the need to administer the solutions to very small and often very sick animals. The solutions (or suspensions) are given the same time every day, and immediately after the flavin is administered the diet is made available to the animal.[6]

1.2. Biological Activity for *Lactobacillus casei*

The principal aspects of the use of *L. casei* for the microbiological assay for riboflavin have gone largely unchanged since they were described by Snell and Strong.[103] Detailed procedures for the assay have been presented in the book *Methods of Vitamin Assay*[4] and are discussed in detail in Chapter 2. The procedure and the preparation of reagents as described in *Methods of Vitamin Assay* are satisfactory for the analysis of riboflavin, but they present shortcomings when used for evaluation of the biological activity of analogs of riboflavin. If prepared

---

[5]Polyethylene tubing, PE-60, connected to a 1 ml tuberculum syringe by means of a No. 20 needle.

[6]The diet, being the same diet the animal ate during the deprivation period, does not introduce a new variable.

as described in this reference, both the basal medium and the inoculum contain traces of riboflavin and, while the quantities may be small, they can be significant in terms of a high blank. In the assay of riboflavin, a high blank due to riboflavin, if not too high, is relatively unimportant. However, this small amount of riboflavin can be very important when an effort is made to determine the growth-promoting or inhibitory properties of an analog. The small amount of riboflavin means that the response to the analog may be more apparent than real; it may be a response due to the influence of the combination of riboflavin and the analog. These factors are especially important if the analog is one of low potency as either a growth stimulant or an inhibitor. For example, if the blank is nearly two ml N/10 sodium hydroxide and the addition of an analog causes the production of sufficient lactic acid to require 4 ml N/10 alkali to neutralize the medium, caution should be exercised in ascribing activity to the analog.

The commercially available, so-called riboflavin-free, riboflavin assay medium is not suitable for use in the evaluation of analogs of riboflavin. The material can be used with marginal success for routine riboflavin assays where turbidemetry is used, but because of its high blank value and its limited range of response it is less well suited for titratimetic use or for use when an analog is to be studied in the presence of low concentrations of riboflavin.

We make use of additional adsorption and photolytic procedures to eliminate substantially riboflavin from the basal medium with the end result that the sensitivity of the test system to the activity of riboflavin analogs is greatly increased.

1.3. Scope of Compounds To Be Described

Since the classical studies of flavin syntheses done by Kuhn and Karrer and their co-workers, which culminated in the synthesis of riboflavin, a relatively large number of analogs of riboflavin have been synthesized which differed from riboflavin in respect to the form, number, or position of the substituents on the benzene ring portion of the molecule or with respect to the glycityl portion of the molecule. While a large number of flavins have been synthesized,[75] relatively few have been subjected to detailed studies to evaluate their biological activity. Among those that have been studied to reveal biological activity, some have been inactive in the test systems and some have shown extremely low potency in terms of biological activity. Limited space will necessitate a considerable degree of selectivity in the discussion of compounds of these two groups, but reference might well be made to some of them during discussions of findings.

Undoubtedly one of the most important aspects of studies directed toward the evaluation of the biological activity of any compound, particularly when part of the aim is to relate chemical structure to biological activity, is that the composition, structure, and purity of the compound to be studied must be known with absolute certainty. There are time-honored procedures available to responsible chemists for establishing that a compound meets these criteria. Analogs of riboflavin that have not met these criteria will not be included among those discussed in this chapter. It is well to remember that the absorption spectrum of flavins is associated with the isoalloxazine portion of the molecule and that it cannot be taken as proof of identity of the flavin. Similarly, chromatography cannot be used to establish purity but only homogenity of the material that responds to the means of viewing or detection. Infrared spectra cannot be used to establish purity of the flavin to the degree required. [72]

In the following portions of this chapter, a variety of ways in which biological activity has been studied will be described. In some instances, these observations will be as definitive as in the case of the rat and *L. casei*, but in other cases, while they may provide interesting information, the findings may have little to do with the overall vital economy of riboflavin as a metabolic essential.

2. DERIVATIVES OF RIBOFLAVIN

There are two groups of compounds derived from riboflavin. One group, described in a general way, would include all those compounds resulting from such chemical reactions which would add structural groups to the molecule but would not alter the basic structure of the vitamin. Riboflavin-5'-phosphate or 2', 3', 4', 5'-tetrabutyrate and several other compounds of this sort have been prepared. Since any biological activity that these derivatives might possess would be a function of the riboflavin molecule, they are not within the scope of this chapter. It is interesting to note that conversion to riboflavin *in vivo* does not necessarily occur. For example, while the administration of riboflavin tetrabutyrate cures riboflavin deficiency in the rat, the administration of riboflavin tetrapalmitate does not correct the deficiency. [111] The other group would include other flavins derived from riboflavin (I) by a modification of the basic riboflavin structure.

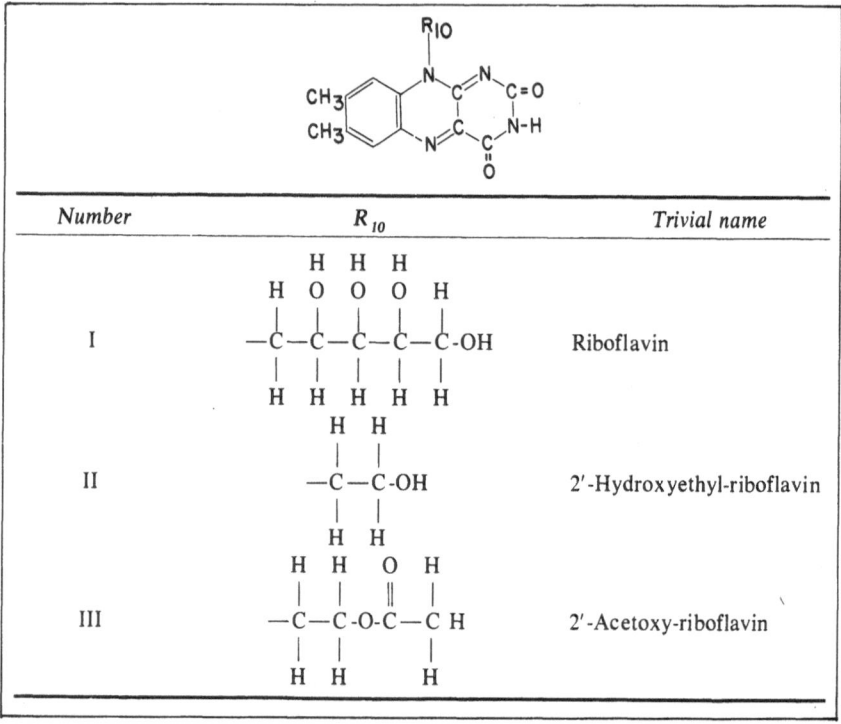

Fig. 2. Basic structure for derivatives of riboflavin.

Fall and Petering[19] prepared 7,8-dimethyl-10-(2'-hydroxyethyl)-isoalloxazine (II) and 7,8-dimethyl-10-(2'-acetoxyethyl) isoalloxazine (III). In spite of their claims that compounds II and III were potent antagonists of riboflavin in *L. casei* and the rat, the only information provided was as a personal communication to Lane *et al.*[82] They report having observed inhibition of the growth of *L. casei* and the rat when flavin III was administered with riboflavin in a ratio of 100:1. Whether the inhibition observed was 10% or 100% we do not know nor do we know what constituted the normal value for either. They reported that flavin II was only one-tenth as active as flavin III as an inhibitor for *L. casei* and that it possessed only one-fourth the inhibitory activity of III for the rat. Later Lane *et al.*[83] demonstrated that flavin II had an inhibition index (I.I.)[7] of approximately 480, which makes it a low-potency

---

[7] Inhibition Index.

$I.I = [$(analog at $\frac{1}{2}$ max. growth, μg (in presence of riboflavin providing max. growth, μg)$]$/(riboflavin providing max. growth, μg) $\times$ (riboflavin, mol. wt.)/(analog mol. wt.).

antagonist. In all instances, the antagonism could be reversed by increasing the ratio of riboflavin to flavin II or to flavin III. Flavin II had previously been synthesized by another route by Karrer et al.[36] and had been isolated as a bacterial decomposition product of riboflavin by Miles and Stadtman.[87]

Lane et al,[82,83] studied these materials as potential anticancer agents in the rat and man; a more detailed discussion is found in Chapter 8.

3. ISOMERS OF RIBOFLAVIN

When the glycityl (penityl) side chain at position 10 is D-ribityl, the flavin is riboflavin. It is interesting in a historical sense that the

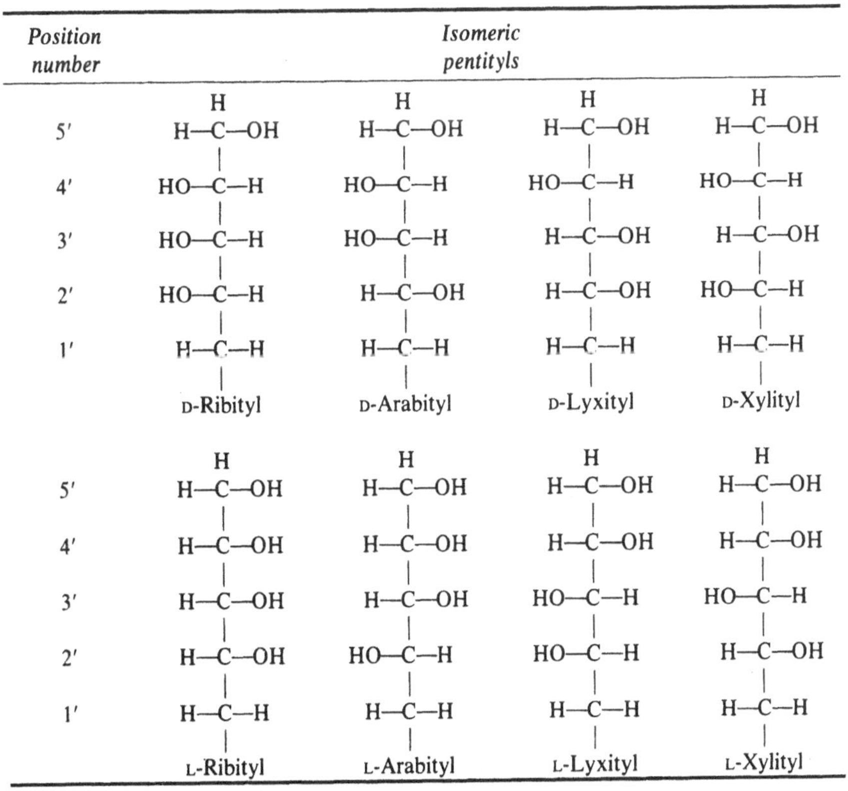

Position number	Isomeric pentityls			
5'	H H—C—OH	H H—C—OH	H H—C—OH	H H—C—OH
4'	HO—C—H	HO—C—H	HO—C—H	HO—C—H
3'	HO—C—H	HO—C—H	H—C—OH	H—C—OH
2'	HO—C—H	H—C—OH	H—C—OH	HO—C—H
1'	H—C—H	H—C—H	H—C—H	H—C—H
	D-Ribityl	D-Arabityl	D-Lyxityl	D-Xylityl
5'	H H—C—OH	H H—C—OH	H H—C—OH	H H—C—OH
4'	H—C—OH	H—C—OH	H—C—OH	H—C—OH
3'	H—C—OH	H—C—OH	HO—C—H	HO—C—H
2'	H—C—OH	HO—C—H	HO—C—H	H—C—OH
1'	H—C—H	H—C—H	H—C—H	H—C—H
	L-Ribityl	L-Arabityl	L-Lyxityl	L-Xylityl

Fig. 3. The eight isomeric pentityl side chains.

identity of the glycityl side chain was not known until riboflavin had been synthesized.

The eight isomeric pentityl side chains of interest in this connection are shown in Fig. 3. They are arranged to emphasize the differences in configuration of the hydroxy groups in the chains.

3.1. Modifications of Side Chain at Position 10

3.1.1. L-Riboflavin (IV)

Within a matter of months after riboflavin had been synthesized, Karrer et al.[39] reported the synthesis of L-riboflavin, and that it was devoid of riboflavin-like activity when administered in quantities of 20 μg/day to riboflavin-deficient rats.

3.1.2. D-Araboflavin (V)

There is serious doubt that D-araboflavin possesses any vitamin-like activity in spite of two reports in the early literature that it produced a growth response in rats.[43,107] The growth response that appears to have been observed in only a few animals may have been due to one of two causes. If severe criteria are not used to establish that an animal is riboflavin deficient, unexpected gains in weight can be a frequent occurrence. Another possibility is that, due to the procedure used to synthesize D-araboflavin by those who found it active, an Amadori rearrangement may have occurred which would have led to the production of a small amount of D-riboflavin as a contaminant of the D-araboflavin,[59],8 for when D-araboflavin was synthesized by procedures precluding the rearrangement it was devoid of vitamin-like activity. In only one other case has vitamin-like activity been found for D-araboflavin, and that in barely detectable activity as a stimulant for *L. casei*.[104] The D-araboflavin used in this study was obtained from Karrer, who had found it active for rats.

Using a synthetic basal medium, Shorb[100] found D-araboflavin devoid of either vitamin-like or inhibitory activity for *L. casei* (ATCC 7469) and *L. lactis* (ATCC 8000). Snell *et al.*[105] found D-araboflavin to be neither vitamin-like nor inhibitory for the growth of the chick

---

8The same argument has been proposed for the activity shown by L-araboflavin as a result of a failure to comprehend the Amadori rearrangement and a mistake in Weygand's definitive paper on the Amadori rearrangement. See Lambooy[75] for clarification.

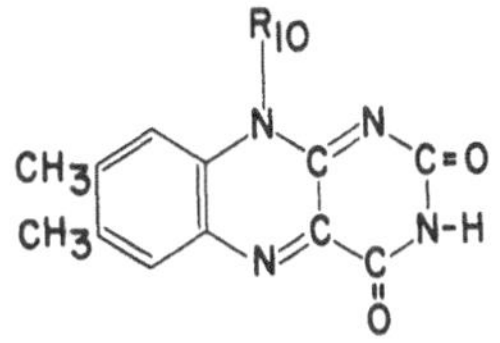

Number	R_{10}	Trivial name
IV	L-Ribityl	L-Riboflavin
V	D-Arabityl	D-Araboflavin
VI	L-Arabityl	L-Araboflavin
VII	D-Lyxityl	D-Lyxoflavin
VIII	L-Lyxityl	L-Lyxoflavin
IX	D-Xylityl	D-Xyloflavin

Fig. 4. Basic structure for isomers of riboflavin.

when added in quantities of 2.5–40 mg/kg to a ration containing 1 mg/kg riboflavin.

While on an earlier occasion Karrer et al.[43] had proposed that D-araboflavin possessed activity for the rat, later they[108] ascribed riboflavin antagonistic activity to it. The basal diet they used in the later study appears to have been inadequate since, when supplemented with 7 μg riboflavin per day, the animals did not show good growth and some actually died.

3.1.3. L-Araboflavin (VI)

When Kuhn and Weygand[52] first synthesized and tested L-araboflavin in the riboflavin-deficient rat, they found that the growth response produced was so exceptional that they reported the material to be identical with lactoflavin. Some time later, Kuhn et al.[54] were more conservative and reported the activity of L-araboflavin to be equivalent to one-third of the activity of riboflavin; 15 μg and 30 μg of L-araboflavin produced the same responses in the riboflavin-deficient rat as were produced by 5 μg and 10 μg, respectively, of riboflavin. Von Euler et al.[107] also reported that L-araboflavin possessed vitamin-like properties. They administered the material to groups of 2, 3, and 5 riboflavin-deficient rats in amounts of 10 μg, 20 μg, and 40 μg, per day, respectively, for from 20–45 days. In each group one animal died but may have gained weight, and one animal showed no weight gain but may have lived. That their material did indeed have vitamin-like activity was confirmed by von Euler and Karrer,[108] but it is interesting to note in this case that in spite of its activity it appeared to interfere with the utilization of riboflavin to a small extent.

L-Araboflavin was shown to have barely detectable stimulatory activity for *L. casei* when in the presence of 0.005 μg/ml riboflavin.[109]

3.1.4. D-Lyxoflavin (VII)

On the basis of the two reports of studies devoted to D-lyxoflavin, it is devoid of biological activity. Shorb[100] found it to possess neither stimulatory nor inhibitory properties for *L. casei* and *L. lactis*, and Snell *et al.*[105] found it without activity in the chick.

3.1.5. L-Lyxoflavin (VIII)

The study of the biological activity of L-lyxoflavin received a great deal of attention for a short period of time. The stimulus for the interest was understandable; Pallares and Garza[91] reported that they had isolated L-lyxoflavin from human myocardium. They also reported the synthesis of the material, but the analytical values found for their product and the absence of a mixed melting point of the tetracetyl derivative of the synthetic and natural material left room for doubt about its identity.[9] Doubt was raised by Gardner *et al.*[23] as to whether L-lyxoflavin existed in the heart at all, but by then the stage was set for considerable effort.

Emerson and Folkers[17, 18] were able to demonstrate that L-lyxoflavin had no riboflavin activity for the riboflavin-deficient rat. They did pose an interesting question: If L-lyxoflavin is a naturally occurring vitamin it might well not be suitable to satisfy the need for riboflavin of a riboflavin-deficient rat. They then made use of a diet devoid of animal protein and containing 0.5% of desiccated thyroid powder which they proposed as a diet useful for revealing the activity of unknown vitamins. Why this diet, which was designed primarily as a vitamin B_{12}-deficient diet, was supposed to be useful for this purpose was never made very clear, and animals consuming the diet responded to a spectrum of compounds[16,66] although the response to vitamin-B_{12} (the animal protein factor) was always exceptionally good. When rats maintained on this thyroid-containing diet were given 150 μg L-lyxoflavin per day for 15 days they did show better growth than those receiving no L-lyxoflavin.

The most definitive work done with L-lyxoflavin in the rat was accomplished by Cooperman *et al.*[11] They used a purified, riboflavin-

---

[9] An unequivocal synthesis of L-lyxoflavin, 7,8-dimethyl-10-(1'-L-lyxityl)isoalloxazine, can be found reported by Heyl *et al.*[29]

deficient diet and found that in a prophylatic test, whether the animals received 7 μg, 35 μg, or 70 μg of L-lyxoflavin per day, they all showed the same growth rate; it was half-way between the growth of groups of animals receiving 3.5 μg and 7 μg per day, respectively, of riboflavin. In a curative test of the riboflavin-deficient rat, 70 μg per day of L-lyxoflavin was better than no flavin but not as beneficial as 3.5 μg per day of riboflavin. They concluded that L-lyxoflavin had limited effectiveness in replacing riboflavin in rats receiving a riboflavin-deficient diet but that in the presence of small amounts of riboflavin it provided some growth stimulus.

The methods used to examine the biological activity of L-lyxoflavin for *L. casei* were not especially well standardized. When Cooperman et al.[11] used the Snell and Strong[103] medium, they found that in the presence of 0.1 μg riboflavin per tube, the presence of 0.02-5 μg L-lyxoflavin per tube caused stimulation (ratio of riboflavin to lyxoflavin being from 1:0.2 to 1:50). When the tubes contained as much as 50 μg L-lyxoflavin, the growth of the organism was inhibited (ratio of 1:500); at 150 μg per tube (ratio of 1:1500) the growth of the organism was approximately 50% of the growth in the presence of 0.1 μg riboflavin per tube (I.I. = 1500). At 250 μg per tube of L-lyxoflavin, the effect of the 0.1 μg riboflavin per tube was completely inhibited.

That L-lyxoflavin has no activity for *L. casei* was confirmed by Snell et al.[105]; they found that, in their hands, whether they used Snell's medium or a synthetic medium made no difference. They also in part confirmed Coopermen et al.[11] in that L-lyxoflavin had activity in the presence of riboflavin.

Lactobacillus lactis (ATCC 8000) like *L. casei* requires an exogenous source of riboflavin, but it has not been used extensively as a test organism. L-Lyxoflavin stimulates the growth of *L. lactis* at all quantities used and at no concentration has it been found to be inhibitory. The response of the organism is dependent on the concentration of L-lyxoflavin and the length of time incubation is continued. If the time of incubation is 22 hr, 100 μg L-lyxoflavin produces the same growth response given by 0.05 μg riboflavin; 1 mg L-lyxoflavin is equivalent to 0.3 μg riboflavin. However, if the incubation is continued for 40 hr, 100 μg L-lyxoflavin is equivalent to 3 μg riboflavin. When low concentrations of L-lyxoflavin are used, the differences are very clear also. Thus, when incubated for 20, 40, and 144 hr, 1 μg L-lyxoflavin is equivalent to 0.09, 0.16, and 0.43 μg riboflavin, respectively. The fact that L-lyxoflavin can serve as the sole flavin for *L. lactis* was also reported by Snell et al.[105]; they reported that this flavin was, however, only one-third to one-tenth as potent as riboflavin.

Briuns *et al.*,[8] Cooperman *et al.*,[11] and Snell *et al.*[101] all agree that L-lyxoflavin has no activity for the chick. The latter workers showed that when L-lyxoflavin was present with riboflavin in amounts 2.5–10 times that of riboflavin it stimulated growth, but if present at 40 times or greater the amount of riboflavin it inhibited growth. The inhibition could be reversed by additional riboflavin.

3.1.6. D-Xyloflavin (IX)

At the time they described the first synthesis of riboflavin, Karrer *et al.*[38] also reported the synthesis of D-xyloflavin and that it had been tested for activity in the riboflavin-deficient rat. They neglected to report the results of the tests on D-xyloflavin. It is interesting that, when Kuhn *et al.*[53] reported the total synthesis of D-riboflavin, they stated that L-araboflavin was about one-third as active as D-riboflavin and that D-xyloflavin was found to be less active than L-araboflavin; somewhat later Kuhn[55] stated that D-xyloflavin is distinctly less active than L-araboflavin.

3.2. Modification of Positions of Substituents on Aromatic Ring

3.2.1. Isoriboflavin

Isoriboflavin (Fig. 5) possesses a substituent on the aromatic ring that is in a position other than 7 or 8. Since the compound is the only one of this class to possess biological activity, it is worthy of some discussion. The compound was made available as a by-product of the Tishler synthesis of riboflavin.

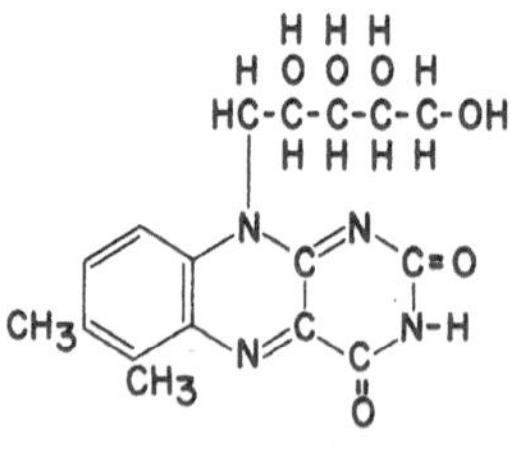

Fig. 5. Isoriboflavin [6,7-dimethyl-10-(1'-D-ribityl)isoalloxazine].

Emerson and Tishler[14] found that when 2 mg per day of isoriboflavin was given to riboflavin-deficient rats they showed less weight gain than those receiving no flavin. Since these riboflavin-deficient controls gained 15 g in 28 days, they were not deficient in the same critical sense we have advocated. When 10 μg riboflavin was given with the 2 mg isoriboflavin each day, the animals grew at twice the rate shown by the deficient controls. The growth shown in this latter group was approximately 50% of that shown by animals receiving 10 μg per day of riboflavin, a fact that demonstrated the inhibitory activity of the isoriboflavin. Rats receiving 40 μg per day of riboflavin showed the same weight gain as shown by those receiving 40 μg riboflavin and 2 mg isoriboflavin; this result shows that the 40 μg per day of riboflavin completely reversed the inhibitory action of the isoriboflavin.

Because of the differing procedures used, the details of the response of *L. casei* in the presence of isoriboflavin differs from laboratory to laboratory. Sarett[97] showed that isoriboflavin provided no stimulus for *L. casei* when it was the sole flavin available to this organism. It did provide considerable stimulus when the ratio of riboflavin to isoriboflavin varied from 1:400 to 1:100, and undoubtedly the ratio might have gone to much lower values except that the largest quantities tested were 10 μg isoriboflavin and 0.1 μg riboflavin per tube. Snell *et al.*[105] found isoriboflavin to be devoid of activity when used alone but in the presence of minimal amounts of riboflavin the growth of the organism was stimulated. The stimulation increased when the ratio of riboflavin to isoriboflavin varied from 1:1 to 1:10 but no further stimulation was produced up to a ratio of 1:4680. It is also true that at this very high ratio no inhibition occurred.

Shorb[100] found that when no riboflavin was present in the medium 1 μg isoriboflavin was equivalent to 0.038 μg riboflavin for *L. casei* and 0.002 μg riboflavin for *L. lactis*.

3.2.2. Other Modifications of Position

Kuhn *et al.*[60] synthesized four flavins to explore the importance of the positions of the methyl groups. They synthesized 6, 8-dimethyl-10-(1'-D-ribityl)-, 6,8-dimethyl-10-(1'-L-arabityl)-, 7,9-dimethyl-10-(1'-D-ribityl)-, and 7,9-dimethyl-10-(1'-L-arabityl) isoalloxazine. None of these was found to be active for the riboflavin-deficient rat when administered at 40 μg per day, and none was found to have "coferment factor" activity when added to the apoenzyme of the "yellow enzyme" (see Biological Activity of Flavins in Other Systems, Section 6).

4. HOMOLOGS OF RIBOFLAVIN

The flavins to be described under homologs of riboflavin differ from the parent structure of riboflavin by multiples of —CH_2— units in the substituents at positions 7 and 8. It is among these flavins that we find the two compounds that are not only remarkable in terms of their biological activity but are unique in that they are the only synthetic analogs of any of the B-complex vitamins which possess true vitamin-like actions in mammalian tissue. In this group is also to be found the only known potent, truly competitive antagonist of riboflavin, an antagonist that mimics in considerable detail the deficiency state induced by riboflavin deprivation.

4.1. 7-Methyl-flavin (X)

The first report[37] of the biological activity of this homolog was credited to von Euler and Malmberg, who found that in daily doses of 10-20 μg the material had "good" activity. A report containing a bit more quantitative information[61] indicated that 10 μg per rat per day was insufficient to permit survival of the animals since all died in 2-6 weeks. When 20 μg per rat per day was given the growth rate

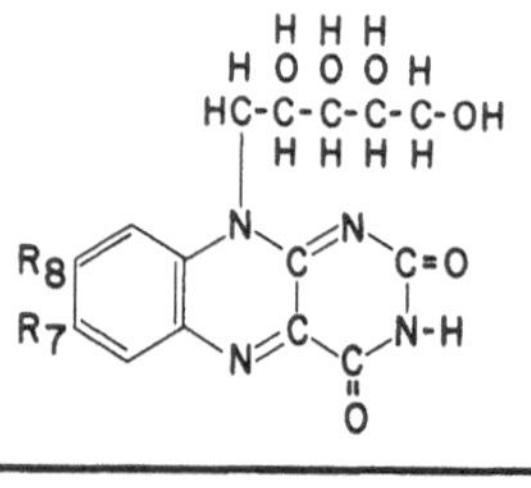

Number	R_7	R_8	Trivial name
X	CH_3—	H—	7-Methyl-flavin
XI	H—	CH_3—	8-Methyl-flavin
XII	C_2H_5—	H—	7-Ethyl-flavin
XIII	H—	C_2H_5—	8-Ethyl-flavin
XIV	C_2H_5—	CH_3—	7-Ethyl-8-methyl-flavin
XV	CH_3—	C_2H_5—	7-Methyl-8-ethyl-flavin
XVI	C_2H_5—	C_2H_5—	7,8-Diethyl-riboflavin

Fig. 6. Basic structure for homologs of riboflavin.

was 40 g in 30 days.[10] Because this is approximately the rate of growth we observe when deficient rats are administered 3 μg riboflavin per rat per day, one might estimate the activity of the homolog to be 15% of that of the vitamin.

Fortunately, we can place reliance on the report of the activity for 7-methyl-flavin for *L. casei* and *B. lactis acidi*.[104] This homolog can serve as the sole flavin in the metabolism of these organisms, and it possesses approximately 40% of the potency of riboflavin for this purpose.

Kuhn *et al.*[61] showed that this flavin possessed considerable activity as a coferment for the yellow enzyme (see Section 6, Biological Activity of Flavins in Other Systems).

4.2. 8-Methyl-flavin (XI)

The animal studies made with 8-methyl-flavin (XI) have the same inadequacies that characterized the work on 7-methyl-flavin (X). Karrer *et al.*[39] reported that at daily doses of 10–20 μg the average growth response was 1.3 g per day. This amount is about the same as shown for 7-methyl-flavin (X) and is equivalent to about 15% of the potency of riboflavin. Later in the same year[40] it was reported to have excellent vitamin B_2 activity, scarcely less than the vitamin itself, and still later Karrer and Strong[37] stated that the 8-methyl-flavin had good B_2 activity. These last two reports and still another[41] are all based on the first one, and there is little evidence that it actually has substantial riboflavin-like activity.

The studies by Snell and Strong[104] show that the homolog can serve as the sole flavin in the metabolism of *L. Casei* and *B. lactis acidi;* for both organisms it possesses approximately 75% of the activity displayed by riboflavin.

4.3. 7-Ethyl-flavin (XII)

The synthesis of 7-ethyl-flavin (XII) was undertaken[2] because of a desire to explore the role of the ethyl groups in positions 7 and 8; 7,8-diethyl-riboflavin (XVI) had been found to possess remarkable biological properties. Making use of rats that were unusually deficient in

---

[10]Other information in this report suggests that a "group" may have consisted of two animals.

riboflavin and, therefore, unusually sensitive to its administration, Aposhian and Lambooy found that 7-ethyl-flavin was devoid of growth-promoting activity and that it was a low-potency antagonist of riboflavin with an inhibition index of approximately 400. [71]

It was found that *L. casei* could utilize 7-ethyl-flavin, that as a replacement for riboflavin it possessed 3% of the activity of the vitamin throughout limiting concentrations (*loc. cit.*), and that even at ratios of homolog to riboflavin as high as 9000:1 the compound possessed no inhibitory properties for this organism. [2]

The mutant strain of *L. casei* which has been discovered and isolated in our laboratory is able to utilize the 7-ethyl-flavin as well as it can be utilized by the "stock" strain of the organism. [74]

4.4. 8-Ethyl-flavin (XIII)

8-Ethyl-flavin (XIII) has been reported as being capable of stimulating a growth response in riboflavin-deficient rats but such activity was not sustained. [42,43]

4.5. 7-Ethyl-8-methyl-flavin (XIV)

Our observations that 7-ethyl-flavin (XII) (see Section 4.3) was a low-potency and 7,8-diethyl-riboflavin (XVI) (see Section 4.7) a high-potency antagonist of riboflavin, coupled with the suggestive evidence that 8-methyl-flavin (XI) possesses approximately 15% of the potency of riboflavin for the rat, brought into question the report [43] that 7-ethyl-8-methyl-flavin had full activity for riboflavin-deficient rats when 10 μg per day was administered. Since the knowledge of the biological activity of this homolog was critical to our study of the metabolism of 7,8-diethyl-riboflavin (XVI) and there was reason to question the specificity of the synthetic procedure used for the earlier preparation, the unambiguous synthesis of 7-ethyl-8-methyl-flavin was undertaken. [69]

The homolog 7-ethyl-8-methyl-flavin is one of the only two synthetic analogs of any of the B-complex vitamins which are able to replace the natural vitamin, in this case riboflavin, in the metabolism of mammalian tissue. The homolog has 47% of the potency of riboflavin for growth and food utilization and is able to serve as the sole flavin in the metabolism of the rat. [72] It is to be emphasized that when the phrase "sole flavin in the metabolism of the rat" is used, it means just that; there is no other discernable flavin to be found in the tissues of these animals and, indeed, none is required. In all visually observable characteristics, rats maintained on the homolog as their dietary flavin are indistinguishable from those maintained on riboflavin.

When it appeared that none of the usual means for establishing biological activity would distinguish between this homolog and riboflavin, it was decided to evaluate the material with respect to its ability to support reproduction and it was found that it was unable to do so. [49,70] While this work will be reviewed in Chapter 12, the following new information is appropriately given here.

While it was true that the homolog would not support normal reproduction when it was the only flavin available to the rat, when 1.6 mg riboflavin (7% of total flavin) and 20.8 mg homolog (93% of total flavin) were added per kilogram of diet, the young survived. The female young produced by the females maintained on a diet containing 20.8 mg and 1.6 mg homolog and riboflavin/kg, respectively, were weaned. The female weanlings of this second generation were fed a diet containing the same quantity of homolog but only 0.8 mg/kg riboflavin until adulthood and then bred; most of the young that they produced survived. When weaned, the females of this third generation were fed a diet containing the same amount of homolog but only 0.4 mg/kg riboflavin until adulthood and then bred; approximately half of the young produced survived, but they were distinctly abnormal. Their movement and behavior suggested that they were blind but this seems to have been ruled out by their response to a cue light. They appeared to have difficulty maintaining equilibrium; they would climb the sides of their cage but could not regain the floor except to fall. They learned to "bar press" for food but their learning rate was slower than that of normal animals. As adults they were sluggish, moved their heads from side to side almost continuously when at rest, and walked in an ungainly manner. The weaned females from this fourth generation were fed a diet containing the same amounts of homolog but only 0.2 mg/kg riboflavin until adulthood and then bred. None of the young produced by these females survived. The females were also abnormal in that they appeared to lack the necessary instinctual maternal behavior; because of this the reasons for the nonsurvival of the young remain uncertain. [80 a]

The influence of this homolog on the succinic acid dehydrogenase activity of fetal tissue will be discussed later under this section.

The fact that the reproductive failure of females on diets containing only the homolog could be corrected by the addition to the diet of a small fraction of the total biologically active flavin as riboflavin suggested that the failure of the young to survive might be due to an enzyme inadequacy, but the excellent health of the female and her ability

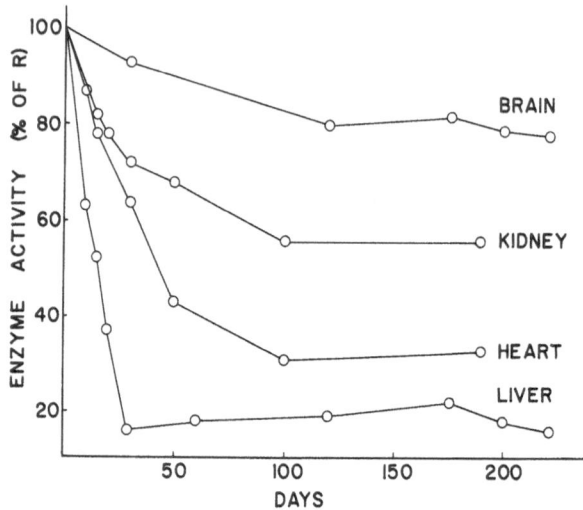

Fig. 7. Succinic acid dehydrogenase activities in tissues of growing rats fed from weaning, a diet containing 7-ethyl-8-methyl-flavin as the sole flavin. The enzyme activities are expressed as percentages of the activities of the same tissues of animals fed a diet containing an equivalent amount of riboflavin. The experimental details were essentially those reported by Kim and Lambooy[47] and Hill and Lambooy.[30]

to bring litter after litter to term made it difficult to select an enzyme for study. For reasons given in Section 1, General Background Information, we decided to turn our attention to the enzymes intimately involved in energy production.

Weanling rats were fed diets containing only homolog or riboflavin as the flavin component, and the SDH activity was determined periodically for the hearts, kidneys, and livers of the two groups of animals. Figure 7 shows in graphic form the time rate of change of the SDH activities in the tissues of the homolog-fed animals with respect to the activities of the same tissues in the riboflavin-fed animals.

The evidence strongly suggested that the coenzyme form of the homolog was able to replace riboflavin in the enzyme at a rate that was reasonably consistent with the half-life of the mitochondria, at least in the liver. It is understood that the actual half-life would indeed, be shorter than the indicated 14 days because the values observed would be summations of the residual riboflavin-containing enzyme and the new homolog-containing enzyme. [47]

The half-life of the heart and kidney mitochondria are not as readily estimated by this means, but a rough approximation might be a half-life of 40 days for the heart and 100 days for the kidney. Assuming that these values are certainly in the correct order and that the extremely slow rate of cell division in the brain reduces the need for new mitochondria in this tissue, one might expect a similar study to show that the half-life of brain mitochondria was much longer than those of the other tissues studied. The time course of change of the SDH activity for the mitochondria of the brain tissue of animals subjected to the same experimental procedure is also shown in Fig. 7. From the original data it is possible to estimate that the half-life of brain mitochondria might be of the order of 500 days. [30]

The profound effect of the homolog on the SDH activity of the liver was obviously well tolerated by the rats; while the depression of activities for the heart and kidney was impressive, it also represented no apparent threat to the animals in spite of the relatively enormous energy requirements of these latter two tissues. It was decided to study the SDH activities of the hearts, kidneys, and livers of the fetuses produced by females being fed diets containing riboflavin, the homolog, or a mixture of riboflavin and homolog (7% and 93%, respectively, of the total flavin) and of the same tissues of the females from which the fetuses had been taken.

The results showed that SDH activities of the hearts, kidneys, and livers of the fetuses produced by the riboflavin-fed females were 54, 36, and 64%, respectively, of the corresponding tissues in the riboflavin females; while the enzyme activities in the same tissues of the fetuses produced by the homolog-fed females were 7, 8, and 6%, respectively, of the same standard tissues.

The fetuses from females fed a diet containing the homolog–riboflavin mixture had SDH activities for the hearts, kidneys, and livers which were 30, 21, and 27%, respectively, of the corresponding tissues in the riboflavin females. The addition of only 7% of the total flavin as riboflavin causes the SDH activities of these tissues to be increased to values that are approximately 440, 260, and 450%, respectively, of the values found for the homolog fetuses. [49]

The nonsurvival of the newborn of the homolog females may also be due, in part, to the influence of the homolog–coenzyme on brain mitochondrial activity. Figure 7 shows that the SDH activity of the brain tissue remains high during the homolog administration from weaning age. In the case of the fetuses of the homolog females, the fetal brain must make its SDH holoenzyme from the available flavin, in this case, homolog, and as a result the brain tissue possesses only approximately 17% of the value found for the brain tissue of the riboflavin female. [30]

Reducing equivalents are also fed into the electron transport chain via the electron transport-linked DPNHD, and, in a quantitative sense, this enzyme is more important than SDH. The uniqueness of the relative inability of the homolog-coenzyme to be used by SDH is emphasized by the finding that the homolog and riboflavin are used equally well by the DPNHD of the heart, kidney, and liver tissue.[49]

Liver flavokinase phosphorylates this homolog at the same rate as it phosphorylates riboflavin. Other similarities in relation to the coenzyme role of this homolog are illustrated by the finding that, while the liver mitochondria of rats fed the homolog diet contain approximately 60% of the normal quantity of acid-extractable flavin, the percentage of the flavin in the form of the F'-AD[11] is about 91%. Under conditions of riboflavin deprivation, the total acid-extractable flavin falls to approximately 23% of normal, but, in this case as well as in the case of the animal receiving adequate vitamin, FAD accounts for 94% of the total.[13a]

The role of this homolog in the coenzyme form in the liver mitochondria has been studied relatively extensively. We have found that, while it functions in all reactions related to energy production, it appears that it serves better in this capacity for the DPN-mediated substrates than it does for those whose path of substrate oxidation enters the respiratory chain beyond the DPNHD site. Liver mitochondria prepared from rats whose sole flavin was 7-ethyl-8-methyl-flavin showed reduced state 3 respiratory rates for several substrates when compared with the rates that were shown by the mitochondria isolated from rats containing only riboflavin. Respiratory rates of the following substrates were reduced to from 90% to 49% of normal: pyruvate (PYR), α-ketoglu- terate (KG), β-hydroxybutyrate (HOB), lauroyl carnitine (LC), α-gly- cerolphosphate (GP) and succinate in the present of rotenone (S + R). However, the efficiency of utilization of the flavin present in the mitochondria is more significant in terms of the physiological response. When expressed in this way, that is, as oxygen consumed per unit of flavin, it is found that HOB and S + R are oxidized at 80–90% of the rate in the mitochondria from the normal animal; the other substrates are all oxidized at essentially normal rates or above. As stated before, the riboflavin-deficient animal's tissues utilize riboflavin with remarkable efficiency; oxidation of the above substrates range from 136 to 372% of normal.[13a]

The relationship between respiration and oxidative phosphorylation has been studied to some extent with regard to the influence of riboflavin deficiency.[7,9] As a frame of reference for our study of the influence

---

[11]The abbreviations F'-AD and F'-MN are used to indicate that the flavin portion of the coenzyme is derived from a flavin other than riboflavin.

of analogs of riboflavin on vital processes, we have studied the respiration rates, the P:O ratios, and the respiratory control ratios (RCR) for a series of substrates to help locate specific areas of malfunction in the reducing-equivalent transfer from such substrates to the electron transport chain. We have found that the P:O ratios for the liver mitochondria from animals receiving adequate riboflavin, animals receiving inadequate riboflavin, and animals utilizing the homolog, for the following sub-strates—PYR, KG, HOB, LC, GP, and S + R—are all essentially the same except that the P:O ratio for succinate in the homolog mitochondria is statistically significantly reduced. This reduction might have been a reasonable expectation in view of the remarkable influence the homolog has on SDH activity in the liver. These values were obtained by the study of mitochondrial preparations that possessed respiratory control ratios indicative of mitochondrial integrity. This is a matter of considerable importance because we have observed that, with mitochondria completely uncoupled with regard to all of the other substrates, oxidation of succinate in the presence of rotenone always proceeds with typical oxidation rates and P:O and RCR values.[13a]

Mitochondria obtained from the livers of animals provided with adequate riboflavin, insufficient riboflavin, and adequate homolog were studied to assess their susceptibility to high-amplitude swelling induced by the addition of inorganic phosphate at 1 and 2 mM concentrations.[34]

The mitochondria obtained from rats utilizing 7-ethyl-8-methyl-flavin showed swelling patterns that could not be distinguished from those shown by the mitochondria from the normal rat.[13a]

Kensler et al.[45] showed that riboflavin provided rats protection against hepatoma induction by means of 4-dimethylaminoazobenzene. The role of riboflavin in providing this protection has not been satisfac-torily defined, but its action cannot be denied. When equimolar amounts of the homolog and riboflavin were compared, it was found that the homolog provided little protection against the induction of hepatomas by azo dyes.[76]

Considerable effort has been expended in trying to relate riboflavin utilization and the growth of neoplasms.[46] While this subject will be dealt with in detail in Chapter 11, it is necessary to give it some attention at this time.

7-Ethyl-8-methyl-flavin is not an antagonist of riboflavin in any sense; it is a vitamin-like homolog of riboflavin which possesses somewhat less than optimal properties in some biochemical roles when used as the biologically essential flavin. Thus, while it does not cause regression of previously established neoplasms, it has caused a retardation of the growth rate of slice fragments of Walker rat carcinoma 256 implanted in the inguinal region of the rat. Since these rats are devoid of riboflavin, clearly the homolog is not inhibiting the action of riboflavin; it is simply not serving the biochemical needs of the tumor for growth as well as riboflavin does when it is available.[46]

The previous observations that 7-ethyl-8-methyl-flavin serves as an inefficient coenzyme for SDH in the heart, kidney, and liver prompted us to investigate its influence on the SDH activity of the Walker carcinoma 256 to see if the retarded growth of the tumor could be correlated with the activity of this enzyme involved in energy production. The results of these studies have confirmed our expectations; the activity of SDH in viable tumor tissue was found to be less than half of that found in riboflavin-deficient animals and less than a fifth of that found in animals receiving adequate riboflavin.[95]

In addition to the respiratory enzymes, two nonrespiratory enzymes were studied. The D-amino acid oxidase (DAAO) and the xanthine oxidase (XO) enzyme activities were studied in the kidneys and livers of animals whose sole tissue flavin was riboflavin or 7-ethyl-8-methyl-flavin. The activities of these enzymes have been found previously by other investigators to be reduced in tissues of rats that were made riboflavin deficient, that were, for this reason, malnourished and in ill health, and that were certain to die.[12,94] The homolog 7-ethyl-8-methyl-flavin served as an effective replacement for riboflavin in other enzyme reactions and it was of obvious interest to study these two enzymes in animals that had received a riboflavin replacement and that were in excellent health.

The D-amino acid oxidase activity in the kidney and liver of the rats whose tissue flavin was 7-ethyl-8-methyl-flavin, expressed as percentage of the activity found for the corresponding tissue in rats receiving adequate riboflavin, was normal and approximately three-fourths of normal, respectively. While the reduction in the liver is highly significant, it appears to cause no metabolic difficulties for the rat since the animal thrives.

The results obtained for xanthine oxidase in these two tissues led to extensive modifications of the preparation of the enzyme, assay procedures for the enzyme, and studies of the stability of the enzyme. When the enzyme activities for the kidney and the liver of the homolog-animal were compared with those of the normal animal as described above, it was found that the kidney activity was slightly reduced and the liver activity was reduced to half.[13b]

7-Ethyl-8-methyl-flavin can serve as the sole flavin in *L. casei* and in *B. lactis acidi.*[68,72,103] For the former organism it possesses 100% of the activity of equivalent amounts of riboflavin up to the concentration of 26.6×10^{-11} moles/ml. At higher concentrations its activity reaches a plateau at about 90% of that shown by equivalent amounts of riboflavin.

The mutant form of *L. casei*,[12] which appears to differ from the "stock" form in that it has decreased specificity of its flavin phosphorylating mechanism, is able to use 7-ethyl-8-methyl-flavin as efficiently as it is used by the "stock" organism.[74,98]

4.6. 7-Methyl-8-ethyl-flavin (XV)

When it was observed that the biological activity of 7-ethyl-8-methyl-flavin (XIV) could not have been predicted on the basis of the activities of 7-ethyl-flavin (XII) and 8-methyl-flavin (XI), our attention was quite naturally drawn to 7-methyl-8-ethyl-flavin (XV). It has been reported earlier in this chapter that 7-methyl-flavin (X) appeared to have approximately 15% of the potency of riboflavin for the growth of the rat. 8-Ethyl-flavin (XIII) had been reported to stimulate a small growth response in the riboflavin-deficient rat but the activity was not sustained. Information about the biological activity of 7-methyl-8-ethyl-flavin was also critical to our study of the metabolism of 7,8-diethyl-riboflavin (XVI) because, among other things, we still had identified no component of the molecule to which we could ascribe the potent antagonistic properties. In order that 7-methyl-8-ethyl-flavin might be studied, it was synthesized[69] by unequivocal procedures.

The homolog 7-methyl-8-ethyl-flavin is one of only two synthetic analogs of any of the B-complex vitamins that are able to replace the natural vitamin in the metabolism of mammalian tissue; 7-ethyl-8-methyl-flavin (XIV) is the other. 7-Methyl-8-ethyl-flavin has 36% of the potency of riboflavin for growth and food utilization and is able to serve as the sole flavin in the metabolism of the rat.[72]

Information concerning the inability of this homolog to support normal reproduction in the rat will be found in Chapter 12.

Weanling rats were fed a diet containing 7-methyl-8-ethyl-flavin in place of riboflavin, and the SDH activity was determined periodically for the hearts, kidneys, and livers. When these activities were expressed as percentages of the activities of the same tissues from animals fed a diet containing riboflavin, it was found that the changes that took place resembled the findings with the isomeric 7-ethyl-8-methyl-flavin (XIV). The SDH activity was decreased in each tissue with the rate of fall being most rapid in the liver and the least rapid in the heart, but in neither tissue was the depression as extreme as had been found true with the 7-ethyl-8-methyl-flavin. After 50 days of the diet the activities

---

[12] For the origin of this mutant see Section 5.2.2, 7-Chloro-8-methyl-flavin (XXII).

for the heart, kidney, and liver had fallen to approximately two-thirds of normal, and these activities were maintained essentially at this level until assays were discontinued at the 124th day.[13]

It is evident, and it must be emphasized repeatedly, that observations made on the whole animal cannot be translated to the tissue and enzyme levels with much quantitative reliability. We note that, while in terms of overall metabolic efficiency as expressed in growth and food utilization 7-ethyl-8-methyl-flavin has 47% of the potency of riboflavin, 7-methyl-8-ethyl-flavin has only 36%. In terms of the activity of the coenzyme forms of these two flavins, we find that, while of equal effectiveness for the kidney, the 7-methyl-8-ethyl-flavin coenzyme F'-AD is much more effective for the heart and the liver where the relative values of two-thirds of normal are greatly increased over the values of 32% and 10%, respectively, for the 7-ethyl-8-methyl-flavin. Contrasts of this sort will be more the rule than the exception when comparing these two flavins, as the case with flavokinase emphasizes.

Liver flavokinase phosphorylates 7-methyl-8-ethyl-flavin at only 12% of the rate it phosphorylates 7-ethyl-8-methyl-flavin and riboflavin. It would appear that the rate of phosphorylation of a flavin has little relationship to how successfully an animal would utilize the material. While the liver mitochondria of rats fed 7-methyl-8-ethyl-flavin contain approximately two-thirds of the normal quantity of acid-extractable flavin, the percentage of the flavin the form of F'-AD is 95%; under identical circumstances FAD is 94% whether the animals receive adequate riboflavin or are deprived of riboflavin.[13a]

The role of this homolog in the coenzyme form in the liver mitochondria has also been studied relatively extensively. Mitochondria prepared from rats whose only tissue flavin was 7-methyl-8-ethyl-flavin showed reduced state 3 respiratory rates for several substrates, when compared with the rates shown by mitochondria isolated from animals whose tissue flavin was riboflavin. Respiratory rates for the following substrates were reduced to from 90% to 47% of normal: PYR, KG, HOB, LC, GP, and S + R, all of which values are essentially equal to or greater than those found for the isomeric 7-ethyl-8-methyl-flavin. The efficiency of utilization of the flavin in the mitochondria show that, in terms of oxygen consumed per unit of flavin, 7-methyl-8-ethyl-flavin is used more efficiently than riboflavin when the animal is provided with adequate amounts of the vitamin.

The P:O ratios for the liver mitochondria from animals receiving adequate riboflavin, animals receiving inadequate riboflavin, and animals utilizing 7-methyl-8-ethyl-flavin, for the following substrates, PYR, KG, HOB, LC, GP, and S + R, are all essentially the same. These values were obtained by the study of mitochondrial preparations that possessed respiratory control ratios indicative of mitochondrial integrity.

The mitochondria obtained from the livers of rats whose only tissue flavin was 7-methyl-8-ethyl-flavin showed a pattern of susceptibility to high-amplitude swelling induced by the addition of inorganic phosphate, which was superimposable on the patterns shown by mitochondria obtained from the livers of the normal rat.[13a]

The homolog 7-methyl-8-ethyl-flavin, an efficient replacement for riboflavin in many biochemical roles, was able to support the growth of Walker carcinoma 256 in animals possessing only this homolog in their tissues as well as growth of the carcinoma was supported in animals whose tissue flavin was the vitamin.[46]

The SDH activity of the viable tissue of the Walker carcinoma 256 was 47% of the activity shown by the tissue isolated from hosts whose tissue flavin was riboflavin; yet the rate of growth of the tumor was the same in these two groups. The SDH activity found for the homolog group (47%) was about the same as found in the viable tissue from tumors isolated from rats maintained on a riboflavin-deficient diet where the value was found to be 42% of normal.[95] However, in the case of the deficient animal, the tumor grows at approximately 50% of the normal rate.[1,46]

The homolog 7-methyl-8-ethyl-flavin provided little protection against the induction of hepatomas by azo dyes when provided as the only flavin available to the rat.[76]

The D-amino acid oxidase activity in the kidney and liver of the rats whose tissue flavin was 7-methyl-8-ethyl-flavin expressed as percentage of the activity found for the corresponding tissue in rats receiving adequate riboflavin was approximately 60% and 40%, respectively. While both of these reductions are large and highly significant, the reduced enzyme activity appears to cause no metabolic difficulties for the rat.

When the xanthine oxidase activities for the kidney and liver of the homolog animal were compared with those of the normal animal as described above, it was found that the kidney activity was approximately 150% and the liver activity approximately 60%, respectively, of the normal values. The reason for this remarkable increase is the subject for further study.

The homolog 7-methyl-8-ethyl-flavin can serve as the sole source of flavin for *L. casei* and for this organism it possess 100% of the activity of equivalent amounts of riboflavin up to a concentration of 26.6×10^{-11} moles/ml. At higher concentrations its activity reaches a plateau about 90% of that shown by equivalent amounts of riboflavin.[68,72]

The mutant strain of *L. casei* which we have isolated in our laboratory is able to utilize the 7-methyl-8-ethyl-flavin as efficiently as it is used by the "stock" *L. casei* organism.[74]

4.7. 7,8-Diethyl-Riboflavin (XVI)

Diethyl-riboflavin was not only the first potent riboflavin antagonist in the rat to have been reported, but it was the first compound structurally related to riboflavin which possessed inhibitor properties for one test organism (rats) and vitamin-like properties for another test organism (lactobacilli).

When diethyl-riboflavin was administered as the only flavin in the diet fed to riboflavin-deficient rats, the animals responded differently depending on the quantity of flavin administered. If the quantity administered is small (3 μg–60 μg/day), the deficient rats will maintain their weights or show small gains over periods of weeks. When intermediate quantities are given (8 μg–32 μg/g food), very large gains are made during the first few days of supplementation but these animals fail to survive. At still higher doses (2 mg/day), there is no growth response and 60% of the test animals fail to survive a 21-day test period. Not only is it the most potent antagonist of riboflavin in the classical sense (weight gain) to have been described, but it is the only one that has

TABLE I. *Net Weight Gained by Groups of Weanling Rats Given Riboflavin, Diethyl-Riboflavin, or Mixtures of Different Quantities of Riboflavin and Diethyl-Riboflavin to Show Competitive Relationship*

Group number	Daily supplement[a]	Number of animals[b]	Net gain in weight ± S.E.[c,d]
1	Flavin deficient	10	0 ± 2
2	2.0 mg D	13	−2 ± 2
3	75 μg R[e] + 0.5 mg D	9	31 ± 2
4	150 μg R + 1.0 mg D	9	32 ± 3
5	225 μg R + 1.5 mg D	10	29 ± 2
6	300 μg R + 2.0 mg D	10	26 ± 5
7	300 μg R	10	55 ± 4

[a] Administered by stomach tube in 0.5 ml of 6% gum acacia immediately before being fed. The diet was the riboflavin-deficient diet described in the text. R, riboflavin; D, diethyl-riboflavin.
[b] Average initial weight was 43 ± 2 g.
[c] Duration of experiment was 21 days.
[d] An estimate of the standard error of the mean.
[e] The ratio of R to D was constant.

been demonstrated to be a truly competitive inhibitor in the rat. Table I presents the data from which it can be concluded that the homolog has an I.I. of 6 (Lambooy and Aposhian[65] and unpublished observations).

The riboflavin-deficient rats given the intermediate quantities of diethyl-riboflavin not only show a growth response, but they showed recovery of most of the visually observable manifestations of the deficiency. This fact was also true of the animals receiving the high doses of the homolog if they survived longer than 14 days of the 21-day test period. This is the first instance cited in which there is an apparent separation of the flavin's influence on (a) food consumption and weight gain, (b) survival, and (c) gross physical appearance.

The homolog is a potent agent for the induction of riboflavin deficiency or a condition that simulates such deficiency. It appears that the most likely explanation for the following events is that the large amounts of diethyl-riboflavin replace riboflavin from the tissues to the extent of its excess tissue stores or that displacement of riboflavin from a limiting enzyme or a critical tissue occurs.[65]

Normal young rats were placed on a riboflavin-deficient diet and separate groups of these normal animals were given 6% gum acacia solution (flavin deficient group), 2 mg/day diethyl-riboflavin for 1, 2, and 5 days. The growth responses for the three latter groups were very different, during a period of 28 days, from that shown by the group receiving the flavin-free supplement. The treated groups grew at a very rapid rate for approximately twice as many days as they had received the diethyl-riboflavin and then, having become riboflavin deficient, lost the weight gained during the remaining days of the test period. The group that had received the homolog for 5 days gained 21 g during the first 10 days, and then, being riboflavin deficient, lost weight until at the 28th day it had returned to its pretreatment weight. The group receiving the gum acacia solution, or the animals on the deficient diet, had continued to gain and was still gaining weight at 35 days.[67]

Although the teratogenic effects of galactoflavin (see Section 5.1.1., XVII) will be discussed in detail in Chapter 9, it is necessary to make reference to it at this time as an introduction to the following study. Since galactoflavin has been described as an inhibitor of riboflavin and its teratogenic activity ascribed to this property (see Chapter 9), one might anticipate that diethyl-riboflavin, an extremely potent antagonist of riboflavin in the rat, might also bring about the production of birth defects. Because diethyl-riboflavin is phosphorylated by the rat, while galactoflavin is not, one might expect more extensive teratogenic action.

Groups of pregnant rats were given 2 mg/day of diethyl-riboflavin for 1-5 days during the period of days 10-14 of gestation. Other groups were given 2-12 mg/day of diethyl-riboflavin for each of the days 7-11 of gestation. During the days when the homolog was given, the animals were fed a riboflavin-deficient diet, but before and after this period they were fed a diet containing 10 mg/kg of the vitamin. The fetuses were removed by section for examination on day 21.

The first groups showed no changes from normal in numbers, no gross defects, and no skeletal abnormalities. The groups given the homolog during days 7-11 showed no changes from normal in numbers, no gross defects, and no skeletal abnormalities. However, in the 12 mg/day group some changes were noted. Seven of 12 animals died because of the toxic action of the homolog, a result found to be unrelated to the pregnancy of the animals. Of the remaining five animals, two produced normal litters, two resorbed their litters, and one had no living young at the time of section. This raises several interesting questions concerning the forms and mechanisms of antagonistic action. By good fortune it was galactoflavin, a compound of little interest as an inhibitor, that became readily and widely available to investigators of teratology.

A study of the influence of diethyl-riboflavin on the SDH activities of the heart, kidneys, and liver could not be undertaken in the same way it was done for 7-ethyl-8-methyl-flavin (XIV) and 7-methyl-8-ethyl-flavin (XV). Since it is an antagonist of riboflavin and not a vitamin-like replacement for riboflavin, it would not become the metabolically active tissue flavin of the animals receiving it. This is not to say that the diethyl riboflavin would not assume a coenzyme role in some reactions, but the fact that it is lethal means it does not satisfy all metabolic reactions for the rat. Thus, rather than start with weanling animals so as to saturate their tissues with the homolog, one must start with adult rats whose tissues are saturated with riboflavin. Our aim was to discover what influence diethyl-riboflavin would have on the SDH activities of tissues in which the coenzyme of the SDH was still FAD so far as we knew.

Groups of normal animals that had been grown to adulthood (about 200 g) on a diet containing adequate riboflavin were continued on that diet, or the diet was changed to one containing an equivalent amount of diethyl-riboflavin; the animals were fed their respective diets for 13 weeks and then the assays were performed on members of both groups at the same time. During this period of time the group receiving riboflavin continued to grow while the homolog group continuously lost weight. The actual study included an additional group that received an equivalent amount of a mixture of the two flavins, 95% diethyl-riboflavin and 5% riboflavin, a combination determined as the minimum amount of riboflavin required to prevent the animals from losing or gaining weight. Table II shows the growth response of these animals.

TABLE II. Net Weight Gained by Groups of Adult Rats Fed Diets Containing Riboflavin, Diethyl-Riboflavin, or Mixtures of the Two Flavins[a]

Group number	Quantity of flavin per kilogram diet[b]	Number of animals	Net gain in weight ± S.E., weeks[c]		
			6	9	13
1	20 mg R	11	58 ± 5	77 ± 5	97 ± 7
2	21.5 mg D	12	−30 ± 3	−41 ± 4	−47 ± 7[d]
3	20.4 mg D[e] 1.0 mg R	12	2 ± 4	−4 ± 6	6 ± 6
4	19.4 mg D 2.0 mg R	12	25 ± 4	37 ± 6	
5	18.3 mg D 3.0 mg R	12	45 ± 5	66 ± 8	

[a] Average weight of rats at start of experiment, 204 ± 1.
[b] R, Riboflavin; D, Diethyl-riboflavin.
[c] Estimate of the standard error of the mean.
[d] Only eight animals of this group survived. In all other groups, all survived.
[e] Ratio of moles of D to moles of R for Groups 3, 4, and 5 are 18.7, 9.1, and 5.7, respectively.

When the activities for the tissues from the animals that received riboflavin are expressed as 100%, the activities for the diethyl-riboflavin group were approximately 80% for the heart and kidney and 30% for the liver. The activities for the same tissues in the animals receiving the mixture of flavins were approximately 90% and 40%, respectively.[13a]

The activities found for the tissues from the animals receiving homolog mimic the values for animals made riboflavin deficient, except that in the animal made deficient by deprivation, the activities of the heart and kidney do not fall. The small reductions in these two tissues might be due to competition in the utilization of the FAD by SDH but can be due to a number of other factors, for example, apoenzyme lack or failure to deposit protein.[47,48] The activities for the tissues from the group receiving the mixture of flavins may be due to the replacement of the riboflavin lost and destroyed each day or to the fact that the stability of weight necessitates some protein deposition and thus provides a mechanism for scavenging riboflavin during metabolic turnover.[20,81]

The first evidence that enzymatic phosphorylation could be accomplished in vivo, in mammalian tissue, on an analog of riboflavin, and that it could be accomplished on an analog that was a potent antagonist of riboflavin in that tissue was provided by Aposhian and Lambooy.[3]

The phosphorylation of diethyl-riboflavin *in vitro* by rat liver flavokinase is accomplished at a rate that is 65% of that shown by riboflavin.[13a] This fact is significant because, while a large number of molecular forms might be phosphorylated, we have yet to find one that is a potent antagonist of riboflavin which is not phosphorylated.

The influence of diethyl-riboflavin on the acid-extractable flavin content and composition of the liver mitochondria is of considerable interest. The total acid-extractable flavin is approximately 70% of what it is for the animal receiving riboflavin in its diet, and that part of the acid-extractable flavin found in the form of FAD is approximately 95% in both cases. A further point of interest is that the ratio of FAD to FMN plus free flavin is also exactly the same, namely 16.2. How these conditions can prevail in the mitochondrion and be consistent with the severe fall of SDH activity is of interest and will require further study.

In spite of what appears to be a relatively good flavin content of the mitochondria isolated from animals in which riboflavin deficiency had been induced by the use of diethyl-riboflavin, the state 3 respiration rates for a number of substrates is very consistent with the riboflavin-deficient state produced by deprivation of the vitamin. If the respiration rates found for the mitochondria isolated from normal animals receiving riboflavin are considered to be 100%, then the rates for the deficient animal produced by vitamin deprivation and by diethyl-riboflavin administration for the following substrates are in both cases: PYR, about 60%; KG, about 80%; HOB, about 70%; LC, about 30%; GP, about 50%, and S + R, about 70%, respectively. One might conclude that under such circumstances the respiratory control ratios would resemble those of the riboflavin-deficient state, and, indeed, the values are almost identical.

There is, however, an inconsistency between the respiratory rates and the efficiency of utilization of the tissue flavin. As stated above, the mitochondrial flavin content is more suggestive of adequate flavin stores than of riboflavin-deficient stores. The respiration rates of various substrates and the respiratory control ratios for these substrates are suggestive of the riboflavin-deficient state. The efficiency of utilization of the flavin in the oxidation of the substrates resembles much more the normal animal than the riboflavin-deficient animal except in the case of LC and GP, where the efficiencies are approximately 50% and 75%, respectively.

The values for the P:O ratios for the liver mitochondria obtained from animals in which riboflavin deficiency had been induced by diethyl-riboflavin were not different when compared with those obtained from animals made riboflavin deficient by deprivation, nor were they different from the ratios observed for normal mitochondria, for any of the above mentioned substrates.

The liver mitochondria obtained from rats given diethyl-riboflavin show a pattern of susceptibility to high-amplitude swelling induced by the addition of inorganic phosphate that resembled to a striking degree the pattern shown by mitochondria isolated from the animals that had been deprived of the vitamin.[13a]

The homolog 7,8-diethyl-riboflavin can serve as the sole source of flavin for *L. casei* and for *B. lactis acidi*. For *L. casei* the homolog has 100 percent of the activity of equivalent amounts of riboflavin through 8.22×10^{-11} M/ml. At higher concentrations its potency appears to plateau at about 90% of the activity for riboflavin. The reduced activity suggests that the flavoprotein enzymes utilizing F'-MN and F'-AD formed from diethyl-riboflavin are less well able to carry out their metabolic roles in the lactic acid acidified medium than those enzymes utilizing FMN and FAD formed from riboflavin. For *B. lactic acidi* the homolog possesses 100% of the activity of equivalent amounts of riboflavin through approximately 6×10^{-11} moles/ml, but at higher concentrations it possesses only about 90% of the activity shown by riboflavin.[64,65]

The mutant strain of *L. casei* which has been discovered in our laboratory is able to utilize diethyl-riboflavin somewhat more efficiently than it can be utilized by the "stock" strain of the organism.[74]

Diethyl-riboflavin inhibited multiplication of psittacosis virus (sic) (6BC) to a significant degree in concentration of 0.01–0.05 mg/ml and was, in this respect, more potent than antagonists of other vitamins. Even at the lower concentration the homolog also suppressed somewhat the growth of fibroblasts from heart explants without, however, any effect on contractility.[89]

5. ANALOGS OF RIBOFLAVIN

5.1. Modifications of the Side Chain at Position 10

5.1.1. Galactoflavin (XVII)

Emerson *et al.*[15] were the first to report that galactoflavin, which is the trivial name for 7,8-dimethyl-10-(1'-D-dulcityl)isoalloxazine, was an antagonist of riboflavin in the rat. They fed diets that contained either no flavin, riboflavin, galactoflavin, or mixtures of the two flavins

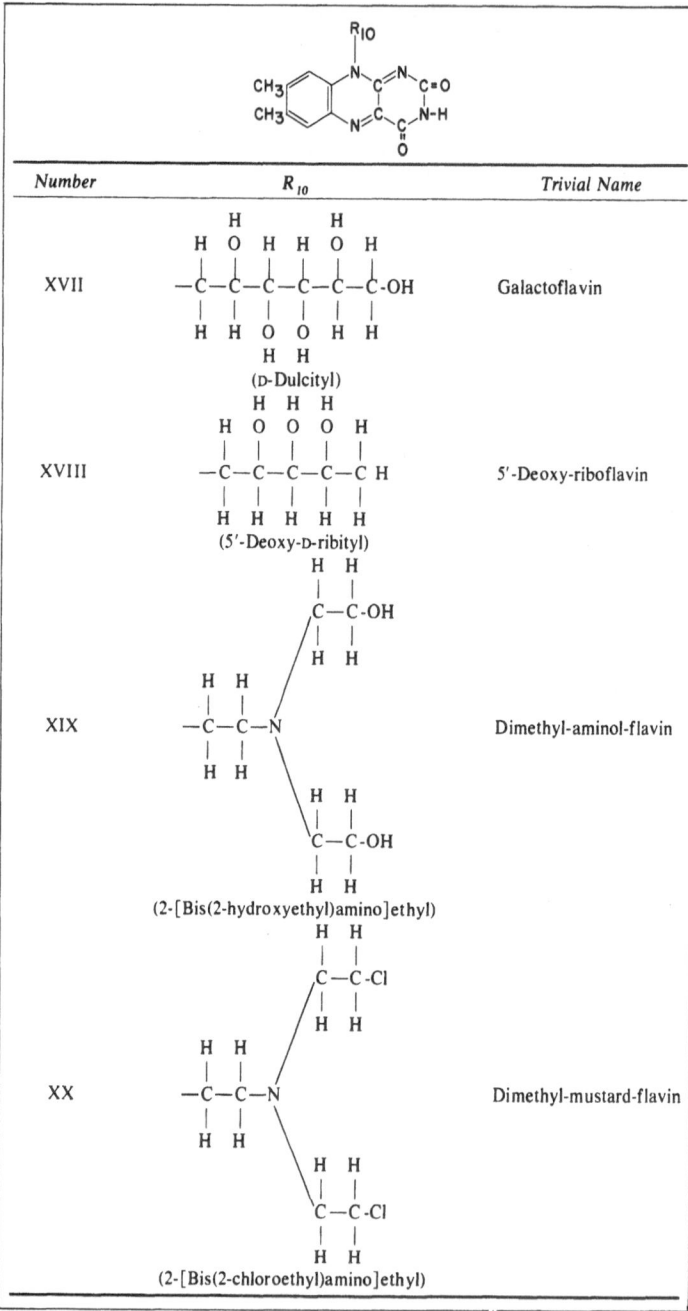

Fig. 8. Basic structure for analogs of riboflavin which are modified at position 10.

to groups of rats that were not made riboflavin deficient before the flavin supplementation began. The animals fed the flavin-free diet showed growth during the 28-day test period; since those receiving either 1.08 or 2.16 mg galactoflavin/day showed no growth during this time, it was assumed that the analog was an antagonist of riboflavin. Only 20-30% of the animals receiving galactoflavin survived the test period, but when 40 μg/day of riboflavin was administered with the 2.16 mg galactoflavin the survival of the animals was assured. When 120 μg/day of riboflavin was added to 2.16 mg galactoflavin, the animals grew to a weight in excess of 50% of the growth observed on 120 μg riboflavin/day. If reasonable estimates are made of the quantitative composition of a mixture of the two flavins which might yield 50% of the growth observed for the quantity of riboflavin alone, the analog has an inhibition index for the rat of approximately 25. Galactoflavin is, therefore, a reversible inhibitor of riboflavin in the rat.

That the flavin requirements of weanling rats could not be satisfied by galactoflavin had been demonstrated and the effects of adding the extremely large quantity of 2 mg galactoflavin/g of diet fed to adult rats was shown vividly by Lane.[84] Adult animals (250 g) lost 82 g in a period of 21 days, while others receiving a riboflavin-deficient diet for this period gained approximately 20 g. It is very clear, of course, that the galactoflavin group consumed very little food during this time; indeed, it is unfortunate that the degree of their general malnourishment must have been severe.

The effect of the administration of galactoflavin on the biochemical competence of the liver mitochondria was studied first by Beyer *et al.*[7] The galactoflavin was fed with the diet at the high concentration of 1 g/kg to adult rats (200-250 g) for either 15 or 28 days. It was observed that after 10 days of the galactoflavin-containing diet the flavin content of the liver mitochondria had been reduced to an average of 34% of normal; after 28 days the concentration was 22% of normal. At the end of the same time intervals, the reductions in flavin content of the mitochondria of animals deprived of riboflavin had reached 54% and 44%, respectively, of the normal value.

Miller *et al.*[88] found that if a riboflavin-deficient diet containing 60 mg galactoflavin/kg was fed to pregnant rats for days 11-15 of the gestation period, the fetuses assayed at day 21 contained only 40% of the concentration of riboflavin found for animals maintained on a diet containing adequate riboflavin during that time. They suggested that galactoflavin might inhibit the synthesis of FAD. Nelson *et al.*[90] also noted congenital malformations in rats treated with galactoflavin.

The respiratory rates of the mitochondria obtained from rats that had been fed the galactoflavin-containing diet for 15 days for the substrates

BOH or glutamate was 65% and 53% of normal, respectively, while that for succinate was normal. The mitochondria had normal P:O ratios for these substrates.[7]

An extensive study of the influence of galactoflavin on nucleotides and enzymes in rat liver was reported by Prosky et al.[92] A significant observation reported was that, while rats fed diets containing galactoflavin and no riboflavin for 5 weeks weighed only 66% as much as those on a riboflavin-deficient diet, there were few biochemical differences observed. However, when the rats that were given galactoflavin (3 mg/100 g body wt) were also given riboflavin (15 μg/100 g body wt), and this group was fed by the matched-weight technique and compared with a group that was given only riboflavin (15 μg/100 g body wt), significant reductions were found in the activities of flavin-containing enzymes and in the flavin concentrations of the liver. When the activities of the enzymes were expressed as percentage of the normal, the influence of the galactoflavin was to reduce glycolic acid oxidase to 9%, DAAO to 4%, and TPNH dehydrogenase to 56% of normal, while DPNH dehydrogenase was unchanged. The FAD and FMN concentrations in the liver were reduced to 33% and 42% of normal, respectively. No coenzyme form or derived form of galactoflavin was found in the tissue, and only traces of galactoflavin were detected. These latter findings have been essentially confirmed.[84]

Galactoflavin in diets at the concentration of 2.5 mg–40 mg/kg in the presence of 1 mg riboflavin/kg was found not to be stimulatory nor inhibitory for the chick.[105]

Shorb[100] reported that galactoflavin alone provided no stimulus and was not inhibitory for L. casei. While Snell et al.[105] confirmed the lack of activity for galactoflavin as the sole flavin for this organism, they found that it both stimulated and was an inhibitor of riboflavin when the latter was present. For example, they found that in the presence of 0.1 μg riboflavin per tube, galactoflavin was stimulatory when 1 μg–70 μg per tube was present, but that as the concentration increased from 70 μg–200 μg per tube it caused inhibition of the utilization of riboflavin. The inhibitory properties could be reversed by additional riboflavin. Lane and Brindley[85] found galactoflavin to have an I.I. for riboflavin in this organism of approximately 310.

Both Shorb[100] and Snell et al.[105] found galactoflavin alone to provide no stimulation for L. lactis, and Shorb found it to possess no inhibitory properties.

5.1.2. Other Modifications

It must be apparent at this point in the review of the biological activity of analogs of riboflavin that no substantial inhibitory or vitamin-like activity is likely to be found among compounds possessing substituents other than D-ribityl in position 10. A few examples will be cited because of special considerations involved in their design and syntheses. Two analogs of this type were discussed under Section 2, Derivatives of Riboflavin.

5.1.2A. 5'-DEOXY-RIBOFLAVIN (XVIII). It had been known for 20 years that to be active riboflavin must be unsubstituted at position 3. It was also known that in *in vitro* systems the 5'-hydroxyl group permitted some activity but that when this hydroxyl group was phosphorylated maximum activity was obtained. Shunk *et al.*[102] synthesized the 5'-deoxy analog of riboflavin to learn to what extent the absence of this essential hydroxyl group would alter the activity of riboflavin. The analog was found to be devoid of riboflavin-like activity, but it did possess inhibitory properties for *L. casei* in which organism it was found to have an I.I. of approximately 150. The reversal of the inhibition by riboflavin prompted the authors to suggest that it was a competitive inhibitor. The essentiality of the 5'-hydroxyl group for this microorganism was thus established.

5.1.2B. DIMETHYL-AMINOL-FLAVIN (XIX). To some people the structure of quinacrine resembles riboflavin.[10,50] One of the significant portions of the structure of quinacrine is the —9-(1-methyl-4-diethylaminobutylamino)— side chain. The supposed resemblance to riboflavin prompted the synthesis of several basically substituted isoalloxazines[10,50,51] as potential antimalarial drugs. None possessed antimalarial activity nor did any show antagonism toward riboflavin. All of the isoalloxazines which have a basic substituent at position 10 have a dialkylaminoalkyl side chain. We interpreted the absence of a hydroxyl group on the side chain at a distance comparable to the terminal hydroxyl group of riboflavin as a possible reason why these basically substituted analogs of riboflavin are inactive. Godfrey[25] molecular models of D-ribityl and 2-[bis(2-hydroxyethyl)amino]ethyl side chain (see XIX) show that they assume comparable steric conformations, and the latter has hydroxyl groups in positions comparable to the 5'-hydroxyl group of riboflavin. To test the essentiality of such a hydroxyl group for antagonistic properties, 7,8-dimethyl-10-{2-[bis(2-hydroxy-ethyl)amino]ethyl}isoalloxazine (XIX) was synthesized by Faulkner and Lambooy.[21]

The analog was found to be a reversible inhibitor of riboflavin for the riboflavin-deficient rat. The quantity of riboflavin required to obtain a 50% reversal of the growth inhibition resulting from the administration of 2 mg/day can be estimated as about 40 μg, resulting in an inhibition index of approximately 50.

Dimethyl-aminol-flavin is biologically inert for *L. casei*; at a ratio of analog to riboflavin of 5000:1, no inhibition took place. The analog was also devoid of antimalarial activity.

5.1.2c. DIMETHYL-MUSTARD-FLAVIN (XX). The availability of dimethyl-aminol-flavin (XIX) provided an opportunity to convert the material to a "two-arm mustard" compound, a class that had shown promise as anticancer agents. This opportunity was attractive not only because of the hope that an active agent might be found but because it provided an excellent opportunity to explore along with others the possible role of the "carrier" molecule in cancer chemotherapy. The analog was found to be especially effective against Walker rat carcinoma 256; 100 percent cures were obtained at doses of 25 mg/kg/day for 5 days, and even when 1.56 mg was used in the same regimen while no cures were observed a 50% prolongation of the survival of the rat was obtained. The material possessed a therapeutic index of 4 for the Walker 256. No cures were observed in the case of L-1210 lymphoid leukemia, but here also levels ranging from 8 to 400 mg/kg/day produced significant increases in survival time.[13] (See Section 5.2.1, Dichlororiboflavin (XXI), and Section 5.3.2, Dichloro-mustard-flavin XXXII).

5.2. Modifications of Substituents at Positions 7 and 8

5.2.1. Dichlororiboflavin (XX)

Dichlororiboflavin (7,8-dichloro-10-(1'-D-ribityl)isoalloxazine)[62] was the first antagonist of riboflavin to be described. To present the information on dichlororiboflavin in a meaningful way, it will be necessary to alter the form of presentation employed in this chapter. In this instance, the early studies, which were microbiological, will appear before the animal studies. The change in the usual order emphasizes that the only reason this analog was often described as a riboflavin antagonist was not related to knowledge of the activity of the material but to the fact that it was the only one on the scene for many years.

Dichlororiboflavin was shown to inhibit *Staphylococcus aureus* and *Streptobacterium plantarum* P32, neither of which require an exogenous source of riboflavin. The results are interesting, although they leave much to be desired in terms of the present concepts of antagonists. The findings for *S. plantarum* will be used as an example. All culture tubes contained 130 μg/ml dichlororiboflavin. Four sets were prepared

---

[13] The screening was done by the Cancer Chemotherapy National Service Center.

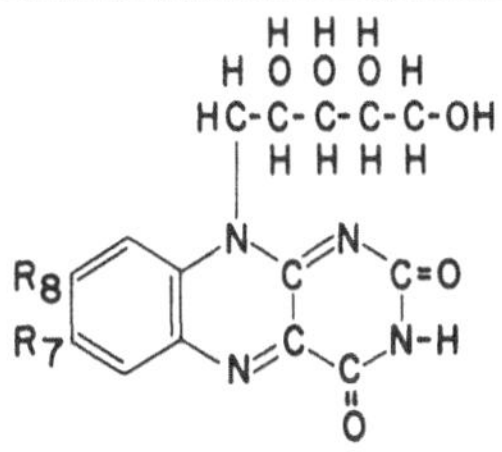

Number	R_7	R_8	Trivial name
XXI	Cl—	Cl—	Dichlororiboflavin
XXII	Cl—	CH_3—	7-Chloro-8-methyl-flavin
XXIII	Cl—	C_2H_5—	7-Chloro-8-ethyl-flavin
XXIV	CH_3—	Cl—	7-Methyl-8-chloro-flavin
XXV	C_2H_5—	Cl—	7-Ethyl-8-chloro-flavin
XXVI	Br—	Br—	Dibromo-riboflavin
XXVII	Br—	CH_3—	7-Bromo-8-methyl-flavin
XXVIII	Br—	C_2H_5—	7-Bromo-8-ethyl-flavin
XXIX	CH_3—	Br—	7-Methyl-8-bromo-flavin
XXX	C_2H_5—	Br—	7-Ethyl-8-bromo-flavin

Fig. 9. Basic structure for analogs of riboflavin which are modified at positions 7 and 8.

and to the tubes of each set riboflavin was added as graded increments through the range of 0.06–8.0 μg/ml. One set of tubes was incubated at 28°C for each time period of 2, 3, 4, and 6 days. The authors then report that 50% of the normal growth was found for each of the above incubation periods at concentration ratios of 1:25, 1:60, 1:130, and 1:165, respectively. These ratios tell us that the longer the organism is in contact with the antagonist, the less inhibited it is by the antagonist.

The authors[62] also report that throughout the concentration range of 0.05–25 μg/ml, dichlororiboflavin provided no vitamin-like stimulus for *B. lactis acidi*, an organism dependent on an exogenous source of riboflavin. Later[110] a report of the use of the same organism showed that at the end of 24 hr the ratio of riboflavin to dichlororiboflavin resulting in 50% of the normal growth was from 1:29 to 1:59.

Although dichlororiboflavin had been known since 1943, no useful information concerning the analog's activity in the rat could be found in the literature.

As a result of our findings relative to 7-chloro-8-methyl-flavin (Section 5.2.2, XXII) and 7-methyl-8-chloro-flavin (Section 5.2.4, XXIV), we were obliged to prepare dichlororiboflavin in a state of indisputable purity for detailed study in the rat. Ironically, dichlororiboflavin was found to be completely inert as a replacement for riboflavin in the riboflavin-deficient rat and as an antagonist of riboflavin in this animal. [73]

The evidence that dichlororiboflavin is inert, possessing neither vitamin-like nor inhibitory properties for *L. casei* has been firmly established. [73,105] In both instances, however, it was found that in the presence of riboflavin at concentrations of both 0.1 and 0.3 μg per tube, the addition of from 1 to 25 μg per tube of dichlororiboflavin produced a very small but measurable increase in the number of cells and acid production. Greater quantities of the analog provided no additional stimulus. In the absence of riboflavin, the analog provides no vitamin-like stimulus for the organism. [74]

The mutant strain of *L. casei* discovered and studied extensively in our laboratory is indistinguishable from the "stock" strain with respect to its response to dichlororiboflavin; neither can utilize it. [74]

Kearney [44] has shown that yeast flavokinase phosphorylates dichlororiboflavin at the same rate it forms FMN from riboflavin, yet Kuhn *et al.* [62] found yeast not to be inhibited by the analog when present in concentrations up to 250 μg/ml.

An additional observation made by Kuhn *et al.* [62] was that the E_0' of dichlororiboflavin (at pH7) was -0.095 V, while under the same conditions the E_0' for riboflavin was -0.185 V. The analog, in its dihydro or reduced form is a considerably weaker reductant than dihydroriboflavin. They state that, "perhaps the dichlororiboflavin cannot functionally replace riboflavin in the cell because the reduced form of the analog is not sufficiently negative to reduce oxygen to hydrogen peroxide." Restated, this is, they believe, the reason dichlororiboflavin does not possess vitamin-like activity, and not, as has sometimes been cited, the reason for its inhibitory activity. There is no evidence that dichlororiboflavin is reduced to the dihydro form in the cell. They did not propose that the more positive E_0' is the reason that the analog is an inhibitor, nor did they propose that the dihydro form of the analog was the inhibitor.

5.2.2. 7-Chloro-8-methyl-flavin (XXII)

The background for the study of this analog, 7-chloro-8-methyl-10-(1'-D-ribityl)isoalloxazine, is linked to the study of its isomeric form, 7-methyl-8-chloro-flavin (Section 5.2.4, XXIV) or 7-methyl-8-chloro-10-(1'-D-ribityl)isoalloxazine, so the background can be given here and thus will serve for both.

Dichlororiboflavin (Section 5.2.1, XXI) was the first and most widely cited antagonist of riboflavin. It had frequently been referred to as a potent antagonist despite the fact that little was known about the biological activity of this analog. It had been shown to bring about a temporary inhibition of two strains of microorganisms which did not require exogenous riboflavin, but the inhibition was not sustained. Ten years later Snell *et al.*[105] showed that dichlororiboflavin was essentially inert in the nutrition of *L. casei.*

As a result of what we had observed in our laboratory, we had arrived at the conclusion that the structure of the riboflavin molecule could not be altered extensively and still retain any substantial vitamin-like or inhibitory activities.[67] We concluded that the activity of dichlorori-boflavin as an antagonist was much overrated and that the lack of significant antagonistic activity when chlorine atoms replaced both methyl groups was probably due to too great a departure from the riboflavin structure. The two most likely structures that resemble dichlororiboflavin but that are not so radically different from riboflavin are 7-chloro-8-methyl-flavin (XXII) and 7-methyl-8-chloro-flavin (XXIV), compounds that represent changes of the methyl groups of riboflavin to chlorine atoms, one at a time.[27]

When groups of riboflavin-deficient rats are administered from 3 to 50 μg 7-chloro-8-methyl-flavin per day for 28 days, the average growth rate of each group is equal to that produced in groups of animals given one-half that quantity of riboflavin. An appreciable number of the rats receiving 50 μg per day fail to survive the 28-day test period. When 500 μg or 2 mg per day are given, all the animals show maximum growth rates but all are dead in 8 days and 4 days, respectively. The growth rates of groups of animals receiving 50 μg/day of either 7-chloro-8-methyl-flavin or riboflavin are the same.

During the administration of 7-chloro-8-methyl-flavin, not only do the animals gain weight rapidly but they also show complete recovery from all visually observable signs of riboflavin deficiency. Ultimately, all animals receiving this analog die, but, while 40 μg riboflavin plus 500 μg of analog per day does not provide protection against the antagonist, 200 μg of riboflavin per day does. To ensure all animals survive the experimental period, we administer only 24 μg of the analog per day; this is equivalent to 12 μg of riboflavin per day for purposes of growth and recovery of external signs of the deficiency.[28]

When 7-chloro-8-methyl-flavin is given to riboflavin-deficient rats as their only dietary flavin, the total body content of riboflavin is increased but the total body concentration of riboflavin is reduced. The increase in riboflavin content is due to the increased food consumption, which causes increased synthesis of riboflavin by the intestinal microorganisms; this riboflavin is absorbed. The fall in concentration of riboflavin is due to the rapid growth of the animal with the resulting dilution of the tissue stores of riboflavin. [77] When administered in quantities related to riboflavin as described above, the beneficial effects of 7-chloro-8-methyl-flavin for the riboflavin-deficient rat in terms of growth, efficiency of food utilization, which is equivalent to that of riboflavin, and the recovery of the visually observable signs of the deficiency, are all due to the biochemical properties of the analog, although no form other than the unaltered analog has been found in the tissues of rats that have received it.

Administration of the analog causes a specific and rapid displacement of riboflavin from the rat's kidneys causing a precipitous fall in both the content and concentration of the vitamin. Associated with this loss of tissue riboflavin is a profound fall in the SDH activity of the kidney. The riboflavin content or concentration is not altered in the heart, but there is a small and significant loss of SDH activity in this organ. The liver shows a substantial gain in riboflavin, and the SDH activity of this organ is not reduced but maintained by the administration of the analog. The analog appears not to be able to provide an F'-AD form that can be utilized by SDH. [81]

Rat liver flavokinase phosphorylates 7-chloro-8-methyl-flavin at a rate that is equal to that for riboflavin. [13a] This fact might seem inconsistent with the failure to find derived forms of the analog in the tissues of rats to which it had been administered. However, derived forms may be destroyed too rapidly to have survived during the efforts to isolate them, since no special precaution was taken beyond what had been taken in identifying the derived forms of riboflavin. That the rate of destruction might be rapid is suggested by the finding that after 24 μg/day had been given for 28 days the analog was not a significant component on chromatograms of the tissue flavins. [81]

The influence of 7-chloro-8-methyl-flavin on the acid-extractable flavin content and composition of the liver mitochondria after the rats had been maintained on a diet containing 10 μg/g of the analog was found to be approximately 70% of what it was found to be for the animals receiving riboflavin in their diet, but it was 200% greater than it was for animals receiving no riboflavin. The part of the acid-extractable flavin that was found in the form of FAD was approximately 90%. This amount was lower than it was for animals receiving either a sufficient or an insufficient amount of riboflavin.

While the flavin content of the mitochondria appears to be relatively high, the state 3 respiration rates for a variety of substrates show a strange pattern. The rates for PYR and KG fall almost halfway between the mitochondria isolated from rats receiving adequate riboflavin and those receiving none. The rates for HOB and GP are very near to those found for the normal animal, while those for LC and S + R are very similar to those for the riboflavin-deficient rat. One might expect that the respiratory control ratios would show comparable inconsistencies and indeed, they do; for PYR, KG, and HOB they are the same as those for the normal animal, while for LC, GP, and S + R they are the same as those for the deficient animal.

The P:O ratios for the liver mitochondria from the 7-chloro-8-methyl-flavin animals group in the same way as they did for the respiratory control ratios. The P:O ratios for PYR, KG, and HOB are the same or nearly the same as those for the normal animal, while those for LC, GP, and S + R are significantly lower than those for the deficient animal.

The efficiency of utilization of the flavin in the oxidation of the above referenced substrates resembles much more closely those of the normal animal than those of the deficient animal, although the rates for HOB and LC are only about 70% of normal. [13 a]

As a replacement for riboflavin in the metabolism of L. casei, 7-chloro-8-methyl-flavin is inert when used as the sole flavin available to the organism, but as an inhibitor of the utilization of riboflavin by this organism, it is a potent inhibitor with an I.I. of 76. During the course of these inhibition studies Haley[26] observed that in a medium containing 2.5 µg 7-chloro-8-methyl-flavin and 0.01 µg riboflavin/ml, instead of the anticipated complete inhibition there was, after 48 hr, some barely visible growth of the organism. This apparent escape from inhibition was explored sufficiently to suggest that the phenomenon was due to the emergence of a mutant form.[28]

Scala and Lambooy[98] continued the study and showed that, by continued subculturing of L. casei in media containing progressively increased amounts of the analog in the presence of very small amounts of riboflavin, one could finally remove the riboflavin altogether and the 7-chloro-8-methyl-flavin could serve as the organism's sole flavin source. The mutant and the stock strains utilize riboflavin equally well.

It was shown that the mutant strain possessed a decreased or altered specificity of its flavin phosphorylating mechanism because it could phosphorylate either riboflavin or 7-chloro-8-methyl-flavin. The "stock" strain could not phosphorylate the analog to the F'-MN, but the "stock" strain could utilize either the enzymatically or chemically synthesized F'-MN or 7-chloro-8-methyl-10-(1'-D-ribityl)isoalloxazine-5'-phosphate.

Interesting evidence for the presence of the mutant strain is shown by the production of more acid than could be produced by the utilization of riboflavin alone in tubes containing 2.5 µg–15 µg of the analog in addition to the 0.30 µg riboflavin in the routine procedure used to study riboflavin inhibition in *L. casei*. This additional acid production is due to the appearance and culturing of the mutant strain of *L. casei*, which can utilize the analog as well as riboflavin for its flavin requirements.

The mutant strain can utilize the analogs 7-methyl-8-chloro-flavin (Section 5.2.4, XXIV) and 7-bromo-8-methyl-flavin (Section 5.2.7, XXVII) as its sole flavin also. At present the only way this mutant can be identified is by its ability to utilize these three flavins, and if they had not been available for study the existence of the mutant would not have been revealed.[74]

The possibility that 7-chloro-8-methyl-flavin might be a chemo-therapeutically interesting antagonist was explored minimally. It was found not to inhibit *Candida albecans, Hemophilus pertussia, Mycobacterium tuberculosis, Bacillus subtilis, Aerobacter aerogenes, Staphylococcus aureus, Salmonella paratyphosa* A, and *Escherichia coli*.

5.2.3. 7-Chloro-8-ethyl-flavin (XXIII)

The reason for the synthesis of 7-chloro-8-ethyl-10-(1'-D-ribityl)isoalloxazine was to determine what effect the modification of the methyl group in position 8 to an ethyl group would have on the activity of the analog already possessing a chloro group in position 7.[79]

When 7-chloro-8-ethyl-flavin is administered to riboflavin-deficient rats in quantities varying from 50 μg to 250 μg/day, all groups grow but only 40% of a group that received 150 μg day and 10% of a group that received 250 μg/day survived the 28-day test period. While the growth response was appreciable, large quantities of the analog were required and it appears that this analog possesses only 10% of the activity of the 7-chloro-8-methyl-flavin (XXII) and about 5% of the activity of riboflavin for growth.

Since the analog promotes growth of the riboflavin-deficient rat, it is, as stated before, difficult to demonstrate potential antagonistic properties. However, the analog does possess inhibitory properties and this can be demonstrated by the effect the analog has on the utilization of riboflavin when both are given simultaneously to a riboflavin-deficient rat. The administration of 250 μg of the analog and 20 μg of riboflavin per day reduces the growth response to the latter to what would normally be produced by the administration of 10 μg of the vitamin, but half of the animals fail to survive the 28-day test period. The toxic effects of 250 μg of the analog per day are completely counteracted by 40 μg of riboflavin per day; the growth response to the riboflavin is, however, reduced to 85% of the normal response.

During the administration of 7-chloro-8-ethyl-flavin it was observed, as in the case of 7-chloro-8-methyl-flavin, that the riboflavin-deficient rats showed complete recovery from the visually observable signs of the deficiency.

As a replacement for riboflavin in the metabolism of *L. casei*, 7-chloro-8-ethyl-flavin, like 7-chloro-8-methyl-flavin (XXII) is inert when used as the sole flavin available to the organism. As an inhibitor of the utilization of riboflavin by this organism, it is a strong reversible inhibitor with an I.I. of 100.

As was found to be true in the case of 7-chloro-8-methyl-flavin (XXII), more acid was produced in tubes containing low levels of analog and riboflavin in the routine procedure used to study riboflavin inhibition in *L. casei* than could have been produced by the utilization of the riboflavin alone. Presumably, this additional acid is produced by the mutant strain of *L. casei* discovered and isolated in our laboratory.[79]

5.2.4. 7-Methyl-8-chloro-flavin (XXIV)

The reason for the decision to synthesize the analog of riboflavin 7-methyl-8-chloro-10-(1'-D-ribityl)isoalloxazine has been presented under Section 5.2.2, 7-Chloro-8-methyl-flavin (XXII). When 25 or 50 μg/day 7-methyl-8-chloro-flavin is administered to a riboflavin-deficient rat, it stimulates no growth response. When the quantity of this analog is increased to 0.5–1.0 mg/day, it has significant growth-promoting properties. The activity of 1 mg/day of the analog is equivalent to approximately 5 μg/day of riboflavin and, therefore, the analog possesses about 0.5% of the activity of the vitamin for growth of the rat.

The analog does have inhibitory properties that can be observed in the effect it has on the utilization of riboflavin when the two are given simultaneously. The administration of 500 μg/day of the analog with 20 μg riboflavin reduces the growth response of the latter to what would normally be produced by the administration of 10 μg/day of the vitamin.

The remarkable improvement in the visually observable signs of the deficiency when 7-chloro-8-methyl-flavin (XXII) was given was not observed when this analog was given. There was some improvement, but since it was not dramatic it was hard to quantitate. An estimate would be that most of the animals showed some improvement but that probably not more than 20% were considerably improved.

This analog appears to be essentially nontoxic for the rat in that the administration of 2 mg/day for 28 days was not lethal. This lack of toxicity is like that of dichlororiboflavin (XXI), but it is in sharp contrast to the extreme toxicity of 7-chloro-8-methyl-flavin (XXII).

That the E_0' for dichlororiboflavin (XXI) of itself is the reason why it is unable to act as a riboflavin replacement appears to be an over-simplification. 7-Methyl-8-chloro-flavin has an E_0' that is still more positive than that of dichlororiboflavin. The evidence for its having a more positive E_0' is that it is reduced to a poised "rhodoflavin" state when it is autoclaved with the basal medium used for the growth of *L. casei*. The partially reduced form of the analog can be readily returned to its fully oxidized state and it can also be reduced to the leucoflavin form. While there was no substantial evidence that it was necessary to do so, to insure reproducibility the flavin and the media were always mixed after sterilization.

This analog is the most potent inhibitor of riboflavin in the metabolism of *L. casei* to be described to date; the I.I. in this microorganism is 59. As a replacement of riboflavin as the sole flavin in the metabolism of this organism 7-methyl-8-chloro-flavin is inert. [73] 7-Methyl-8-chloro-flavin was found not to be inhibitory toward the list of clinically significant pathogens listed under 7-chloro-8-methyl-flavin (Section 5.2.2, XXII).

This analog can be utilized to suppress the growth of the "stock" strain of *L. casei* while the mutant we have discovered emerges. Once available the mutant of *L. casei* can utilize this analog as well as it utilizes riboflavin. The mutant isolated by the use of 7-methyl-8-chloro-flavin can utilize the analogs 7-chloro-8-methyl-flavin (Section 5.2.2, XXII) and 7-bromo-8-methyl-flavin (Section 5.2.7, XXVII) as its sole flavin also. [74]

5.2.5. 7-Ethyl-8-chloro-flavin (XXV)

The reason for the synthesis of 7-ethyl-8-chloro-10-(1'-D-ribityl)isoalloxazine was to determine what effect the modification of the methyl group in position 7 to an ethyl group would have on the activity of the analog that already had a chloro group in position 8. [79]

Riboflavin-deficient rats receiving various quantities up to 1 mg/day of this analog showed no increase in food consumption, no growth response, and no improvement in their appearance. The analog is inert for the rat either as a vitamin replacement or as an antagonist of riboflavin.

As a replacement for riboflavin in the metabolism of *L. casei*, 7-ethyl-8-chloro-flavin is inert when used as the sole flavin available to the organism. When made available to the organism in the presence of riboflavin throughout the range where the ratio of analog to riboflavin was 10:1 to 70:1, the material is exceedingly stimulatory. At ratios of analog to riboflavin of from 80:1 to 150:1 the material is inhibitory: At one point it causes a 50% reduction in the normal acid production by the microorganism and from this ratio we can derive an I.I. of approximately 100. The response to 7-ethyl-8-chloro-flavin is similar to that obtained with 7-chloro-8-methyl-flavin (XXII) rather than that obtained from 7-methyl-8-chloro-flavin (XXIV), to which it is more closely related.

In the case of this analog, as was found to be true for 7-methyl-8-chloro-flavin, the compound has an E_0' that is sufficiently positive so that it is reduced to a "poised" rhodoflavin state when autoclaved with the basal medium used for the growth of *L. casei*. The partially reduced form of 7-ethyl-8-chloro-flavin can be readily reoxidized or reduced to the appropriate forms. The medium and analog were always mixed after autoclaving.[79]

5.2.6. Dibromo-riboflavin (XXVI)

The analog of riboflavin 7,8-dibromo-10-(1'-D-ribityl)isoalloxazine is hardly worthy of mention. Very limited work has been done to evaluate the biological activity of this analog. Weygand *et al.*[110] tested a number of halogen-substituted analogs of riboflavin as potential inhibitors of riboflavin in *Streptobacterium plantarum* P-32, and related them to the activity of dichlororiboflavin (Section 5.2.1, XXI). Dibromo-riboflavin was found to possess only 10–25% of the potency of dichlororiboflavin as an inhibitor in this organism. As indicated above, dichlororiboflavin possesses questionable inhibitory properties. In the report that dibromo-riboflavin supports the growth of *L. casei*, it should be recognized that the supposed "growth" is equivalent to that produced by 1/1000 the amount of riboflavin.[112]

5.2.7. 7-Bromo-8-methyl-flavin (XXVII)

The remarkable biological properties of 7-chloro-8-methyl-flavin (XXII) prompted us to synthesize and study 7-bromo-8-methyl-10-(1'-D-ribityl)isoalloxazine. It was found that 7-bromo-8-methyl-flavin mimicked 7-chloro-8-methyl-flavin in biological activity except that it was substantially less toxic.[22]

When groups of riboflavin-deficient rats were administered 5–50 μg 7-bromo-8-methyl-flavin per rat per day for 28 days, the average growth rate of each group was equal to that produced in groups of animals given one-half the amount of riboflavin. Since the molecular weight of the analog is greater than that of 7-chloro-8-methyl-flavin, this means that it is even more potent for the stimulus of growth of the riboflavin-deficient rat than 7-chloro-8-methyl-flavin. In the case of

7-bromo-8-methyl-flavin, the rats tolerated 50 μg/day with no fatalities; at 250 μg/day 33% and at 500 μg/day 67% of the animals failed to survive the 28-day test period although they showed very impressive weight gains. As had been true of the corresponding chloro compound, those that survived showed complete recovery from the visually observable signs of the deficiency. Animals receiving 500 μg/day of the analog grew at the same rate as those receiving 500 μg/day of analog and 40 μg per day of riboflavin, for 15 days. After this time the animals of the former group died (67 percent dead at 28 days), while those in the latter group continued to grow and all survived. The stimulus provided by 50 μg/day of the analog plus 10 μg/day of riboflavin is very nearly additive.[22]

When 7-bromo-8-methyl-flavin is the only flavin made available to *L. casei*, it is devoid of activity, but as an inhibitor of the utilization of riboflavin by this organism it is a strong reversible inhibitor with an I.I. of 137.

If we had synthesized this analog before we synthesized 7-chloro-8-methyl-flavin, it would as readily have led us to the discovery of the mutant form of *L. casei*. Again it was found that more acid was produced than could be accounted for by the riboflavin alone in tubes containing 5-35 μg 7-bromo-8-methyl-flavin in addition to 0.3 μg riboflavin, in the routine procedure used to study riboflavin inhibition in *L. casei*.[22] Under such circumstances, a true inhibition index cannot be obtained because any replication of the organism will mean the emergence of some of the mutant form and these, far from being inhibited by the analog, utilize it.[28]

The mutant strain of *L. casei* has been isolated from the "stock" strain by the use of 7-bromo-8-methyl-flavin, and it can utilize 7-chloro-8-methyl-flavin (XXII) and 7-methyl-8-chloro-flavin (XXIV) as its sole flavin also.[74]

5.2.8. 7-Bromo-8-ethyl-flavin (XXVIII)

Just as we pursued the investigation of the influence of the interchange of the methyl and ethyl groups with the chlorine atom, we have synthesized for study 7-bromo-8-ethyl-10-(1'-D-ribityl)isoalloxazine.[80]

When 7-bromo-8-ethyl-flavin is administered in quantities of 25-100 μg per day to riboflavin-deficient rats, it stimulates excellent growth; however, the animals' appearance is not improved as consistently as was observed in the corresponding methyl analog, although more improvement is found as the quantity of analog administered is increased. At 250 μg, 500 μg, and 1 mg/day, 30, 90, and 100% of the animals die before the end of the 28-day test period, yet when these quantities are administered, all animals show a prompt return to normal appearance. The administration of 10 μg/day of riboflavin with 500 μg per day of the 7-bromo-8-ethyl-flavin did not protect the animals against the lethal properties of this compound, but 40 μg/day of riboflavin did.

When 7-bromo-8-ethyl-flavin is the only flavin made available to *L. casei*, it is inert; however, when made available with riboflavin, it is a strong, reversible inhibitor with an I.I. of 140. In the case of this analog as in the case of 7-chloro-8-methyl-flavin (XXII) and 7-bromo-8-methyl-flavin (XXVII), more acid is produced than could be accounted for by the riboflavin alone in tubes containing 1-28 μg 7-bromo-8-ethyl-flavin in addition to the 0.3 μg riboflavin, in the routine procedure used to study riboflavin inhibition in *L. casei*.[80]

5.2.9. 7-Methyl-8-bromo-flavin (XXIX)

Just as it was considered to be of interest to synthesize for testing the bromo analog of 7-chloro-8-methyl-flavin (XXII), it was also thought to be of interest to synthesize for testing 7-methyl-8-bromo-10-(1'-D-ribityl)isoalloxazine, the bromo analog of 7-methyl-8-chloro-flavin (XXIV).[78]

The growth response of the riboflavin-deficient rat when this analog is administered in quantities of 50 μg-2 mg/day is very similar to that shown by the 7-methyl-8-chloro-flavin; the gains were not large but they were substantial and significantly increased over the growth shown by the animals receiving no flavin. However, two differences did appear: 7-methyl-8-bromo-flavin stimulated growth when smaller quantities of the analog were given, and the administration of quantities of 250-2 mg/day brought about almost complete recovery in the appearance of the deficient animals. As in the case of the corresponding chloro analog, this analog must also be considered to be an antagonist of riboflavin, because, while it and riboflavin both stimulate growth of the riboflavin-deficient rat, when both are administered (500 μg of analog and 10 μg of riboflavin per day), the growth is less than would be obtained from the riboflavin alone.

It was found that 7-methyl-8-bromo-flavin was like 7-methyl-8-chloro-flavin (XXIV) and 7-ethyl-8-chloro-flavin (XXV) in that the E_0' was sufficiently positive as to show the unusual susceptibility to reduction as described before (Section 5.2.4).

The analog 7-methyl-8-bromo-flavin is devoid of either vitamin-like or riboflavin-antagonistic activity for *L. casei*. This is a remarkable departure from expectations because 7-methyl-8-chloro-flavin (XXIV) was the most potent antagonist of riboflavin to have been described.[78]

5.2.10. 7-Ethyl-8-bromo-flavin (XXX)

As the last of the series of analogs in which the methyl, ethyl, chloro, and bromo groups have been used in nearly all possible combinations 7-ethyl-8-bromo-10-(1′-D-ribityl)isoalloxazine will be discussed. The analog is essentially inert as a riboflavin replacement for the riboflavin-deficient rat and as an antagonist of riboflavin in this animal. When administered in quantities of 100–500 µg/day, while producing no significant increase in weight it did cause a moderate improvement in the appearance of the deficient animals.

When 7-ethyl-8-bromo-flavin is the only flavin available to *L. casei* it has no vitamin-like properties, but when it is made available to this microorganism with riboflavin it is a weak reversible inhibitor with an I.I. of 250. The activity for *L. casei* in the presence of riboflavin is noteworthy in one respect: We have observed that, as in the case of 7-chloro-8-methyl-flavin (XXII), 7-bromo-8-methyl-flavin (XXVII), and 7-chloro-8-ethyl-flavin (XXIII), more acid was produced throughout certain ranges of concentrations than could be accounted for by the riboflavin present in the tubes. While this stimulatory property was not observed in the case of 7-methyl-8-chloro-flavin (XXIV) or 7-methyl-8-bromo-flavin (XXIX), it was found to be true in the case of 7-ethyl-8-bromo-flavin (XXX), as had been found in the case of 7-ethyl-8-chloro-flavin (XXV). When the ratio of 7-ethyl-8-bromo-flavin to riboflavin is in the range of 15:1 to 130:1, a considerable excess of acid is produced. The implication would be that these two analogs, along with those possessing the halogen in the 7- position, also permit the early emergence of the mutant form of *L. casei*, but this must be shown to be true.

It was found that 7-ethyl-8-bromo-flavin was like 7-methyl-8-chloro-flavin (XXIV), 7-ethyl-8-chloro-flavin (XXV), and 7-methyl-8-bromo-flavin (XXIX) in that the E_0' was sufficiently positive to show the unusual susceptibility to reduction as described under 7-methyl-8-chloro-flavin (Section 5.2.4, XXIV).[80]

5.3. Modifications of Side Chain at Position 10 and the Substituents at Positions 7 and 8

5.3.1. Dichloro-sorbityl-flavin (XXXI)

Holly *et al.*[31] reported on the carcinolytic activity of 7,8-dichloro-10-(1′-D-sorbityl)isoalloxazine, a compound that caused the regression of established lymposarcoma implants in C3H mice. This observation

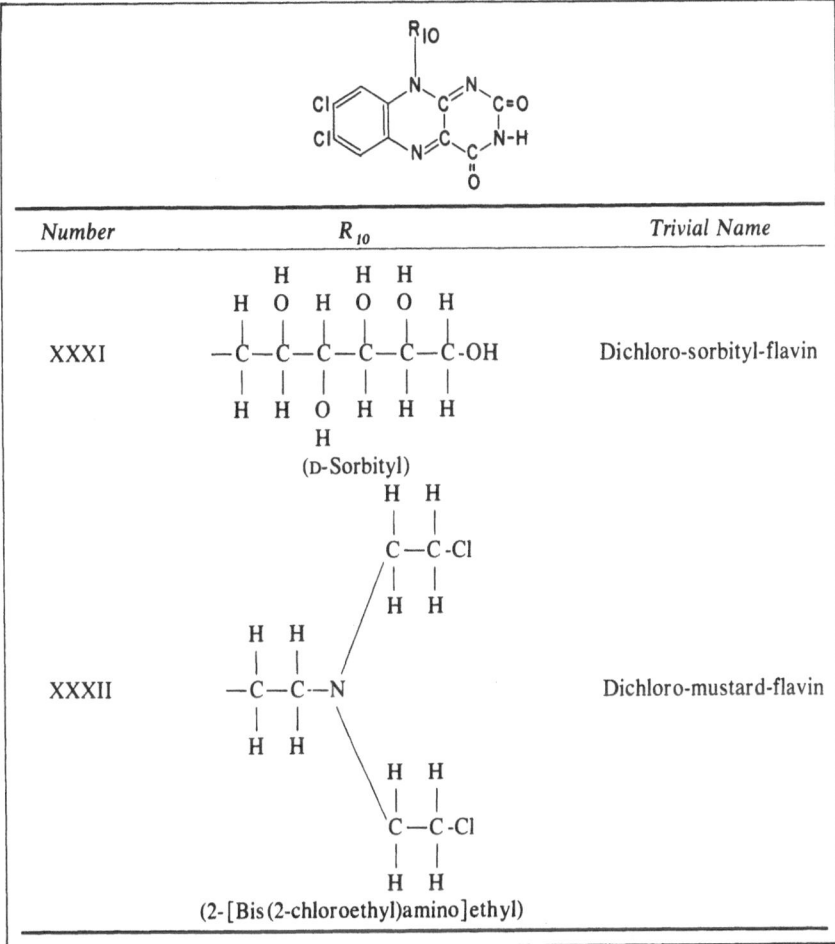

Fig. 10. Basic structure for analogs of riboflavin which are modified at positions 7, 8, and 10.

resulted in the rapid production of several modifications of this basic structure.[32,101] The modifications consisted of using a variety of glycityl side chains at position 10, chlorine atoms at positions 7 and 8, or one chlorine atom at position 7. Of those tested, in addition to dichloro-sorbityl-flavin, only two others showed some activity, namely dichlororiboflavin and 7-chloro-sorbityl-flavin.

Several of these analogs were tested for antagonistic activity in *L. casei* and only dichloro-sorbityl-flavin was tested in the rat. In all cases the results showed the compounds to be inert. The absence of inhibitory properties was probably due to these compounds possessing structures that were too unlike that of riboflavin.

5.3.2. Dichloro-mustard-flavin (XXXII)

Earlier in this chapter (Section 5.1.2c) a description was given of the activity of dimethyl-mustard-flavin (XX). This analog possessed the basic riboflavin structure except that the side chain at position 10 was designed to provide a "two-arm mustard." It was found that this analog was especially effective against Walker rat carcinosarcoma 256. At the time these results were available our attention was attracted to the possibility that molecules that were modifications of naturally occurring or biologically active materials might provide a "carrier" molecular structure that would gain cellular entrance for the anticancer agent, but suitable examples were not readily available.

It is interesting in this connection that riboflavin is biologically active; dimethyl-mustard-flavin (XX) is an active anticancer agent. Dichlorori-boflavin (XXI) is devoid of biological activity; dichloro-mustard-flavin is devoid of anticancer activity.

5.4. Miscellaneous Modifications

As stated at the beginning of this chapter, a number of factors were taken into consideration in the selection of compounds to be discussed. Only one other analog of riboflavin which does not fit any of the above categories of analogs is of interest—2-thioriboflavin. This analog has the same structure as riboflavin except that the oxygen at position 2 has been replaced by a sulfur atom. Berezovskii and Melniko-va[6] reported that 2-thioriboflavin had riboflavin activity similar to that of the vitamin itself as shown by animal growth experiments.

6. BIOLOGICAL ACTIVITY OF FLAVINS IN OTHER SYSTEMS

6.1. Warburg's "Old Yellow Enzyme"

It should be recalled that the interest in analogs of riboflavin, although some of this interest was not intentionally directed toward the synthesis of analogs, started in 1934, only 2 years after the discovery of the "yellow enzyme" by Warburg and Christian and 1 year after Theodor Wagner-Jauregg had isolated pure riboflavin. In 1934 Theorell showed that the highly purified old yellow enzyme contained one phosphate group that was associated with the coenzyme portion of the molecule and that was shown by Kuhn's group to be in the form of riboflavin-5'-phosphate. Kuhn and Rudy[56] developed a technique using the biochemical activity of the combination of the apoenzyme portion of the old yellow enzyme and a variety of flavins, to characterize essential features of the latter for biological activity.

The ability of the various flavins or derivatives of flavins to combine with the apoenzyme was determined by loss of fluorescence; the catalytic activity of the potential pseudoholoenzyme was then determined by its ability to oxidize either Neuberg's ester or Robinson's ester as measured by the decolorization of methylene blue or by oxygen consumption. Preparations resulting from combinations of the apoenzyme and FMN from natural sources or FMN of synthetic origin yielded holoenzymes that were indistinguishable in activity.

The technique was used in a variety of ways. The combination of L-araboflavin-5'-phosphate and the apoenzyme produced a holoenzyme that possessed 33% of the activity of the holoenzyme prepared from FMN in the decolorization procedure and 61% for oxygen consumption.[58]

Another important finding occurred in the demonstration that the 5'-phosphate group and an unsubstituted 3 position were essential for binding to the apoenzyme,[57] since no activity was retained if the 3 position was substituted, thus preventing it, as they thought at the time, from providing an attachment site to the protein. They also found that the 5'-phosphate group was not essential for activity but was essential for truly catalytic activity. If large amounts of riboflavin, 12-60 times the amount of a catalytic quantity of FMN were added, sufficient association took place between the apoenzyme and the riboflavin by virtue of the unsubstituted 3 position to cause oxygen consumption of the order of 50% of that shown when FMN was added. They also showed that when large and equal amounts of L-araboflavin (VI) or riboflavin were used, the oxygen consumption of the preparation for the former was 60% of that for the latter, but that the same amount of D-araboflavin (V) did not produce an enzymatically active combination.

Some additional observations were made. An active "coenzyme" function was found to be provided by riboflavin-5'-sulfate; when based on equal riboflavin content, it was 30% as active as FMN. The triacetyl and tetraacetyl derivatives of FMN were inactive, as was the riboflavin homolog possessing no methyl groups in position 7 and 8.[60,61]

6.2. The Riboflavin-Deficient Egg

In 1954, Maw[86] reported the discovery of a mutant strain of single-comb white leghorn chickens that, on a diet containing adequate riboflavin, produced eggs so deficient in the vitamin that all of the embryos died between day 10 and day 14 of incubation. Injection of riboflavin into the fertile eggs permitted the embryos to survive and the eggs to hatch. This defect occurred in birds homozygous for a recessive gene (rdrd). The recessive gene alters the renal reabsorption mechanism for free riboflavin, and the vitamin absorbed from the food is rapidly excreted in the urine. This disorder is discussed in Chapter 4.

These deficient eggs provide independent, closed systems for the assay of riboflavin analogs. The ability of analogs to replace riboflavin in such eggs can be measured as increased survival time of the embryo. Antagonistic activity toward riboflavin can be studied because all of the eggs contain some riboflavin. Antagonistic activity would result in the death of embryos before those in the control group die. Dr. E. G. Buss kindly gave us a number of these eggs some years ago, and we conducted a pilot study using some of our analogs. Not enough work was done at that time to provide firm quantitative data but with no reference to quantities of the analogs used, the following general results were obtained. It is interesting to compare the results obtained in avian tissue with those obtained in mammalian tissues and in microorganisms.

When no flavin was administered, all embryos died from day 6 to day 14. All embryos died during the same time span when either 7-ethyl-flavin (XII), 7-chloro-8-methyl-flavin (XXII), or 7-methyl-8-chloro-flavin (XXIV) was injected. When small quantities of 7,8-diethyl-riboflavin (XVI) were injected, the average life of the embryo was increased, while 7-methyl-8-ethyl-flavin (XV) and large quantities of 7,8-diethyl-riboflavin shortened the average life of the embryos. Both riboflavin (I) and 7-ethyl-8-methyl-flavin (XIV) permitted most embryos to live longer than 19 days and many of both groups pipped and hatched.[99]

7. STRUCTURE-ACTIVITY RELATIONSHIPS

The most specific characteristics of the structure of a flavin which are involved in its ability to link to protein are located in that portion of the molecule extending from the 5'-hydroxy group to the 3-imino group. The relative importance of these two sites has been discussed under Section 6.1, Warburg's "Old Yellow Enzyme." Since these two sites represent the extremes of that portion of the molecule, it is not surprising to find that only limited alterations can be tolerated in the polyhydroxy side chain at position 10 without sacrifice in the ability of the flavin to link to protein. The influence of phosphorylation of the 5'-hydroxy group does not reduce the significance of the above argument, and it seems a safe assumption that for biological activity as a vitamin-like agent or a vitamin antagonist some form of flavin-protein binding must take place.

Maintenance of the integrity of this portion of the molecule directs our attention to the side chain at position 10, since the remainder of the basic structure is determined by its being an isoalloxazine. It was possible to state at one time[63] that, with the exception of L-araboflavin (V), only those flavins that can serve as a sole source of flavin for *L. casei* are capable of supporting growth in animals. This activity was possible only if a flavin was a D-ribityl derivative and if it was substituted in either the 7 or 8 positions or both by a methyl group or by an ethyl group. This generalization must be broadened in the light of recent findings.

With these considerations in mind, the fact that L-araboflavin and riboflavin could both bind to protein and possess biological activity calls attention to the stereoconfiguration about the 2'-hydroxy group of the side chain at position 10. It is interesting to note that it was also possible to state[67] that flavins known to date that have appreciable activities either as vitamin-like agents or antagonistic agents have a common configuration about the 2'-position. Thus, in addition to D-ribityl, L-arabityl, L-lyxityl, and D-xylityl, shown in Fig. 3, we find D-dulcityl (galactoflavin, XVII) and D-sorbityl (dichloro-sorbityl-flavin XXXI) showing the same configuration about the 2'-position. Kuhn and Rudy[57] observed that the configuration about this position was one of the points of similarity between riboflavin and L-araboflavin and suggested that it might be of importance for the activity of the latter. It is of further interest that Kuhn *et al.*[53] stated that the sugar-like side chain in riboflavin could, from chemicophysical considerations, be of the arrangement of L-arabityl, D-ribityl, L-lyxityl, or D-xylityl. It is not inconsistent with the above specifications that 5'-deoxy-riboflavin (XVIII) and 2'-hydroxyethyl-riboflavin (II) are weak inhibitors or that L-lyxoflavin (VIII) is a very weak inhibitor. The former conclusion that for significant potency as a vitamin-like agent or an inhibitory agent the D-ribityl side chain at position 10 must be retained is still valid today.

While the substituents in positions 7 and 8 have little influence on the flavin's ability to link to the protein, such substituents do have a pronounced influence on the oxidation–reduction potential of the compound.[67] At one time we thought we would be able to produce subtle changes in the redox potential of flavins by modifications of the substituents at positions 7 and 8 and that this would provide us with a series of compounds in which redox potential could be correlated with biological activity. It quickly became obvious that the hope of establishing such a correlation was misdirected since 7-methyl-8-chloro-flavin (XXIV) had an E_0' that was certainly greater than 0.09 V more positive than the E_0' for riboflavin. Dichlororiboflavin has an E_0' that is 0.09 V more positive than the E_0' for riboflavin, and it is inert in both rats and *L. casei*. The above 7-methyl-8-chloro-flavin (XXIV), which is even more positive than dichlororiboflavin, is an inhibitor in rats and the most potent antagonist of riboflavin in *L. casei* to be described to date. Yet, a mutant strain of *L. casei* can utilize it as efficiently as it can riboflavin.

Other flavins have redox potentials that are greater than 0.09 V more positive than the E_0' of riboflavin. Of these, 7-ethyl-8-chloro-flavin (XXV) is inert for the rat but a potent inhibitor in *L. casei*. 7-Ethyl-8-bromo-flavin (XXX) improves the visually observable signs of riboflavin deficiency in the animal, but it is not an inhibitor for the rat while it is an inhibitor for *L. casei*. Finally, for purposes of further illustration, 7-methyl-8-bromo-flavin (XXIX) provides excellent growth and recovery of the appearance of the riboflavin-deficient rat and is an inhibitor in this animal, while it is inert for *L. casei*.

The interpretation of what is meant by biological activity of flavins in rats and *L. casei* will require considerable modification. In the case of the rat, we have shown that it might involve, to a considerable degree independently, growth, improved appearance, survival, reproduction, and inhibition of the beneficial influence of riboflavin. In the case of *L. casei*, we may observe support of multiplication of cells (growth) or the inhibition of the utilization of riboflavin for that purpose. We must also consider the activity of the flavins for the new mutant strain of *L. casei* which can use many more flavins for growth than are active for the normal strain. While we have found several flavins capable of inhibiting the use of riboflavin by the "stock" strain of the microorganism, we have not yet found an agent that can inhibit the utilization by the mutant strain of any of the biologically active flavins for the mutant strain.

We have pointed out that two of the flavins described are able to replace riboflavin in the metabolism of the rat. The fact that this is true raises interesting questions concerning the role of SDH in such animals and the way the flavins must be covalently bound to the apoenzyme of SDH. Walker and Singer[109] have recently shown that FAD appears to be linked to the protein of SDH by a methylene bridge ($-CH_2-$) formed from the methyl group at position 8 and attached to the number 3 nitrogen of the histidyl portions of the amino acid chain of the protein.

Riboflavin—(8)—CH_2—N—(3)—histidyl

If this is the case one can visualize that 7-ethyl-8-methyl-flavin (XIV) might readily form a similar bond. However, this flavin permits the SDH activities of the heart, kidneys, and liver to fall to 33%, 56%, and 9%, respectively, of the normal values. The isomeric 7-methyl-8-ethyl-flavin (XV) would seem unable to form such a bond with the protein but might be able to do so as shown.

TABLE III. *Biological Activities of Flavins Possessing a* D-*Ribityl Chain at Position 10 and Various Substituents at Positions 7 and 8*

Flavin number	Position 7	8	Growth	Rat Appearance	Inhibitor	L. casei Growth	Inhibitor	Mutant growth
XI	H—	CH_3—	+ᵃ			+		
XIII	H—	C_2H_5—	±			+		
X	CH_3—	H—	+			+		
I	CH_3—	CH_3—	+	+	Oᵇ	+	O	+ᶜ
XV	CH_3—	C_2H_5—	+	+	O	+	O	+
XXIV	CH_3—	Cl—	+	±	Iᵈ	O	I	+
XXIX	CH_3—	Br—	+	+	I	O	O	
XII	C_2H_5—	H—	O	O	I	+	O	+
XIV	C_2H_5—	CH_3—	+	+	O	+	O	+
XVI	C_2H_5—	C_2H_5—	+	+	I	+	O	+
XXV	C_2H_5—	Cl—	O	O	O	O	I	
XXX	C_2H_5—	Br—	O	+	O	O	I	
XXII	Cl—	CH_3—	+	+	I	O	I	+
XXIII	Cl—	C_2H_5—	+	+	I	O	I	
XXI	Cl—	Cl—	O	O	O	O	O	O
XXVII	Br—	CH_3—	+	+	I	O	I	+
XXVIII	Br—	C_2H_5—	+	+	I	O	I	
XXIV	Br—	Br—				O		
	Isoriboflavinᵉ		O	O	I	O		
XVII	Galactoflavinᵉ				I	O	I	

ᵃThe + means positive response in the riboflavin-deficient rat with no quantitative dimensions.
ᵇThe O means tested but no activity; blank spaces mean unknown.
ᶜActivity for the mutant strain of *L. casei.*
ᵈThe I means an inhibitor of riboflavin in the test organism.
ᵉThese two flavins have been added to the table for comparative purposes.

Flavin—(8)—CH—N—(3)—histidyl
|
CH₃

This form would appear to be less easily attained than the normal form of bonding, yet the 7-methyl-8-ethyl-flavin provides for considerably more SDH activity for the heart, kidneys, and liver where the enzyme was found to be no less than two-thirds of the normal values.[13]

It is obvious that a similar bond could not be formed between flavins possessing chlorine or bromine atoms in position 8, but 7-methyl-8-chloro-flavin is active for the mutant strain of *L. casei*. The answer is, of course, that *L. casei* does not contain SDH. We cannot make the same statement for rats where several flavins possessing halogens in position 8 promote growth and the normal appearance of the riboflavin-deficient rat. It must be concluded that the growth that occurs and the improvement in appearance are not dependent on SDH, or that the SDH is able to confiscate most of the residual riboflavin in the tissues when these flavins are used, or that these events take place only as long as SDH covalently bound to FAD is still present and active in the tissues. Recent work[81] appears to support the latter possibility.

The flavins of significant biological activity as vitamin-like materials or antagonistic material are collected in Table III, where they are summarized in such a way as to minimize space and the expenditure of words.

8. REFERENCES

1. Aposhian, H. V., and Lambooy, J. P. 1951. Retardation of growth of Walker rat carcinoma 256 by administration of diethyl-riboflavin, *Proc. Soc. Exptl. Biol. Med.* **78**:197–199.

2. Aposhian, H. V., and Lambooy, J. P. 1954. The synthesis of 6-ethyl-9-(D-1′-ribityl)isoalloxazine, *J. Am. Chem. Soc.* **76**:1307–1308.

3. Aposhian, H. V., and Lambooy, J. P. 1955. The *in vivo* synthesis of diethyl-riboflavin phosphate, *J. Am. Chem. Soc.* **77**:6738.

4. Association of Vitamin Chemists. 1966. "Methods of Vitamin Assay," 3rd ed., pp. 147–158, Interscience Publishers, Inc., New York.

5. Bebawi, G. M., Kim, Y. S., and Lambooy, J. P. 1970. A study of the carcinogenicity of a series of structurally related 4-dimethylaminoazobenzenes, *Cancer Research* **30**:1520–1524.

6. Berezovskii, V. M., and Melnikova, L. M. 1961. Allo- and isoalloxazine series. III. Synthesis of thioriboflavin and thioanalogs of alloxazines, *Zh. Obschek. Khim.* **31**:3827–3831 (*Chem. Abstr.* **57**:11290 (1962)).

7. Beyer, R. E., Lamberg, S. L., and Neyman, M. A. 1961. The effect of riboflavin deficiency and galactoflavin feeding on oxidative phosphorylation and related reactions in rat liver mitochondria, *Can. J. Biochem. Physiol.* **39**:73–88.

8. Briuns, H. W., Sunde, M. L., Cravens, W. W., and Snell, E. E. 1951. Growth promoting activity of L-lyxoflavin, *Proc. Soc. Exptl. Biol. Med.* **78**:535-536.
9. Burch, H. B., Hunter, F. E., Combs, A. M., and Schutz, B. A., 1960. Oxidative enzymes and phosphorylation in hepatic mitochondria from riboflavin-deficient rats, *J. Biol. Chem.* **235**:1540-1544.
10. Burkett, A. 1947. Basically substituted isoalloxazines, *J. Am. Chem. Soc.* **69**:2555.
11. Cooperman, J. M., Marusich, W. L., Scheiner, J., Drekter, L., De Ritter, E., and Rubin, S. H. 1952. A critique of biological activity of L-lyxoflavin, *Proc. Soc. Exptl. Biol. Med.* **81**:57-62.
12. Decker, J. E., and Byerrum, R. W. 1954. The relationship between dietary riboflavin concentration and the tissue concentration of riboflavin containing coenzymes and enzymes, *J. Nutr.* **53**:303-312.
13. Dombrowski, J. J., and Lambooy, J. P. 1973. The reduction of succinic dehydrogenase in the rat by 7-methyl-8-ethylflavin, *Arch. Biochem. Biophys.* **159**:378-382.
13a. Dombrowski, J. J., and Lambooy, J. P., to be published.
13b. Dombrowski, J. J., Hill, W. A., and Lambooy, J. P., to be published.
14. Emerson, G. A., and Tishler, M. 1944. The antiriboflavin effect of isoriboflavin, *Proc. Soc. Exptl. Biol. Med.* **55**:184-185.
15. Emerson, G. A., Wurtz, E., and Johnson, O. H. 1945. The antiriboflavin effect of galactoflavin, *J. Biol. Chem.* **160**:165-167.
16. Emerson, G. A., Brink, N. G., Holly, F. W., Koniuszy, F. R., Heyl, D., and Folkers, K. 1950. Vitamin B$_{12}$. VIII. Vitamin B$_{12}$-like activity of 5,6-dimethylbenzimidazole and tests on related compounds, *J. Am. Chem. Soc.* **72**:3084-3085.
17. Emerson, G. A., and Folkers, K. 1951a. Tests with lyxoflavin for vitamin activity, *J. Am. Chem. Soc.* **73**:2398-2399.
18. Emerson, G. A., and Folkers, K. 1951b. Vitamin activity for lyxoflavin. *J. Am. Chem. Soc.* **73**:5383-5386.
19. Fall, H. H., and Petering, H. G. 1956. Metabolic inhibitors. I. 6,7-Dimethyl-9-formylmethylisoalloxazine, 6,7-dimethyl-9-(2'-hydroxyethyl)-isoalloxazine and derivatives. *J. Am. Chem. Soc.* **78**:377-380.
20. Faulkner, R. D., and Lambooy, J. P. 1961. Intestinal synthesis of riboflavin in the rat, *J. Nutr.* **75**:373-378.
21. Faulkner, R. D., and Lambooy, J. P. 1963. Synthesis and biological activity of 7,8-disubstituted isoalloxazines. Synthesis of nitrogen mustard derivatives, *J. Med. Chem.* **6**:292-294.
22. Faulkner, R. D., and Lambooy, J. P. 1966. Synthesis and biological activity of 7-bromo-8-methyl-10-(1'-D-ribityl)isoalloxazine, an analog of riboflavin, *J. Med. Chem.* **9**:495-497.
23. Gardner, T. S., Wenis, E., and Lee, J. 1951. L-Lyxoflavin, *Arch Biochem. Biophys.* **34**:98-104.
24. Garnjobst, L., and Tatum, E. L. 1956. A temperature sensitive riboflavin-requiring mutant of *Neurospora crassa*, *Amer. J. Botany* **43**:149-157.
25. Godfrey, J. C. 1959. Accurate molecular models. *J. Chem. Educ.* **36**:140-143.
26. Haley, E. E. 1954. The synthesis and biological activity of compounds structurally related to riboflavin and vitamin B$_{12}$. Dissertation, The University of Rochester, Rochester, New York.
27. Haley, E. E., and Lambooy, J. P. 1954. The synthesis of 6-chloro-7-methyl-9-(1'-D-ribityl)isoalloxazine and 6-methyl-7-chloro-9-(1'-D-ribityl)isoalloxazine, *J. Am. Chem. Soc.* **76**:5093-5096.
28. Haley, E. E., and Lambooy, J. P. 1960. The biological activity of 6-chloro-7-methyl-9-(1'-D-ribityl)isoalloxazine, *J. Nutr.* **72**:169-176; 481.

29. Heyl, D., Chase, E., Koniuszy, F. R., and Folkers, K. 1951. Synthesis of lyxoflavin, *J. Amer. Chem. Soc.* **73:**3826-3827.

30. Hill, W. A., and Lambooy, J. P. 1970. The effect of a vitamin-like homolog of riboflavin on succinic acid dehydrogenase activity of brain, *Proc. Soc. Exptl. Biol. Med.* **134:**922-925.

31. Holly, F. W., Peel, E. W., Mozingo, R., and Folkers, K. 1950. Studies on carcinolytic compounds. I. 6,7-Dichloro-9-(1'-D-sorbityl)-isoalloxazine, *J. Am. Chem. Soc.* **72:**5416-5418.

32. Holly, F. W., Peel, E. W., Cahill, J. J., Koniuszy, F. R., and Folkers, K. 1952. Carcinolytic compounds. III. 9-1'-Glycityl)-isoalloxazines, *J. Am. Chem. Soc.* **74:**4047-4048.

33. Huber, H., and Verzar, F. 1938. Phosphorylierung von Riboflavin durch Darmschleimhautextrakte und die Wirkung von Jodessigsaure darauf, *Helv. Chim. Acta* **21:**1006:1009.

34. Hunter, F. E., and Smith, E. E. 1967. Measurement of mitochondrial swelling and shrinking—high amplitude, *in:* "Methods in Enzymology" R. W. Estabrook and M. E. Pullman, eds., Vol. 10, pp. 689-696, Academic Press, New York.

35. Iwatsubo, M., Nishimoto, S., and Hiraoka, K. 1956. Inhibition of amino acid oxidase. Effect of methyl group of isoalloxazine, *Osaka Daigaku Zassi* **8:**699-701. (*Chem. Abstr.* **51:**3712 (1957)).

36. Karrer, P., Schlittler, E., Pfachler, K., and Benz, F. 1934. Weitere Synthesen Lactoflavin-ahnlicher Verbindungen II, *Helv. Chim. Acta* **17:**1516-1523.

37. Karrer, P., and Strong, F. M. 1935. Flavinsynthesen VIII. Synthese des 6-Methyl-9-(d,1'-ribityl)-iso-alloxazine und weitere synthetische Versuche in der Flavinreihe, *Helv. Chim. Acta* **18:**1343-1351.

38. Karrer, P., Schopp, K., and Benz, F. 1935. Synthesen von Flavinen IV. *Helv. Chim. Acta* **18:**426-429.

39. Karrer, P., Solomon, H., Schopp, K., Benz, F., and Becker, B. 1935. Synthesen von drei weiteren Stereoisomeren des Lactoflavins, *Helv. Chim. Acta* **18:**908-910.

40. Karrer, P., Solomon, H., Schopp, K., and Benz, F. 1935. Synthetische Flavine VII, *Helv. Chim. Acta* **18:**1143-1146.

41. Karrer, P., von Euler, H., Malmberg, M., and Schopp, K. 1935. Die biologische Wirkungen des 7-Methyl-9-(d,1'-ribityl)-isoalloxazine, *Svensk. Kem. Tidskr.* **47:**153-154.

42. Karrer, P., 1936. Über einige naturlich vorkommende, biochemisch bemerkenswerte Pigmente, *Helv. Chim. Acta* **19:**E33-E48.

43. Karrer, P., and Quibell, T. H. 1936. Synthesen einiger neuer Flavine, *Helv. Chim. Acta* **19:**1034-1042.

44. Kearney, E. B. 1951. The interaction of yeast flavokinase with riboflavin analogues, *J. Biol. Chem.* **194:**747-754.

45. Kensler, C. J., Sugiura, K., Young, N. F., Halter, C. R., and Rhoads, C. P. 1941. Partial protection of rats by riboflavin with casein against liver cancer caused by dimethylaminoazobenzene, *Science* **93:**308-310.

46. Kim, Y. S., Aposhian, M. M., and Lambooy, J. P. 1966. The influence of homologs of riboflavin on the growth of Walker rat carcinoma 256. *Cancer Research* **26:**1344-1348.

47. Kim, Y. S., and Lambooy, J. P. 1967. Use of a riboflavin homolog in the reduction of succinic dehydrogenase in the tissues of healthy rats, *Arch. Biochem. Biophys.* **122:**644-647.

48. Kim, Y. S., and Lambooy, J. P. 1969. Biochemical and physiological changes in the rat during riboflavin deprivation and supplementation, *J. Nutr.* **98:**467-476.

49. Kim, Y. S., and Lambooy, J. P. 1971. Induction of a specific enzyme inadequacy in infant rats by the use of a homolog of riboflavin, *J. Nutr.* 101:819-830.

50. King, F. E., and Acheson, R. M. 1946. New potential chemotherapeutic agents. Part V. Basically substituted isoalloxazines, *J. Chem Soc.* 681-685.

51. Kipnis, F., Weiner, N., and Spoerri, P. E. 1947. 9-(Dialkylaminoalkyl)-isoalloxazines, *J. Am. Chem. Soc.* 69:799-800.

52. Kuhn, R., and Weygand, F. 1934. Synthetisches Vitamin B₂. *Ber.* 67:2084-2085.

53. Kuhn, R., Reinemund, K., Kaltschmidt, H., Strobele, R., and Trischmann, H., 1935. Synthetisches 6,7-Dimethyl-9-ribo-flavin, *Naturwiss.* 23:260.

54. Kuhn, R., Rudy, H., and Weygand, F. 1935. Über die zücker-ahnliche Seitenketta des Lactoflavins, *Ber.* 68:625-634.

55. Kuhn, R. 1936. Lactoflavin (Vitamin B₂), *Angew. Chem.* 49:6-10.

56. Kuhn, R. and Rudy, H. 1936. Katalytische Wirkung der Lactoflavin-5'-phosphorsaure; Synthese des gelben Ferments, *Ber.* 69:1974-1977.

57. Kuhn, R., and Rudy, H. 1936. Lactoflavin als Co-Ferment; Wirkstoff und Trager, *Ber.* 69:2557-2567.

58. Kuhn, R., Rudy, H., and Weygand, F. 1936. Über die Bildung eines kunstlichen Ferments aus 6,7-Dimethyl-9-1-araboflavin-5'-phosphorsaure, *Ber.* 69:2034-2036.

59. Kuhn, R., and Weygand, F. 1937. Die Amadori-Umlagerung, *Ber.* 70:769-772.

60. Kuhn, R., Desnuelle, P., and Weygand, F. 1937. Zur Spezifität des Lactoflavins; die Bedeutung der Stellung der Methylgruppen, *Ber.* 70:1293-1301.

61. Kuhn, R., Vetter, H., and Rzeppa, H. W. 1937. Zur Spezifität des Lactoflavins; Ersatz des Methylgruppen durch den Tetramethylene und Trimethylene Ring, *Ber.* 70:1302-1314.

62. Kuhn, R., Weygand, F., and Moller, E. F. 1943. Über einen Antagonisten des Lactoflavins, *Ber.* 76:1044-1050.

63. Lambooy, J. P. 1950. The synthesis of 6,7-diethyl-9-(D-1'-ribityl)isoalloxazine, *J. Am. Chem. Soc.* 72:5225-5228.

64. Lambooy, J. P. 1951. Activity of 6,7-diethyl-9-(D-1'-ribityl)isoalloxazine for *Lactobacillus casei*, *J. Biol. Chem.* 188:459-462.

65. Lambooy, J. P., and Aposhian, H. V. 1952. The biological activity of diethyl-riboflavin, *J. Nutr.* 47:539-560.

66. Lambooy, J. P., and Haley, E. E. 1952. Additional *o*-phenylenediamines tested for vitamin B₁₂ activity, *J. Am. Chem. Soc.* 74:1087-1088.

67. Lambooy, J. P. 1955. Riboflavin antagonists, *Amer. J. Clin. Nutr.* 3:282-290.

68. Lambooy, J. P. 1957. Synthesis and activity for *Lactobacillus casei* of 6-ethyl-(methyl)-7-methyl-(ethyl)-9-(1'-D-ribityl)isoalloxazine, *Federal Proc.* 16: 208.

69. Lambooy, J. P. 1958. The synthesis of 6-ethyl-7-methyl-9-(1'-D-ribityl)isoalloxazine and 6-methyl-7-ethyl-9-(1'-D-ribityl)isoalloxazine, *J. Am. Chem. Soc.* 80:110-113.

70. Lambooy, J. P. 1958. The biological activity of 6-ethyl-7-methyl- and 6-methyl-7-ethyl-9-(1'-D-ribityl)isoalloxazine, *Biochem. Biophys. Acta* 29:221.

71. Lambooy, J. P., and Aposhian, H. V. 1960 The biological activity of 6-ethyl-9-(1'-D-ribityl)isoalloxazine, *J. Nutr.* 71:182-187.

72. Lambooy, J. P. 1961. Growth promoting properties of 6-ethyl-7-methyl-9-(1'-D-ribityl)isoalloxazine and 6-methyl-7-ethyl-9-(1'-D-ribityl)isoalloxazine, *J. Nutr.* 75:116-126.

73. Lambooy, J. P., Scala, R. A., and Haley, E. E. 1961. The biological activities of 6-methyl-7-chloro-9-(1'-D-ribityl)isoalloxazine and dichlororiboflavin, *J. Nutr.* 74:466-472.

74. Lambooy, J. P. 1966. The utilization of riboflavin antagonists by a mutant of *Lactobacillus casei*, *Arch. Biochem. Biophys.* 117:120-124.

75. Lambooy, J. P. 1967. The alloxazines and isoalloxazines, *in:* "Heterocyclic

Compounds," (R. C. Elderfield, ed.), Vol. 9, Chap. 2, pp. 118-223, John Wiley & Sons, Inc., New York.

76. Lambooy, J. P. 1970. Riboflavin protection against azo dye hepatome induction in the rat, *Proc. Soc. Exptl. Biol. Med.* **134:**192-194.
77. Lambooy, J. P., Scala, R. A., and Homan, E. 1970. Nondisplacement of rat tissue riboflavin by 7-chloro-8-methyl-flavin and the stimulation of intestinal synthesis of riboflavin, *J. Nutr.* **100:**883-892.
78. Lambooy, J. P., 1972. Synthesis and biological activity of 7-methyl-8-bromo-10-(1'-D-ribityl)isoalloxazine, an analog of riboflavin, *Proc. Soc. Exptl. Biol. Med.* **141:**948-952.
79. Lambooy, J. P., and Lambooy, J. P. 1973. Syntheses and biological activities of 7-ethyl-8-chloro-10-(1'-D-ribityl)isoalloxazine and 7-chloro-8-ethyl-10-(1'-D-ribityl) isoalloxazine, analogs of riboflavin, *J. Med. Chem.* **16:**765-771.
80. Lambooy, J. P. 1974. Syntheses and biological activities of 7-ethyl-8-bromo-10-(1'-D--ribityl)isoalloxazine and 7-bromo-8-ethyl-10-(1'-D-ribityl)isoalloxazine, analogs of riboflavin, *J. Med. Chem.* **17:**227-231.
80a. Lambooy, J. P., to be published.
81. Lambooy, J. P., Smith, C. D., and Kim, Y. S. 1971. Utilization of 7-chloro-8-methyl-flavin in the rat and its specific antiriboflavin action in the kidney, *J. Nutr.* **101:**1137-1146.
82. Lane, M., Fahey, J. L., Sullivan, R. D., and Zubrod, C. G. 1958. The comparative pharmacology in man and the rat of the riboflavin analogue 6,7-dimethyl-9-(2'-acetoxyethyl)isoalloxazine, U-2112, *J. Pharmacol. Exptl. Therap.* **122:**315-326.
83. Lane, M., Petering, H. G., and Brindley, C. O. 1959. Synthesis, pharmacology and clinical trial of the riboflavin analogue sodium-6,7-dimethyl-9-(2'-hemisuccinox-yethyl)isoalloxazine U-6538. *J. Natl. Cancer Inst.* **22:**349-361.
84. Lane, M. 1964. Studies on the mechanism of the growth-inhibitory action of galactoflavin in rats, *Cancer Res.* **24:**1811-1813.
85. Lane, M., and Brindley, C. O. 1964. Laboratory and clinical studies with the riboflavin antagonist, galactoflavin, *Proc. Soc. Exptl. Biol. Med.* **116:**57-61.
86. Maw, A. J. G. 1954. Inherited riboflavin deficiency in chicken eggs, *Poultry Sci.* **33:**216-217.
87. Miles, H. T., and Stadtman, E. R. 1955. Isolation and characterization of 6,7-dimethyl-9-(2'-hydroxyethyl)isoalloxazine as a bacterial fermentation product of riboflavin, *J. Am. Chem. Soc.* **77:**5746-5747.
88. Miller, Z., Poncet, I., and Takacs, E. 1962. Biochemical studies on experimental congenital malformations: flavin nucleotides and folic acid in fetuses and liver from normal and riboflavin-deficient rats, *J. Biol. Chem.* **237:**968-973.
89. Morgan, H. R. 1954. Factors related to the growth of psittacosis virus (strain 6BC) IV. Certain amino acids, vitamins, and other substances, *J. Exptl. Med.* **99:**451-460.
90. Nelson, M. M., Baird, C. D. C., Wright, H. V., and Evans H. M. 1956. Multiple congenital abnormalities in the rat resulting from riboflavin deficiency induced by the antimetabolite galactoflavin, *J. Nutr.* **58:**125-134.
91. Pallares, E. S., and Garza, H. M. 1949. Isolation of L-lyxoflavin from the human myocardium, *Arch. Biochem.* **22:**63-65.
92. Prosky, L., Burch, H. B., Bejrablaya, D., Lowry, O. H., and Combs, A. M. 1964. The effects of galactoflavin on riboflavin enzyme and coenzyme, *J. Biol. Chem.* **239:**2691-2695.
93. Pulver, R., and Verzar, F. 1939. Die Phosphorylierung von Riboflavin durch Darmschleimhaut, *Enzymologia* **6:**333-336.
94. Ramakrishnan, S. V., Srinivasan, V., and Nedungadi, T. M. B. 1961. Studies on

the combined and relative influence of dietary protein and riboflavin in flavoprotein enzymes, *J. Nutr.* **75**:443-446.

95. Ringenberg, L. K., and Lambooy, J. P. 1973. Succinic acid dehydrogenase activity of Walker rat carcinoma 256 when utilizing riboflavin homologs, *Proc. Soc. Exptl. Biol. Med.* **143**:1211-1214.

96. Rudy, H. 1935. Enzymatische Phosphoryleirung des Lactoflavin. *Naturwiss.* **23**:286-287.

97. Sarett, H. P. 1946. The effect of riboflavin analogs upon the utilization of riboflavin and flavin adenine dinucleotide by *Lactobacillus casei*, *J. Biol. Chem.* **162**:87-97.

98. Scala, R. A., and Lambooy, J. P. 1958. Utilization of the riboflavin inhibitor 6-chloro-7-methyl-9-(1'-D-ribityl)isoalloxazine by *Lactobacillus casei*, *Arch. Biochem. Biophys.* **78**:10-14.

99. Shaffner, C. S., and Lambooy, J. P., to be published.

100. Shorb, M. S. 1952. Growth-promoting activity of L-lyxoflavin for *Lactobacillus lactis*, *Proc. Soc. Exptl. Biol. Med.* **79**:611-614.

101. Shunk, C. H., Koniuszy, F. R., and Folkers, K. 1952. Studies on carcinolytic compounds. IV. 6-Chloro-9-(1'-D-glycityl)-isoalloxazines, *J. Am Chem. Soc.* **74**:4251-4253.

102. Shunk, C. H., Lavigne, J. B., and Folkers, K. 1955. Studies on carcinolytic compounds. V. 6,7-Dimethyl-9-(1'- 5'-deoxy -D-ribityl)isoalloxazine, *J. Am. Chem. Soc.* **77**:2210-2212.

103. Snell, E. E., and Strong, F. M. 1939. A microbiological assay for riboflavin, *Ind. & Eng. Chem., Anal. Ed.* **11**:346-350.

104. Snell, E. E., and Strong, F. M. 1939. The effect of riboflavin and certain synthetic flavins on the growth of lactic acid bacteria. Enzymologia, **6**:186-193.

105. Snell, E. E., Klatt, O. A., Briuns, H. W., and Cravens, W. W. 1953. Growth-promotion by lyxoflavin. II. Relationship to riboflavin in bacteria and chicks, *Proc. Soc. Exptl. Med.* **82**:583-590.

106. Tillotson, J. A., and Sauberlich, H. E. 1971. Effect of riboflavin depletion and repletion on the erythrocyte glutathione reductase in the rat, *J. Nutr.* **101**:1459-1466.

107. von Euler, H., Karrer, P., and Malmberg, M. 1935. Wachstumswirkungen des L-und D- Araboflavins 6,7-Dimethyl-9-(L-resp. D-1'-arabityl)iso-alloxazines, *Helv. Chim. Acta.* **18**:1336-1338.

108. von Euler, H., and Karrer, P. 1946. Iso-alloxazinderivate als Antagonisten des Riboflavins, *Helv. Chim. Acta* **29**:353-354.

109. Walker, W. H., and Singer, T. P. 1970. Identification of the covalently bound flavin of succinate dehydrogenase as 8α-(histidyl) flavin adenine dinucleotide, *J. Biol. Chem.* **245**:4224-4225.

110. Weygand, F., Lowenfeld, R., and Moller, E. F. 1951. Über die Specifität von 6,7-Dichloro-9-*d*-riboflavin als Antagonist des Lactoflavin, *Chem. Ber.* **84**:101-109.

111. Yagi, K., Okuda, J., and Kobayashi, M. 1963. Studies on fatty acid esters of flavins. III. Nutritional and ariboflavinosis-curing effects, *J. Vitaminol.* **9**:168-176.

112. Yang, C. S., Arsenis, C., and McCormick, D. B. 1964. Microbiological and enzymatic assays of riboflavin analogues, *J. Nutr.* **84**:167-172.

RIBOFLAVIN AND CANCER

Richard S. Rivlin

1. INTRODUCTION

Animals and humans with tumors may display profound cachexia during the course of illness. In some instances, weight loss may be an initial manifestation of cancer, occurring before the neoplasm is widespread. Anorexia, nausea, vomiting, and diminished food intake may be important factors in contributing to the development of cachexia in far advanced cancer. In addition, inanition may arise from diminished intestinal absorption, blood loss, tissue ulceration and necrosis, or infection and other factors.[70] Disturbances in the metabolism of lipids, amino acids, carbohydrates, and electrolytes have all been described in patients with cancer, but the precise mechanisms underlying weight loss and malnutrition remain uncertain.[11,13] Tumors have been referred to as "nitrogen traps" that derive their amino acid supplies at the expense of the animal or human host.[23,44] It appears that, when the supplies of dietary nitrogen are limited, tumor competes for them more successfully than normal host tissues.

There is considerable experimental evidence that the initiation and further development of tumors in animals may be dependent to some

RICHARD S. RIVLIN—Department of Medicine, Francis Delafield Hospital and Presbyterian Hospital; and Institute of Human Nutrition, College of Physicians & Surgeons of Columbia University, New York, New York. This work was supported by USPHS grants AM15265 and CA12126 and by the Stella and Charles Guttman Foundation.

extent upon nutritional factors. Transplanted tumors are particularly sensitive to total caloric restriction and frequently have a slowed rate of growth when the intake of food is reduced.[68] In mice of the C3H strain, reduction in caloric intake resulted in a greatly diminished development of spontaneous mammary carcinoma.[73] Similarly, in mice of a strain that has a high incidence of spontaneous lymphoid leukemia, underfeeding of the animals dramatically reduced the overall incidence of the neoplasm and delayed its emergence.[64] Tumors may, however, continue to grow under certain circumstances despite progressive weight loss of the host.[68] Force-feeding of experimental animals with tumors does not necessarily slow the evolution of metabolic alterations in the host, such as anemia and changes in the activities of certain enzymes.[5,66] Similarly, in man metabolic abnormalities such as hypoalbuminemia are not prevented by increasing the dietary intake of nitrogen.[25] There are reports that force-feeding of patients with cancer with diets high in calories and nitrogen may even accelerate the growth of the cancer.[69] These studies suggest that, under certain conditions, dietary factors may be of importance in regulating the growth of tumors, but that other manifestations of cancer appear to be less dependent upon nutritional factors.

The relationship of vitamin metabolism to cancer is equally complex.[58] Vitamins appear to influence the genesis and growth of cancer, but it has frequently been difficult to differentiate the effect of a specific vitamin lack from the accompanying reduction in dietary intake.[68] Not only do vitamins affect the rate of neoplastic growth, but tumors, in turn, may affect the metabolism of vitamins. Vitamins also affect the inactivation of drugs and may influence the response to chemotherapy.[6] The present review considers the various relationships of cancer to a single vitamin, riboflavin.

2. SPONTANEOUS AND TRANSPLANTED CANCERS

The investigations of Morris and Robertson in 1943[50] demonstrated that the growth and spread of spontaneous mammary cancers in mice are markedly diminished in animals that have become riboflavin-deficient. In these studies animals were placed on riboflavin-supplemented or riboflavin-deficient diets as soon as mammary tumors were first observed. The loss of body weight exhibited by these riboflavin-deficient mice during a 9-week period was nearly the same as that of similarly deficient animals that were not bearing tumors. The growth rate of tumors that

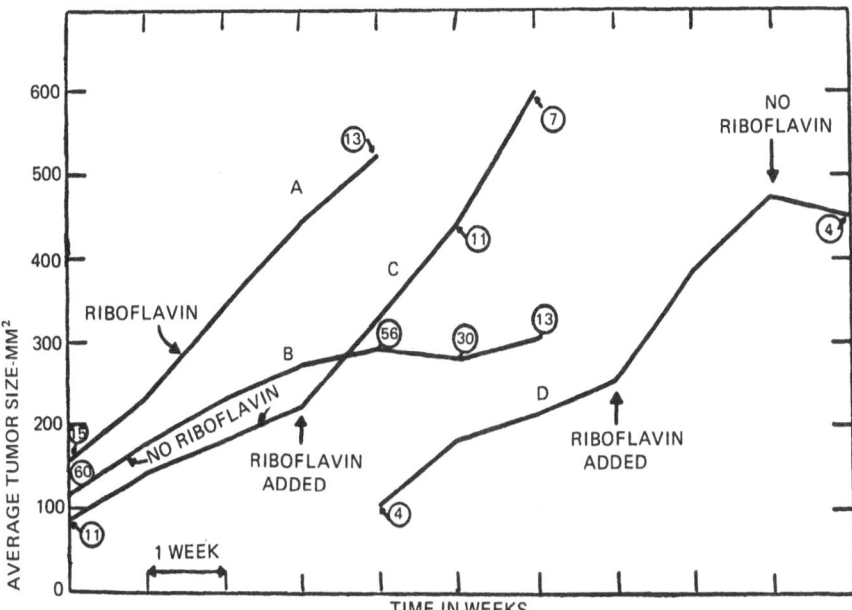

Fig. 1. Average rate of tumor growth in acute riboflavin deficiency. *A*—riboflavin-supplemented; *B*—deficient; *C*—deficient 3 weeks, then supplemented; *D*—deficient 3 weeks, supplemented 2 weeks, then deficient 1 week. The circled numbers are the number of tumors used to obtain the average values. (From Morris[49] with the permission of the publisher.)

appeared in riboflavin-deficient animals, however, underwent a gradual and progressive decrease compared to those tumors grown in mice on a diet containing normal amounts of riboflavin. The decreased rate of tumor growth was most marked in mice during the later stages of deficiency. Riboflavin refeeding of deficient animals rapidly led to a restoration of the normal growth rate of the mammary tumor.

The results of one of these experiments are shown in Fig. 1. In animals on a normal diet (curve *A*), tumor growth increased at a uniform rate throughout the 4-week experimental period. In riboflavin-deficient animals (curve *B*), the decrease in the rate of tumor growth first appeared at 1-3 weeks of deficiency. From 3 to 6 weeks of deficiency, virtually no increase in tumor size occurred. In animals that had received a high riboflavin diet after 3 weeks of riboflavin deficiency (curve *C*), the tumor growth rate showed a rapid recovery after the initial lag in growth and for the following several weeks was at least as great as in normal animals. In a fourth group of animals (curve *D*) fed a deficient diet for 3 weeks, followed by a high riboflavin diet for 2 weeks, and then a low riboflavin diet again, tumor growth rate closely reflected each dietary manipulation.

These studies clearly demonstrated that rates of growth of mammary tumors occurring spontaneously are greatly depressed in riboflavin-deficient animals. Other studies by Morris[49] indicated that the eventual size of spontaneous tumors is less in the deficient than in the control animals. A direct relation was found between the dietary riboflavin content and the number of mammary tumors observed grossly. C3H mice feeding on a regular diet were selected for study shortly after spontaneous tumors were first noted. Animals were placed at random on low and high riboflavin diets; the total quantity of food consumed was essentially the same in all groups, although exact figures were not reported. The results of these experiments are given in Fig. 2. In mice on a high riboflavin diet, the mean number of tumors per animal increased from slightly more than 1.0 to more than 2.5 during the 5-week experimental period. By contrast, in mice on a deficient diet, the average number of tumors per animal did not exceed 1.5 at any time.

A depression of tumor growth has also been observed with pantothenic acid deficiency.[49] Thiamin deficiency did not suppress tumor

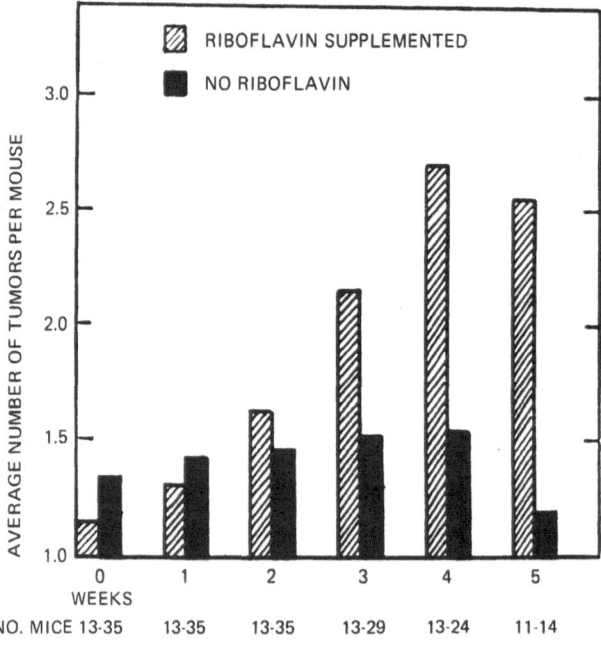

Fig. 2. Average number of tumors per mouse in mice fed riboflavin-deficient and supplemented diets. (From Morris[49] with the permission of the publisher.)

growth when the effect of diminished food intake was taken into account. Pyridoxine deficiency has been reported to produce regression of mouse sarcoma 180 and other tumors [36,45] or to have no effect upon tumor growth. [17] In the latter study, seventeen patients with severely progressive cancers, including carcinoma of the breast, esophagus, larynx, lung, and lymphosarcoma, were treated with a pyridoxine-deficient diet for periods of 10–80 days. Nine of these patients also received a pyridoxine antagonist, 4-deoxypyridoxine, for varying intervals to accentuate the metabolic deficiency state that had been induced in these patients, but no inhibitory effects on tumor growth were noted. [77]

Further investigations concerning the antitumor effects of riboflavin deficiency have used either a deficient diet or structural analogues of riboflavin. In one study, a marked reduction in the size of previously developed lymphosarcoma transplants in mice was observed. [67] The findings of this study differed from the results obtained by Morris [49] in one respect: Accelerated growth of tumors was not observed once the animals had undergone refeeding with riboflavin. Holly et al. [24] showed that several additional isoalloxazine derivatives also cause regression of one form of lymphosarcoma. Studies with a structural analogue of riboflavin, diethyl riboflavin, which antagonizes the biological effects of the vitamin, have shown that this compound diminishes the growth rate of Walker carcinoma in rats. [1] In rats treated with diethyl riboflavin, tumor weight, expressed per body weight, was decreased to two-thirds that observed in normal animals bearing Walker tumors. It is of interest that an analogue of riboflavin, 7-methyl-8-ethyl-flavin, which appears not to produce riboflavin deficiency but instead to replace the vitamin in a variety of biochemical functions, does not inhibit the growth rate of Walker carcinoma. [33]

In a culture medium, the growth and metabolism of ascites tumor cells are inhibited by riboflavin. The addition to the culture medium of small quantities of riboflavin, but not of several related compounds, has been effective in substantially reducing the fermentation rate of these neoplastic cells. This effect appears to be light-mediated, since it is not demonstrable when cells are grown in complete darkness. [74,75] The inhibition of oxidative metabolism by riboflavin in Ehrlich ascites tumor cells was also observed by David et al., [12] who reported changes in the morphology of the cells under electron microscopy in response to the administration of riboflavin. It is not certain how these observations are related to tumor growth in the deficient animal as a whole.

In summary, these studies generally indicate that riboflavin deficiency decreases the rates of growth of a variety of tumors from experimental animals. This is true with respect to certain forms of mammary tumors, lymphosarcoma in mice, and Walker carcinoma in rats. Because tumor weight relative to body weight has been used in the past as the major index of tumor growth, it is not possible to determine from these early reports whether riboflavin deficiency decreases tumor cell size as well as cell number, or whether it produces other morphological changes in the tumors studied. The mechanism of the inhibitory effects of riboflavin deficiency has not been elucidated.

Some evidence exists that experimental riboflavin deficiency may inhibit cancer in man. In an initial study using a derivative of riboflavin, 6,7-dimethyl-9-(2'acetoxyethyl)-isoalloxazine (U-2112), in ten cancer patients, Lane and colleagues[42] observed neither laboratory evidence of riboflavin deficiency nor regression of the tumors. One possible reason for the failure of the drug to produce riboflavin deficiency under these conditions was that, in the doses administered, the drug appeared to undergo rapid and complete degradation. Later, however, Lane[41] reported results in six patients with advanced cancer treated with galactoflavin, in whom manifestations of riboflavin deficiency developed 10–25 days after the start of drug therapy. One patient was believed to have a decrease in tumor size and two others an apparent decrease in tumor growth rate.

Recent observations by this group suggest that riboflavin deficiency induced by dietary means in combination with galactoflavin may be useful in the treatment of certain patients with polycythemia vera and lymphoma.[40] Patients were treated for periods of 1–5 months with this regimen. Partial remissions were obtained in one of the two patients with Hodgkin's disease and in two of the four patients with lymphosarcoma. A prolonged remission was observed in two patients with polycythemia vera. These findings have been discussed in greater detail by Lane in Chapter 9. The long-term implications of the observation that riboflavin deficiency may inhibit certain tumors will be awaited with great interest.

3. CHEMICAL CARCINOGENESIS

A variety of epithelial changes, including atrophy, hyperkeratosis, alopecia, ulceration, and dermatitis, are produced both in animals and in man as a result of riboflavin deficiency. Wynder and Klein[79] documented the histological changes that developed in the epithelium in mice during progressive riboflavin deficiency. The earliest change noted was atrophy of the epithelium of the esophagus and stomach, which developed during the third to fifth week of deficiency. From the seventh to the ninth week of deficiency, epithelial hyperplasia and hyperkeratosis were prominent. The hyperkeratosis led to nearly complete obstruction of the esophageal lumen. The authors concluded that the epidermal atrophy and hyperkeratosis observed in riboflavin-deficient mice may have been related to accompanying starvation, since normal animals with greatly restricted food intake also exhibited these changes. Hyperplasia of the epidermis, however, was not noted in starved animals and appeared to represent a more specific effect of riboflavin deficiency.

In subsequent studies,[78] riboflavin deficiency in young mice was

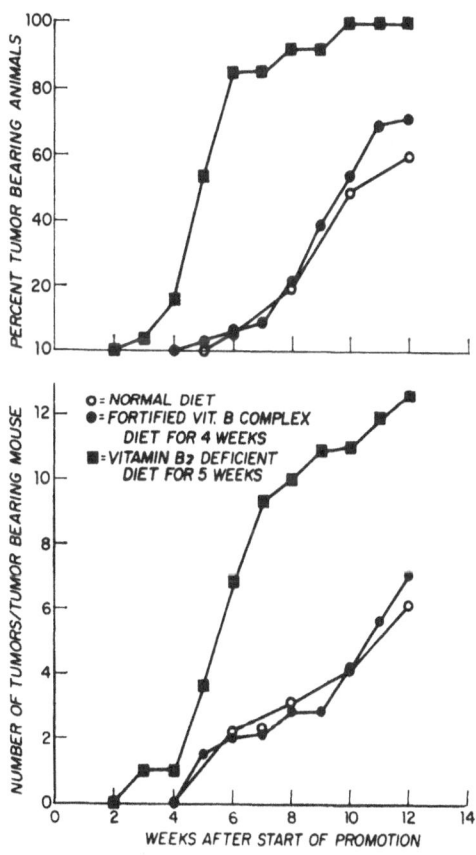

Fig. 3. Cumulative tumor incidence in female Swiss mice (3 weeks old) initiated with DMBA after being put on a normal diet for 4 weeks, a fortified vitamin B complex diet for 4 weeks, or a vitamin B_2-deficient diet for 5 weeks. All mice were put on normal diet after initiation and painted with 1% croton oil twice weekly beginning 10 days after initiation. (From Wynder and Chan[78] with the permission of the publisher.)

observed to increase chemically induced carcinogenesis in the epithelium. These experiments were performed by placing 3- to 4-week-old mice on a riboflavin-deficient diet for a 4-week period, after which they received a normal diet. Papilloma development following local application of 7,12-dimethylbenz[a]anthracene (DMBA) and croton oil was studied in normal animals and in animals at intervals following recovery from riboflavin deficiency. In all the animals that had previously received a deficient diet, skin tumors developed earlier and in greater numbers than in control animals. The results of other experiments, in which tumor development was studied in animals on a normal diet, a riboflavin-deficient diet, and a high riboflavin diet, are shown in Fig. 3. Animals on a normal and on a riboflavin-supplemented diet had nearly an identical number of tumors per animal and equal percentages of tumor-bearing animals. By contrast, in animals on a deficient diet, both the total number of tumors per animal and the percentage of animals that developed tumors were greatly increased. Tumors also arose more rapidly after application of the carcinogen to the skin of animals on a deficient than on a normal or high riboflavin diet: Tumors did not appear until 4 weeks in the animals on a normal or a high riboflavin diet, but were noted after only two weeks on the low riboflavin diet. It is of interest that in animals which underwent caloric restriction alone, the tumor incidence was similar to that of control animals fed a normal diet *ad libitum*.

When the carcinogenic hydrocarbon 7,12-dimethylbenz[a]anthracene (DMBA) was placed on the skin of deficient animals, and a diet containing normal amounts of riboflavin was fed, an increase in skin tumor formation occurred.[10] Under these conditions, there was a marked increase in the activity of aryl hydrocarbon hydroxylase, an enzyme that metabolizes carcinogens. The authors suggested that increased activity of this enzyme could enhance the formation of reactive intermediates of DMBA and lead to increased binding of carcinogenic compounds to DNA. Roe[62] also observed that the feeding of a diet with a very high level of flavin had little if any effect upon inhibiting the development of skin papillomas in mice treated with 9,10-dimethyl-1,2-benzanthracene.

Other systematic investigations of chemical carcinogenesis in relation to riboflavin have largely been restricted to the azo dyes. Numerous reports indicate that hepatic carcinogenesis by azo dyes is potentiated by riboflavin deficiency, and that riboflavin administration to deficient animals inhibits the development of hepatomas.[21,31,38,39,46,51,68] These studies indicate a specific relationship between nutrition and the growth of a tumor in experimental animals.

The accelerated rate of growth of azo dye-induced tumors that occurs in riboflavin deficiency has been observed in animals treated with dietary vitamin restriction alone, with structural analogues of riboflavin, or with a deficient diet in combination with the riboflavin analog.[21,38,46] Each method appears to be suitable provided that the hepatic flavin concentration is significantly depleted below normal levels. The hepatic flavin concentration appears to be the critical factor, and with any given diet the incidence of hepatomas in experimental animals after treatment with azo dyes is inversely proportional to the concentration of riboflavin in liver.[21] Furthermore, a given dose of azo dye carcinogen that is too small to produce tumors in normal animals is highly effective in animals that have been previously treated with a particular riboflavin analog.[51]

More recent studies on the relationship of riboflavin to azo dye carcinogenesis and to succinic dehydrogenase activity[56] have been conducted by Lambooy and colleagues.[4,38,39] Further documentation of the protective effect of riboflavin against a variety of tumors induced by azo dyes has been provided. However, it has also been shown that after treatment of experimental animals with an azo dye carcinogen of extremely high potency—3'-methyl-4'-ethyl-4-dimethyl-aminoazobenzene—riboflavin does not apparently inhibit tumor formation.[4] These findings are also discussed in Chapter 10.

The increased carcinogenicity of azo dyes in riboflavin-deficient animals may be due in part to the fact that the hepatic metabolism of these drugs appears to involve flavin-containing enzymes. The demethylation of 4-dimethyl-aminoazobenzene (DAB) and other azo dyes and the cleavage of the azo linkage are both believed to require flavin cofactors.[47] Suggestive evidence is that the addition of flavins *in vitro* to the tissue preparations greatly enhances the activities of the enzymes degrading the azo dyes. Definitive proof that FAD is the cofactor of these enzymes remains to be obtained, however. The hepatic concentration of FAD is decreased to one-third of normal in riboflavin-deficient animals, and there is therefore less FAD available to stabilize a variety of flavoprotein apoenzymes.[57] It is likely that, under these circumstances, inactivation of the enzymes that degrade azo dyes would occur. As a result of such inactivation, the actual dose of carcinogen delivered to the liver may be greatly increased over that of animals on a normal diet.

The observation that azo dye reductase activity is diminished in livers of riboflavin-deficient rats has been confirmed and extended by Williams *et al.*,[77] who noted considerable enzyme activity in cecal contents. Azo dye reductase activity expressed per milligram protein in cecal contents was in fact six times higher than that in liver, and showed a significant decline in riboflavin-deficient animals. These data suggest that bacterial flora as well as the host liver degrade azo dye carcinogens and that dietary riboflavin regulates enzyme activity at both sites.

In addition to influencing the hepatic activities of enzymes that inactivate azo dyes, riboflavin may influence azo dye carcinogenesis by another mechanism. Tung and Lin[72] observed a quenching effect of two azo dyes, 4-dimethylaminoazobenzene (DAB) and 4-aminoazobenzene (AAB), on riboflavin fluorescence and postulated the formation of a complex between these drugs and riboflavin in aqueous solution. Riboflavin has been effective in solubilizing the azo dyes. These investigators have suggested that the direct complexing of riboflavin with the azo dyes may block their action as carcinogens at the postulated tissue receptor sites. The riboflavin–azo dye complex has not been isolated or characterized further.

Another and perhaps related effect of the administration of azo dyes is to lower the hepatic flavin concentrations[32,46,72] and the activities of FAD-dependent enzymes, such as xanthine oxidase.[76] Kensler *et al.*[76] showed that the total flavin concentration in livers of animals treated with 4-dimethylaminoazobenzene is reduced to less than 60% of that of control animals. Several compounds that are structurally related to DAB, but that are not carcinogens, do not appear to lower the hepatic flavin concentration.[21] The carcinogenicity of a number of azo dyes has in fact been correlated with the extent to which they decrease the flavin levels in liver.[20] The decreased hepatic flavin concentrations that are observed after azo dye treatment may arise by at least two mechanisms:

1. Increased urinary excretion of riboflavin. This has been suggested to occur after treatment with azo dyes.[54] The factors responsible for the riboflavinuria need to be determined more precisely.
2. Enhanced enzymatic degradation of FAD. During a study of the reduced hepatic flavin content produced by DAB, Yang and Sung[81] noted that treatment with this drug lowers the hepatic FAD fraction proportionately more than the hepatic FMN or riboflavin fractions. Rubenchik also observed that FAD was particularly depressed in concentration in DAB-treated animals.[63]

To explore possible mechanisms accounting for the marked depletion of FAD concentration in this tumor, Yang and Sung[81] developed an assay for nucleotide pyrophosphatase which, besides other reactions, catalyzes the degradation of FAD to FMN. The results of assay of the various flavin fractions in normal liver and in hepatic carcinoma

TABLE I. *Nucleotide Pyrophosphatase Activity and Flavin Concentration in Rats Treated with 4-Dimethylaminoazobenzene (DAB)*

	Liver	Carcinoma
Nucleotide pyrophosphatase activity (μm FAD degraded/g tissue/hr)	2.8	8.4
Total flavin conc. (μg/g tissue)	21.77	4.53
FAD conc. (μg/g tissue)	18.91	2.70
FMN + riboflavin conc. (μg/g tissue)	2.86	1.83
Nitrogen (g/100 g tissue)[a]	2.85	2.49

[a] Measured by the micro-Kjeldahl method. (Data are derived from Yang and Sung.[81])

produced by DAB treatment are shown in Table I. Nucleotide pyrophosphatase activity was three times as great in the carcinoma as in the control liver. In the carcinoma, FAD concentration was reduced to one-seventh that of liver, but FMN and free riboflavin concentrations measured together were two-thirds as great as in liver. The total nitrogen concentration was nearly the same in liver and in carcinoma. These authors also found relatively low activity of FAD pyrophosphorylase, which synthesizes FAD from FMN. An increase in the rate of enzymatic FAD degradation relative to synthesis would be expected particularly to diminish the FAD fraction.

In a recent report,[9] riboflavin deficiency reduced the activity of benzpyrene hydroxylase, the hepatic enzyme that metabolizes the carcinogen 3–4 benzpyrene, to less than one-third of that observed in normal animals. These findings have been confirmed and extended by Shargel and Mazel,[65] who noted that the magnitude of the induction of benzpyrene hydroxylase by 3-methylcholanthrene was less in riboflavin-deficient than in normal animals. Others[9,10,80] have reported that hepatic aryl hydroxylase activity is also reduced in riboflavin deficiency and can be increased by riboflavin administration. The suggestion has been made[80] that the increased rate of chemical carcinogenesis in mice recovering from riboflavin deficiency[78] is related to increased aryl hydroxylase activity, because this enzyme may be producing derivatives more active in carcinogenesis than the original compound.

In summary, riboflavin deficiency potentiates carcinogenesis by azo dyes. This effect may be due in part to diminished activities of presumed flavin-dependent enzymes that inactivate the azo dyes. The enhanced growth rates of tumors induced by azo dyes is in sharp contrast to the reduced rates of growth of spontaneously developing and transplanted tumors noted above in riboflavin-deficient animals. Azo dyes, in turn, decrease the hepatic concentration of FAD in host animals.

4. DRUG METABOLISM IN CANCER

The potentiation of azo dye carcinogenesis appears to be one of a number of effects of riboflavin deficiency upon drug metabolism. The observation that the hepatic activity of microsomal NADPH$_2$-cytochrome C reductase, a major drug metabolizing enzyme that has FAD as its cofactor, is reduced in livers of riboflavin-deficient rats[61] has been confirmed recently[65,80] and suggests that the effects of many other drugs both toxic and therapeutic may be enhanced under these conditions. The hepatic activities of drug-metabolizing enzymes appear to be quite variable in riboflavin-deficient animals. The observation that the pharmacological effect of hexobarbital, as measured by sleeping time in mice, is markedly increased in riboflavin-deficient animals, is compatible with diminished drug-metabolizing enzyme activity *in vivo*.[9] Kato *et al.*[30] have shown that many of the drug-metabolizing enzymes are reduced in activity in livers of tumor-bearing animals. If the effects of riboflavin deficiency and of bearing a tumor are additive upon drug metabolism, then it is likely that riboflavin deficiency produced in a tumor-bearing animal would depress drug inactivation rates to an extreme degree. At the present time, knowledge of the metabolism of drugs, in riboflavin-deficient animals bearing transplanted tumors and in nutritionally depleted patients with cancer, is very scanty.

The effects of riboflavin upon folic acid metabolism may have implications for the use of folic acid antagonists in cancer chemotherapy. In riboflavin deficiency, the concentration of folic acid is reduced in serum.[16] Injection of tritium-labeled folic acid to riboflavin-deficient animals results in a much greater fraction of the isotope excreted in urine than that observed in normal animals.[52] Suggestive evidence of an alteration in the metabolism of folic acid in riboflavin deficiency has been the observation that in animals that have received a deficient diet for 11-30 days, the urinary excretion of formiminoglutamic acid (FIGLU) following a histidine load is markedly reduced. The excretion of FIGLU is decreased whether the histidine is administered by the oral, intraperitoneal, intramuscular, or intravenous route.[53] Riboflavin-deficient animals may have a defect in the conversion of folic acid to N^5-methyltetrahydrofolic acid in liver.[26] Riboflavin deficiency appears to decrease the hepatic activities of two enzymes involved in folic acid metabolism, $N^{5,10}$-methylenetetrahydrofolate reductase and N^5-methyltetrahydrofolate transferase; this may result in accumulation in liver of tetrahydrofolate compounds other than N^5-methyltetrahydrofolate.[53] Another group of investigators[7,55] has observed an increase rather than a decrease in the urinary excretion of FIGLU following a histidine load in riboflavin-deficient animals and has suggested that the major defects are in the conversion of folate to tetrahydrofolate, and in tetrahydrofolate dehydrogenase activity. Thus, it is likely that defects in the metabolism of folic acid occur in riboflavin deficiency, since flavin cofactors appear to be involved in certain important metabolic transformations of folic acid. The nature and specificity of these defects require further clarification.

Another effect of riboflavin upon drug metabolism in cancer is that upon the transport of certain drugs into neoplastic cells. Hakala[22] showed that, in Sarcoma 180 cells grown in tissue culture, riboflavin *inhibits* the net rate of uptake of amethopterin (Methotrexate, MTX). Riboflavin in the concentration usually present in tissue culture medium is sufficient to cause this effect. By contrast, Goldman *et al.*[19] reported that riboflavin *enhances* the net transport of methotrexate into L1210 mouse leukemia cells. The differences in the results obtained appear to have been resolved by the subsequent studies of Lichtenstein and Goldman,[43] who reported that riboflavin and methotrexate are involved in two separate processes:

1. Riboflavin competitively inhibits methotrexate influx. Methotrexate and riboflavin were mixed at the moment of contact with cells of

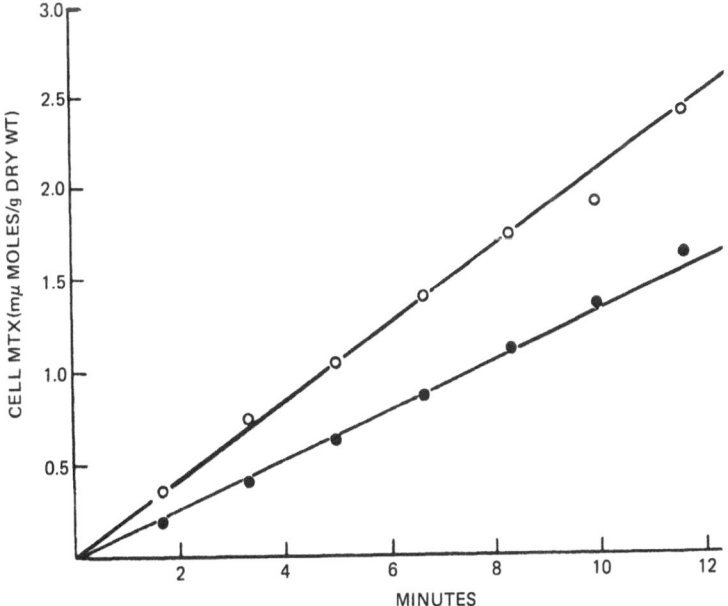

Fig. 4. Time course of uptake of 0.1 μM MTX in the presence (●) and absence (○) of 290 μM RF. Both compounds were mixed together at the instant of exposure to the cells. (From Lichtenstein and Goldman[43] with the permission of the publishers.)

L1210 mouse leukemia grown in cell culture. As shown in Fig. 4, measurements of the time course of uptake of methotrexate revealed that riboflavin at a concentration of 290 μM appreciably inhibited influx of the drug. In subsequent experiments, increasing the riboflavin concentration in the extracellular medium while maintaining a constant methotrexate concentration resulted in progressive reduction in methotrexate influx. Analysis of kinetic data suggested that the mechanism of inhibition was competitive. Later, Goldman[18] reported that the inhibition of influx of methotrexate into the L1210 cells was probably due to the anionic nature of the riboflavin phosphate moiety.

2. Riboflavin appears to undergo a photochemical reaction with methotrexate. In the dark, the spectrum of methotrexate was not affected by the addition of riboflavin to the solution. By contrast, when methotrexate and riboflavin in solution were exposed to light, a spectral shift occurred. These and other experiments suggested that incubation of methotrexate with riboflavin resulted in the production of new compounds the elution pattern of which on column chromatography differed from that of methotrexate.[43]

The degradation products of methotrexate which are produced photochemically have not been characterized fully. They appear to be transported across the cell membrane by a carrier system different from that of methotrexate. In addition, unlike methotrexate, these derivatives are not bound to dihydrofolate reductase. It appears that these two competing processes may govern the net uptake of methotrexate and its derivatives by tumor cells *in vitro* in tissue culture.

Thus, riboflavin may determine to some extent the effectiveness of folic acid antagonists in chemotherapy by regulating the metabolic utilization of folic acid. Additionally, the transport of methotrexate across cell membranes is affected by riboflavin. The regulation of activities of drug-metabolizing enzymes by dietary riboflavin may potentially be of considerable clinical significance.

5. EFFECTS OF CANCER ON TISSUE FLAVIN LEVELS

As noted above, in tumors that have been induced by azo dyes, FAD concentrations are markedly reduced, an effect that may be due in part to increased riboflavin excretion and enhanced FAD degradation.[81] In this instance, a carcinogen has a direct effect upon tissue flavin levels.

A more general effect of cancer on flavin levels was revealed by the studies of Morris and Robertson,[49,50] noted above, who demonstrated for the first time that neoplastic tissue differs from normal tissue in the rate at which total riboflavin concentration decreases with increasing duration of riboflavin deficiency. These investigators observed that in mammary tumors grown in riboflavin-deficient mice, the flavin levels in the tumor decrease at a much slower rate than that recorded in either liver or muscle of the host animal. It was suggested that the time at which the greatest decrease in tumor flavin levels occurs—the third to fifth week of vitamin deficiency—corresponds to the point at which the tumor growth rate is first observed to decrease. In this study, neoplastic tissue compared to normal tissues exhibited a relative resistance to riboflavin deficiency. These studies comprised measurements of the total riboflavin content of the various tissues and did not distinguish among FAD, FMN, and free riboflavin.

Clinical studies on riboflavin metabolism have demonstrated that patients with cancer tend to excrete lower than normal amounts of total riboflavin in urine.[28] Measurements of total urinary riboflavin excretion of 1000 patients with a wide variety of malignancies, including cancer of the stomach, breast, skin, uterus, and lung, and in other nonneoplastic diseases, was reported by Kagan.[28] He observed that patients with cancer, regardless of the site of origin or whether the lesion is primary or metastatic, excrete virtually no riboflavin in urine in 80% of the cases, whereas the great majority of normal individuals have detectable amounts of the vitamin in urine. Furthermore, administration of an oral dose of riboflavin results in markedly less urinary excretion of riboflavin in cancer patients than in normal individuals. These results are compatible with increased uptake and/or increased retention of riboflavin by neoplastic tissue but do not exclude other effects, such as altered intestinal absorption, or greater uptake and binding by host tissues. Unfortunately, the actual quantity of riboflavin excreted in the urine was not indicated in this report, nor was the dietary intake of the vitamin regulated in the patients studied.

In a clinical study of patients with cancer of the larynx, the concentration of riboflavin in urine and blood was determined before and after the administration of a load of riboflavin.[34] Results were then compared with those obtained in patients with benign diseases of the larynx, including chronic laryngitis, laryngeal papillomas, and fibromas, as well as in normal subjects. In the patients with cancer, the plasma concentration of riboflavin was one-half as great and the urinary excretion one-third as great as in the other groups of patients. After receiving a riboflavin load, the patients with cancer had lower concentrations of the vitamin both in plasma and urine then those of patients with benign disorders. The plasma concentrations of riboflavin could be correlated with the stage of the disease in the patients with laryngeal cancer: after effective treatment, riboflavin concentrations increased to normal, and in patients in whom treatment was unsuccessful or in whom disease reoccurred, riboflavin concentrations in plasma remained at a low level. More recently, these workers have shown that riboflavin concentrations in blood and urine of patients with tumors of the maxilla are also substantially depressed below those of normal individuals.[35] Patients with infectious diseases of the maxilla had blood and urinary riboflavin concentrations that were intermediate between those of normal individuals and of patients with maxillary tumors.

In animals that have received transplants of sarcomas, epitheliomas, and ascites hepatomas, riboflavin excretion may increase initially, but it decreases below normal when the tumor growth has become more advanced.[71] The effects of transplanted tumors upon the flavin concentrations of host tissues were measured by Aptekar,[2] who reported that in rats that had received transplants of ascites hepatoma, the concentration of FAD was reduced approximately one-third in liver and slightly less in kidney and heart. The FMN and riboflavin concentrations in the organs of normal and of tumor-bearing animals did not differ from one another. Transplantation of four other tumors, including several varieties of sarcomas, had no effect upon the tissue concentration of FAD, FMN, or riboflavin. In mice that had received transplants of hepatoma and sarcoma, FAD concentrations were decreased by one-quarter in host kidney and liver, but riboflavin and FMN concentrations in these organs were not altered.[3]

In a recent study,[60] suspensions of Novikoff hepatoma, rapidly growing, undifferentiated tumor, were transplanted[27] into the peritoneal cavity of normal and of riboflavin-deficient rats. Animals were sacrificed at intervals after transplantation, and simultaneous measurements were made of the concentrations in tumor of FAD, FMN, and riboflavin. As shown in Table II, the FAD concentrations in tumor in contrast to those in liver were completely unaffected by riboflavin deficiency. FMN concentrations in tumor grown in riboflavin-deficient rats were decreased appreciably below levels in tumor grown in normal animals, but the concentration of FMN in the tumor of deficient animals (36% of normal) was still decreased significantly less ($p < 0.001$) than in liver (20% of normal) of these animals.

In tumor grown in deficient animals (Table II), free riboflavin concentrations were greatly diminished to 16% of those measured in tumor from normal animals. The proportional decrease in free riboflavin

TABLE II. Concentrations of Riboflavin, FMN, and FAD in Novikoff
Hepatoma Grown Intraperitoneally in Normal and Riboflavin Deficient Rats

Group	Number of animals	Riboflavin	FMN	FAD
Normal	22	$100.0 \pm 23.1\%$[a]	$100.0 \pm 17.7\%$[a]	$100.0 \pm 2.9\%$[a]
Riboflavin deficient	32	$16.2 \pm 4.8\%$	$35.5 \pm 3.6\%$	$87.5 \pm 6.4\%$

[a] All values expressed as percentages of the concentrations measured in tumors grown
in normal animals (mean ± s.e.m.). Values in Novikoff hepatoma from normal animals
are:
Riboflavin $0.069 \pm 0.024 \ \mu g/g$ fresh wt.
FMN $0.460 \pm 0.045 \ \mu g/g$ fresh wt.
FAD $1.82 \pm 0.500 \ \mu g/g$ fresh wt.
(Data derived from Rivlin et al.[60])

concentrations in tumor was significantly greater than that of either
FMN or FAD ($p < 0.001$).

These results indicate that the Novikoff hepatoma shows a remarkable resistance to riboflavin deficiency: FAD concentrations are completely
intact and FMN levels are decreased proportionately less than are those
of host liver. Aptekar,[2,3] as noted above, reported a decrease in the
hepatic concentration of FAD in animals bearing one form of ascites
hepatomas, but no change in either FAD, FMN, or riboflavin concentrations in animals bearing other varieties of transplanted tumors.

One physiological mechanism that appears to be involved in the
adaptation of normal animals to riboflavin deficiency is the increase
in hepatic FAD pyrophosphorylase activity. The relatively greater decrease in FMN than in FAD concentrations in liver of deficient
animals [8,9,14,37,48] may be mediated in part by an adaptive increase in
the activity of this enzyme, which converts FMN to FAD.[14] It is of
interest that, in the Novikoff hepatoma grown in riboflavin-deficient
rats, FMN levels decrease proportionately more than FAD levels but
no increase in FAD pyrophosphorylase activity occurs.[59] It is likely,
therefore, that tumor tissue conserves FAD by different mechanisms,
such as more efficient uptake, greater trapping, tighter binding to tissue
flavoprotein apoenzymes, or a decrease in the rate of enzymatic FAD
degradation. Information on these points is not available at present.
The fact that the free riboflavin content of the tumor is depleted to
an extremely low level suggests that one of the mechanisms that permits
tumor to preserve its concentrations of flavin coenzymes required for
vital metabolic processes is to sacrifice the relatively small and dispensable
supply of stored free vitamin.

In additional studies, the rate of formation of ^{14}C-FAD from

[14]C-riboflavin was determined in tumor and liver using newly devised techniques of isotope dilution and ion exchange column chromatography. In tumor from riboflavin-deficient rats, rates of ^{14}C-FAD synthesis were unchanged from that in tumor from nondeficient animals, but radioactivity remaining as ^{14}C-riboflavin in tumor from deficient rats was markedly less than that in tumor from nondeficient rats. The data further suggest that the Novikoff hepatoma apparently maintains its high FAD concentration despite dietary riboflavin restriction by at least two mechanisms: (a) maintaining its own high rate of FAD synthesis, and (b) utilizing nearly completely the dispensable supply of free riboflavin.[15]

The thyroid hormonal regulation of riboflavin-dependent enzymes has been examined in both well-differentiated (Morris hepatoma 7800) and poorly differentiated (Novikoff) hepatomas in rats. The induction by thyroid hormone of the FAD-dependent enzyme, mitochondrial α-glycerophosphate dehydrogenase, five- to tenfold in normal liver, is undetectable in Novikoff hepatoma, is diminished but present (twofold) in Morris hepatoma 7800, and is completely intact in livers of rats bearing either tumor.[27] Karsten *et al.*[29] have also shown no increase in activity of this enzyme in several transplanted hepatomas after treatment with thyroid hormone.

These studies indicate in sum that flavin concentrations and activities of flavoprotein enzymes in tumor tissue are relatively resistant both to hormonal and to nutritional regulation. Neoplastic liver differs from normal liver in the total concentrations and relative amounts of riboflavin and its coenzyme derivatives.

6. SUMMARY AND CONCLUSIONS

The relationship of riboflavin to cancer is intriguing, but many gaps remain in our knowledge. Several studies indicate that riboflavin deficiency inhibits tumor growth in experimental animals and possibly in man, but the precise mechanisms involved have not been elucidated. Azo dye carcinogenesis in liver appears to be a special case in that riboflavin deficiency increases the potency of these drugs in tumor causation, probably in large measure because flavin cofactors are involved in their metabolic degradation. Riboflavin influences uptake of the chemotherapeutic drugs in at least one instance (methotrexate) into neoplastic cells.

Neoplastic liver appears to lack certain mechanisms that regulate riboflavin metabolism in normal tissues. In addition, it is more resistant than normal liver to riboflavin deficiency, as reflected in the relatively higher concentrations of FMN and FAD measured in samples of the Novikoff hepatoma than in the host rat liver. By contrast, the concentration of free riboflavin is greatly depressed in Novikoff hepatoma grown in riboflavin-deficient animals. The loss of this relatively dispensable flavin fraction may be one of the mechanisms that enable tumor to retain the more critical FMN and FAD fractions when dietary riboflavin is diminished. Much remains to be learned about the uptake, turnover, binding, and removal of riboflavin and its derivatives from neoplastic tissue.

7. REFERENCES

1. Aposhian, H. V., and Lambooy, J. P. 1951. Retardation of growth of Walker rat carcinoma 256 by administration of diethyl riboflavin, *Proc. Soc. Exptl. Biol. Med.* **78**:197–199.
2. Aptekar, S. G. 1962. Riboflavin content in the organs of rats with transplanted tumors, *Arkh. Patol.* **24**:45–52.
3. Aptekar, S. G., and Ganetskaia, S. A. 1965. Riboflavin content in the organs of mice with transplanted tumors, *Arkh. Patol.* **27**:63–65.
4. Bebawi, G. M., Kim, Y. S., and Lambooy, J. P. 1970. A study of the carcinogenicity of a series of structurally related 4-dimethylaminoazobenzenes, *Cancer Res.* **30**:1520–1524.
5. Begg, R. W., and Dickenson, T. E. 1951. Systemic effects of tumors in force-fed rats, *Cancer Res.* **11**:409–412.
6. Bertino, J. R., and Nixon, P. F. 1969. Nutritional factors in the design of more selective antitumor agents, *Cancer Res.* **29**:2417–2421.
7. Bovina, C., Landi, L., Pasquali, P., and Marchetti, M. 1969. Biosynthesis of folate coenzymes in riboflavin-deficient rats, *J. Nutr.* **99**:320–324.
8. Burch, H. B., Lowry, O. H., Padilla, A. M., and Combs, A. M. 1956. Effects of riboflavin deficiency and realimentation on flavin enzymes of tissues, *J. Biol. Chem.* **223**:29–45.
9. Catz, C. S., Jachau, M. R., and Yaffe, S. J. 1970. Effects of iron, riboflavin and iodide deficiencies on hepatic drug-metabolizing enzyme systems, *J. Pharmacol. Exptl. Therap.* **174**:197–205.
10. Chan, P. C., Okamoto, T., and Wynder, E. L. 1972. Possible role of riboflavin deficiency in epithelial neoplasia. III. Induction of microsomal aryl hydrocarbon hydroxylase, *J. Natl. Cancer Inst,* **48**:1341–1345.
11. Costa, G., and Weathers, A. P. 1964. Cancer and the nutrition of the host, *J. Amer. Diet. Assoc.* **44**:15–17.
12. David, V. H., Velkov, A. Marx, I., and Velkov, M. 1972. Structure and RNA synthesis-performance of Ehrlich ascites tumor cell nucleus following action of dinitrophenol and riboflavin. *Exptl. Pathol. (JENA)* **7**:36–44.
13. DeWys, W. 1970. Working conference on anorexia and cachexia of neoplastic disease, *Cancer Res.* **30**:2816–2818.

14. Fass, S., and Rivlin, R. S. 1969. Regulation of riboflavin-metabolizing enzymes in riboflavin deficiency, *Amer. J. Physiol.* **217**:988-991.
15. Fazekas, A. G., Chaudhuri, R., and Rivlin, R. S. 1974. Adaptation of a transplantable hepatoma to riboflavin deficiency, *J. Clin. Invest.* **53**:27a (Abstr.).
16. Foy, H., Kondi, A., and Mbaya, V. 1966. Serum vitamin B12 and folate levels in normal and riboflavin-deficient baboons (*Papio anubis*), *Brit. J. Haemat.* **12**:239-245.
17. Gailani, S. D., Holland, J. F., Nussbaum, A., and Olson, K. B. 1968. Clinical and biochemical studies of pyridoxine deficiency in patients with neoplastic diseases, *Cancer* **21**:975-988.
18. Goldman, I. D. 1971. The characteristics of the membrane transport of amethopterin and the naturally occurring folates, *Ann. N. Y. Acad. Sci.* **186**:400-422.
19. Goldman, I. D., Lichtenstein, N. S., and Oliverio, V. T. 1968. Carrier-mediated transport of the folic acid analogue, methotrexate, in the L1210 Leukemia cell, *J. Biol. Chem.* **243**:5007-5017.
20. Griffin, A. C., and Baumann, C. A. 1946. Effect of certain azo dyes upon storage of riboflavin in the liver, *Arch. Biochem.* **11**:467-476.
21. Griffin, A. C., and Baumann, C. A. 1948. Hepatic riboflavin and tumor formation in rats fed azo dyes in various diets, *Cancer Res.* **8**:279-284.
22. Hakala, M. T. 1965. On the nature of permeability of sarcoma-180 cells to amethopterin *in vitro, Biochem. Biophys. Acta* **102**:210-225.
23. Henderson, J. F., and LePage, G. A. 1959. The nutrition of tumors: A review, *Cancer Res.* **19**:887-902.
24. Holly, F. W., Peel, E. W., Mozingo, R., and Folkers, K. 1950. Studies on carcinolytic compounds. 1. 6,7-Dichloro-9-(1'-D-sorbityl)-isoalloxazine, *J. Amer. Chem. Soc.* **72**:5416-5418.
25. Homburger, F., and Young, N. F. 1948. Studies on hypoproteinemia; Hypoproteinemia in patients with gastric cancer; its persistence after operation in the presence of body tissue repletion, *Blood* **3**:1460-1471.
26. Honda, Y. 1968. Folate derivatives in the liver of riboflavin-deficient rats, *Tohoku J. Exptl. Med.* **95**:79-86.
27. Hunt, S. M., Osnos, M., and Rivlin, R. S. 1970. Thyroid hormone regulation of mitchondrial α-glycerophosphate dehydrogenase in liver and hepatoma, *Cancer Res.* **30**:1764-1768.
28. Kagan, Y. A. 1960. Riboflavin determination in the urine of patients suffering from malignant neoplasms, *Khirurg.* **2**:103-108.
29. Karsten, U., Sydow, G., Wollenberger, A., and Graffi, A. 1971. Rat liver glycerophosphate dehydrogenases: Activity changes and induction by thyroid hormone of the mitochondrial enzyme in hepatomas and in precancerous and growing liver, *Acta Biol. Med. Germany* **26**:1131-1140.
30. Kato, R., Takanaka, A., Takahashi, A., and Onada, K. 1968. Drug metabolism in tumor-bearing rats. I. Activities of NADPH-linked electron transport and drug-metabolizing enzyme systems in liver microsomes of tumor-bearing rats, *Japan. J. Pharmacol.* **18**:224-244.
31. Kensler, C. J. 1947. Effect of diet on the production of liver tumors in the rat by N, N-dimethyl-p-aminoazobenzene, *Ann. N. Y. Acad. Sci.* **49**:29-40.
32. Kensler, C. J., Suguira, K., and Rhoads, C. P. 1940. Coenzyme 1 and riboflavin content of livers of rats fed butter yellow, *Science* **91**:623.
33. Kim, Y. S., Aposhian, M. M., and Lambooy, J. P. 1966. The influence of homologs of riboflavin on the growth of Walker rat carcinoma 256, *Cancer Res.* **26**:1344-1348.

34. Kitsmanyuk, Z. D. 1967. Riboflavin content in the blood and urine in patients with cancer of the larynx in dynamics, *Zh. Ushn. Nos. Gozl. Bolez.* **28**:80-83.

35. Kitsmanyuk, Z. D., Derbina, M. M., and Teleshova, V. A. 1973. Thiamine and riboflavin content in patients with tumors and inflammatory diseases of the maxilla, *Stomatologiia (Mosk.)* **52**:91-92.

36. Kline, B. E., Rusch, H. P., Baumann, C. A., and Lavik, P. S. 1943. The effect of pyridoxine on tumor growth, *Cancer Res.* **3**:825-829.

37. Lakhanpal, R. K., Harrill, I., and Bowman, F. 1969. Effect of protein and riboflavin on plasma amino acids and hepatic riboflavin-coenzymes in the rat, *J. Nutr.* **99**:497-501.

38. Lambooy, J. P. 1970. Riboflavin protection against azo dye hepatoma induction in the rat, *Proc. Soc. Exptl. Biol. Med.* **134**:192-194.

39. Lambooy, J. P. 1970. Riboflavin and azo dye induced hepatomas in the rat, *Federation Proc.* **29**:296 (Abstr.).

40. Lane, M. 1971. Induced riboflavin deficiency in treatment of patients with lymphomas and polycythemia vera, *Proc. Amer. Assoc. Cancer Res.* **12**:85 (Abstr.).

41. Lane, M., Alfrey, C. P., Jr., Mengel, C. E., Doherty, M. A., and Doherty, J. 1964. The rapid induction of human riboflavin deficiency with galactoflavin *J. Clin. Invest.* **43**:357-373.

42. Lane, M., Fahey, J. L., Sullivan, R. D., and Zubrod, C. G. 1958. The comparative pharmacology in man and the rat of the riboflavin analogue, 6,7-dimethyl-9-(2' acetoxyethyl)-isoalloxazine, U-2112, *J. Pharmacol. Exptl. Therap.* **122**:315-326.

43. Lichtenstein, N. S., and Goldman, I. D. 1970. Riboflavin-methotrexate interactions. Photochemical reaction and competition for transport in the L1210 mouse leukemia cell, *Biochem. Pharmacol.* **19**:1229-1239.

44. Mider, G. B. 1951. Some aspects of nitrogen and energy metabolism in cancerous subjects, *Cancer Res.* **11**:821-829.

45. Mihich, E., and C. A. Nichol. 1959. The effect of pyridoxine deficiency on mouse sarcoma 180, *Cancer Res.* **19**:279-284.

46. Miller, J. A. 1947. Studies on the mechanism of the effects of fats and other dietary factors on carcinogenesis by the azo dyes, *Ann. N. Y. Acad. Sci.* **49**:19-28.

47. Miller, J. A., and Miller, E. C. 1953. Carcinogenic azo dyes, *Advan. Cancer Res.* **1**:339-396.

48. Miller, Z., Poncet, I., and Takacs, E. 1962. Biochemical studies on experimental congenital malformations: Flavin nucleotides and folic acid in fetuses and livers from normal and riboflavin-deficient rats, *J. Biol. Chem.* **237**:968-973.

49. Morris, H. P. 1947. Effects on the genesis and growth of tumors associated with vitamin intake, *Ann. N. Y. Acad. Sci.* **49**:119-140.

50. Morris, H. P., and Robertson, W. V. B. 1943. Growth rate and number of spontaneous mammary carcinomas and riboflavin concentration of liver, muscle, and tumor of C3H mice as influenced by dietary riboflavin, *J. Natl. Cancer Inst.* **3**:479-489.

51. Mulay, A. S., and O'Gara, R. W. 1968. Enhancing effect of a riboflavin analog on azo-dye carcinogenesis in rats, *J. Natl. Cancer Inst.* **40**:731-735.

52. Narisawa, K., Tamura, T., Honda, Y., Tanno, K., Ohara, K., and Arakawa, T. 1969. Increased urinary excretion of ^{3}H-folic acid injected to rats with riboflavin deficiency or excessive dietary methionine, *Tohoku J. Exp. Med.* **97**:263-268.

53. Narisawa, K., Tamura, T., Tanno, K., Honda, Y., Ohara, K., and Arakawa, T. 1968. Tetrahydrofolate-dependent enzyme activities of the rat liver with riboflavin deficiency, *Tohoku J. Exptl. Med.* **94**:417-430.

54. Okuda, K., and Haruna, K. 1959. Changes of some flavin enzymes in the liver of rat during DAB carcinogenesis, *Gann* **51**:153-158.

55. Pasquali, P., Bovina, C., Landi, L., and Marchetti, M. 1969. Studies on relationships between riboflavin and folate, *Experientia* **25:**1031-1032.

56. Ringenberg, L. K., and Lambooy, J. P. 1973. Succinic acid dehydrogenase activity of Walker Rat Carcinoma 256 when utilizing riboflavin homologs, *Proc. Soc. Exptl. Biol. Med.* **143:**1211-1214.

57. Rivlin, R. S. 1970. Medical Progress: Riboflavin metabolism, *New Eng. J. Med.* **283:**463-472.

58. Rivlin, R. S. 1973. Riboflavin and Cancer: A review, *Cancer Res.* **33:**1977-1986.

59. Rivlin, R. S. and Hornibrook, R. 1970. Disturbances in control of flavin metabolism in neoplastic tissue, *Federation Proc.* **29:**799 (Abstr.).

60. Rivlin, R. S., Hornibrook, R., and Osnos, M. 1973. Effects of riboflavin deficiency upon concentrations of riboflavin, flavin mononucleotide, and flavin adenine dinucleotide in Novikoff hepatoma in rats, *Cancer Res.* **33:**3019-3023.

61. Rivlin, R. S., Menendez, C., and Langdon, R. G. 1968. Biochemical similarities between hypothyroidism and riboflavin deficiency, *Endocrinol.* **83:**461-469.

62. Roe, F. J. C. 1962. Effect of massive doses of riboflavin, and other vitamins of the B group, on skin carcinogenesis in mice, *Brit. J. Cancer* **16:**252-257.

63. Rubenchik, B. L. 1963. Changes in riboflavin content in the course of experimentally induced carcinogenesis in rats, *Vop. Pitan.* **22:**799-802.

64. Saxton, J. A., Boon, M. C., and Furth, J. 1944. Observations on the inhibition of development of spontaneous leukemia in mice by underfeeding, *Cancer Res.* **4:**401-409.

65. Shargel, L., and Mazel, P. 1973. Effect of riboflavin deficiency on phenobarbital and 3-methylcholanthrene induction of microsomal drug-metabolizing enzymes of the rat, *Biochem. Pharmacol.* **22:**2365-2373.

66. Stewart, A. G., and Begg, R. W. 1953. Systemic effects of tumors in force-fed rats. 11. Effect on the weight of carcass, adrenals, thymus, liver, and spleen, *Cancer Res.* **13:**556-559.

67. Stoerk, H. C., and Emerson, G. A. 1949. Complete regression of lymphosarcoma implants following temporary induction of riboflavin deficiency in mice, *Proc. Soc. Exptl. Biol. Med.* **70:**703-704.

68. Tannenbaum, A., and Silverstone, H. 1953. Nutrition in relation to cancer, *Advan. Cancer Res.* **1:**451-501.

69. Terepka, A. R., and Waterhouse, C. 1956. Metabolic observations during the forced feeding of patients with cancer, *Amer. J. Med.* **20:**225-238.

70. Theologides, A. 1972. Pathogenesis of cachexia in cancer. A review and a hypothesis, *Cancer* **29:**484-488.

71. Tscherkes, L. A., and S. G. Aptekar. 1960. Urinary riboflavin excretion in experimental tumours, *Arkh. Patol.* **22:**27-38.

72. Tung, T.-C., and Lin, J.-K. 1964. The interaction of riboflavin with 4-dimethylaminoazobenzene and 4-aminoazobenzene, *J. Formosan Med. Assoc.* **63:**225-233.

73. Visscher, M. B., Ball, Z. B., Barnes, R. H., and Sivertsen, I. 1942. The influence of caloric restriction upon the incidence of spontaneous mammary carcinoma in mice, *Surgery* **11:**48-55.

74. Warburg, V. O., Geissler, A. W., and Lorenz, S. 1967. Wirkung von Riboflavin und von δ-amino-Lävulinsäure auf wachsende Krebszellen *in vitro*, *Hoppe-Seyler's Z. Physiol. Chem.* **348:**1683-1685.

75. Warburg. V. O., Geissler, A. W., and Lorenz, S. 1968. Wirkung von Riboflavin und Luminoflavin auf wachsende Krebszellen, *A. Klin. Chem. Klin. Biochem.* **5:**467-468.

76. Westerfeld, W. W., Richert, D. A., and Hilfinger, M. D. 1950. Studies on xanthine oxidase during carcinogenesis by ρ-dimethylaminoazobenzene, *Cancer Res.* **10:**486-494.

77. Williams, J. R., Grantham, P. H., Yamamoto, R. S., and Weisburger, J. H. 1970. Effect of dietary riboflavin on azo dye reductase in liver and in bacteria of cecal contents in rat, *Biochem. Pharmacol.* **19**:2523-2525.
78. Wynder, E. L., and Chan, P. C. 1970. The possible role of riboflavin deficiency in epithelial neoplasia. II. Effect of skin tumor development, *Cancer* **26**:1221-1224.
79. Wynder, E. L., and Klein, U. E. 1965. The possible role of riboflavin deficiency in epithelial neoplasia. I. Epithelial changes of mice in simple deficiency, *Cancer* **18**:167-180.
80. Yang, C. S. 1974. Alterations of the aryl hydrocarbon hydroxylase system during riboflavin depletion and repletion, *Arch. Biochem. Biophys.* **160**:623-630.
81. Yang, W.-K., and Sung, J.-L. 1966. Riboflavin metabolism in liver diseases. IV. Enzymatic splitting and synthesis of flavin adenine dinucleotide in the p-dimethylaminoazobenzene induced rat liver carcinoma tissue, *J. Formosan Med. Assoc.* **65**:299-305.

12

HORMONAL REGULATION OF RIBOFLAVIN METABOLISM

Richard S. Rivlin

1. INTRODUCTION

The endocrine glands play an important role in the control of various aspects of riboflavin metabolism. The conversion of the vitamin into its active coenzyme derivatives, FMN and FAD, is subject to hormonal regulation. Hormones influence the metabolic utilization of the vitamin, the magnitude of tissue concentrations, the rate of excretion in urine, and, in certain species, the transport of the vitamin in plasma. Disturbances in the metabolism of riboflavin accompany endocrine disorders both in experimental animals and in man.

Riboflavin, in turn, has important effects upon the endocrine system. In riboflavin deficiency, structural and functional changes occur in the endocrine glands. Both the synthesis and the peripheral degradation of certain hormones are altered in riboflavin deficiency. Responses to the administration of hormones may be inhibited or modified in riboflavin deficiency.

RICHARD S. RIVLIN—Department of Medicine, Francis Delafield Hospital and Presbyterian Hospital; and Institute of Human Nutrition, College of Physicians & Surgeons of Columbia University, New York, New York. This work was supported by USPHS grants AM15265 and CA12126 and by the Stella and Charles Guttman Foundation.

This chapter reviews the accumulated knowledge concerning these various vitamin-hormone relationships. Particular attention has been paid to the recent advances that have been made in the understanding of how endocrine control is exerted upon riboflavin metabolism.

2. ANDROGEN AND ESTROGEN

2.1. Glandular Structure in Riboflavin Deficiency

The effects of riboflavin deficiency upon the sex organs of the young male rat were investigated by Shaw and Phillips.[96] As riboflavin deficiency progressed for 4-6 weeks, atrophy of the testes, epididymis, prostate, and seminal vesicles was demonstrable. On microscopic examination, the seminiferous tubules were underdeveloped, with diminished spermatogenesis and a decrease in the rate of cell division. These findings occurred only in riboflavin-deficient animals and were not observed in animals that were subjected to food restriction alone.

In subsequent reports of severely deficient animals, similar findings were observed.[22,23] In chickens that had been made riboflavin deficient by dietary means, semen volume was markedly diminished and, in the late stages of deficiency, was not adequate for satisfactory insemination.[2] In a recent study in which rats received riboflavin-deficient diets for a relatively brief period of 20 days, no change in the size of the seminal vesicles or adrenal glands occurred.[76] Similarly, in mature male white leghorn chickens, relatively mild deficiency of riboflavin did not appear to influence semen volume or sperm metabolism.[60] On the basis of these reports, it is likely that prolonged deficiency of riboflavin is required before atrophy of the male sex organs occurs. The influence of shortages of riboflavin and of other vitamins upon the pathology of the sex organs has been reviewed previously.[103,104]

In female rats, ovarian atrophy results from riboflavin deficiency.[23] Anestrus was produced by a diet that contained no riboflavin or only minute amounts.[26,110] Realimentation of deficient animals with riboflavin alone or with milk restored normal estrus. Disturbances in reproduction and in lactation have also been observed in deficient animals. Deficiency of riboflavin during early pregnancy leads to congenital malformations in the offspring (see Chapter 9). Treatment of pregnant rats with various structural analogues of riboflavin results in poor survival of the newborn animals, even if they appear to be grossly normal (see Chapter 10).

2.2. Estrogenic Effects upon Riboflavin Binding in Plasma

The effects of estrogen upon riboflavin metabolism which have received the most concentrated study are those relating to the regulation of the riboflavin-binding protein in chickens. In an early study, Common et al.[24] administered androgen and estrogen to chickens and determined the plasma and hepatic concentrations of total riboflavin. Estradiol caused a dramatic increase in the plasma concentration of total riboflavin, as shown in Table I. In animals treated with the largest dose of hormone, the total riboflavin levels in serum increased from less than 0.1 μg/ml to more than 5.0 μg/ml. Testosterone proprionate, when given together with estradiol, appeared to blunt somewhat the estradiol-provoked increase in serum riboflavin concentrations. Little, if any, change occurred in the hepatic concentration of riboflavin after administration of either androgen or estrogen.

The effect of estrogen upon increasing the plasma concentration of riboflavin in chickens was subsequently shown to be due to the induction of a specific riboflavin-binding protein. Rhodes[82] first demonstrated that the egg white of chickens contains a specific glycoprotein that has a high affinity for riboflavin, much higher than that for either FMN or FAD. An identical protein is found in egg white, egg yolk, and the serum of laying hens,[35] and is under the control of a single

TABLE I. Effect of Administration of Estradiol and Testosterone upon the Serum and Hepatic Concentrations of Total Riboflavin* in Female Chickens

Animal number	Treatment given		Total riboflavin concentration	
	Estradiol mg/dose	Testosterone, mg/dose	Serum, μg/ml	Liver, μg/ml
1	—	—	0.03	24.4
2	1.0	—	0.62	29.0
3	2.0	—	2.65	24.6
4	4.0	—	5.32	23.3
5	—	0.75	0.17	28.2
6	1.0	0.75	0.07	32.9
7	2.0	0.75	1.45	25.6
8	4.0	0.75	4.94	22.9

White Wyandotte pullets at 82 days of age received a total of six intramuscular injections administered on alternate days. Animals were sacrificed on the second day after the last dose, at 94 days of age.

Total riboflavin* = free riboflavin + FMN + FAD (Ed. note: The method for measuring riboflavin is not stated in the text. Judging from the figures given, it is likely that this method measures not only riboflavin, but FMN and FAD as well.)

(Data are adapted from Common et al.[24] with the permission of the publisher.)

gene.[18] Discussion of a mutant strain of birds which lacks the binding protein virtually completely is given in Chapter 5.

   In addition to genetic control, the riboflavin-binding protein of birds is also subject to endocrine regulation. Following administration of estrogen to female chickens at least 8 weeks of age as well as to normal males,[19,35] the concentration of the riboflavin-binding protein in blood can be increased dramatically. Results of studies in male chickens are shown in Fig. 1.

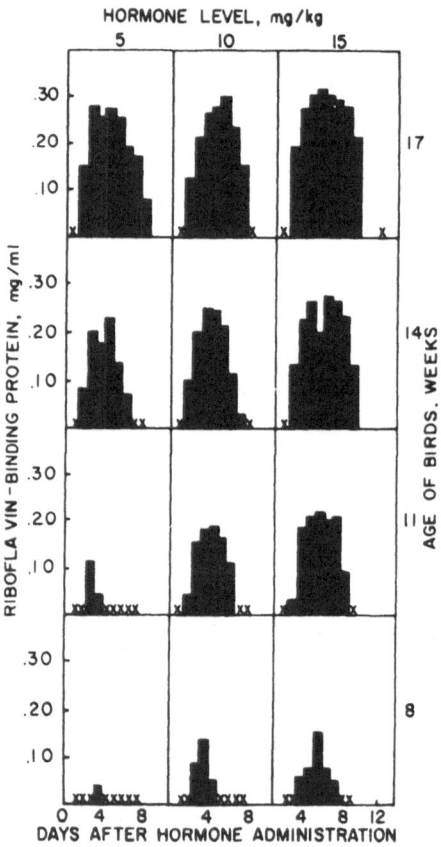

Fig. 1. Effect of administration of 17β-estradiol upon the plasma concentration of riboflavin-binding protein in male chickens. Chickens aged 8, 11, 14, and 17 weeks received an intramuscular injection of the hormone at three dose levels: 5, 10, or 15 mg/kg. The concentration of the riboflavin-binding protein in plasma was determined on the day of injection and on each of the following 9 days. Data shown are the mean values obtained in each group containing three single-comb, white Leghorn chickens per group. (Reprinted from Clagett *et al.*[19] with the permission of the publisher.)

In birds 8 weeks of age treated with the lowest dose of estradiol, the riboflavin-binding protein could be detected at low concentrations in plasma 4 days after administration of the hormone. With increasing doses of estradiol, the protein was detected earlier and at greater concentrations. When older birds were treated similarly, both the magnitude and the duration of the increase in the protein concentration in plasma were progressively greater. In normal female chickens below the age of 8 weeks and in homozygous males with the genetic disorder, no increase in the concentration of the riboflavin-binding protein in plasma was demonstrable.[19,35] It is likely that estradiol induces the synthesis of this specific protein, although the nature of the process has not yet been elucidated. In a further study,[25] the suggestion was considered that the estradiol-provoked increase in serum riboflavin levels might be due to enhanced intestinal absorption. This possibility appears to have been excluded by the finding that estradiol administration did not significantly alter the rate of transport of riboflavin across everted segments of small intestine.

Little is known about the effects of sex hormones upon riboflavin metabolism in man. One point of interest is that human fetal blood contains more free riboflavin and less FAD than does maternal blood.[62] The administration of riboflavin in daily doses of 2-4 mg to a group of anemic, pregnant women already receiving iron and folic acid increased the mean corpuscular riboflavin concentration of both maternal and cord blood, but did not have a significant effect upon the hematocrit.[21] Mechanisms for transport of riboflavin from the maternal to the fetal circulation in man and the role of estrogen and androgen upon plasma binding of the vitamin have not been elucidated.

3. INSULIN AND DIABETES

3.1. Blood Sugar Levels in Riboflavin Deficiency

A relationship between riboflavin and carbohydrate metabolism was suggested by early reports regarding dogs[3] and rats[111] that prolonged deficiency of the vitamin reduces blood sugar concentrations below normal levels. In dogs in late stages of riboflavin deficiency, blood sugar levels were often profoundly low, approaching 20-30 mg/100 ml. These results were not obtained in all riboflavin-deficient animals, however, and it is unclear whether hypoglycemia could be related either

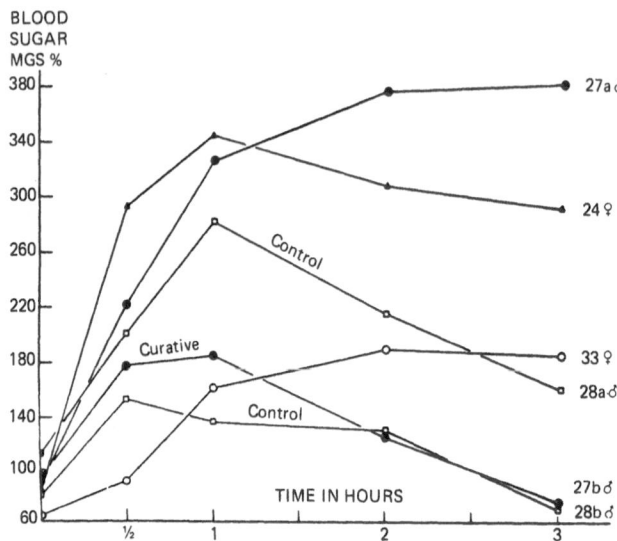

Fig. 2. Results of blood sugar determinations in normal and riboflavin-deficient dogs after receiving 25-50 g glucose by stomach tube. Blood samples were obtained at zero time and for the next 3 hr. The code is as follows:

27a ♂—severely riboflavin deficient

27b ♂—same animal as 27a ♂ studied 78 days after riboflavin repletion

24 ♀—riboflavin deficient, also treated with 5 mg desoxycorticosterone acetate

33 ♀—riboflavin-deficient

28a ♂—normal animal

28b ♂—same normal animal as 28a ♂

(Reprinted from Axelrod, Gullberg, and Morgan[4] with permission of the publisher.)

to the duration or to the severity of the deficient state. In normal rats that were pair-fed to deficient animals, blood sugar levels were completely normal.

In later studies in riboflavin-deficient dogs, fasting blood sugar levels somewhat greater than normal were noted.[4] Oral glucose tolerance tests performed in these animals revealed a diabetic response, with greater and more prolonged elevation of the blood sugar in deficient than in normal animals. The results of some of these experiments are shown in Fig. 2. In one riboflavin-deficient dog (27a) peak blood sugar levels of 380 mg% were obtained 2-3 hr after glucose administration. After refeeding of riboflavin to this animal (27b) the highest blood sugar level was only 180 mg% and was recorded 1 hr after glucose administration. Similar although less dramatic differences were noted between the remainder of the normal and deficient animals in this report. As noted earlier,[3,111] when dogs were in the terminal stages of riboflavin deficiency, blood sugar levels were decreased below normal levels.

3.2. Response to Insulin in Riboflavin Deficiency

Suggestive evidence that insulin regulation of glucose metabolism may be disturbed in riboflavin deficiency was provided by the studies of Ershoff.[34] The change in blood glucose concentration in response to injection of insulin was determined in young female rats receiving

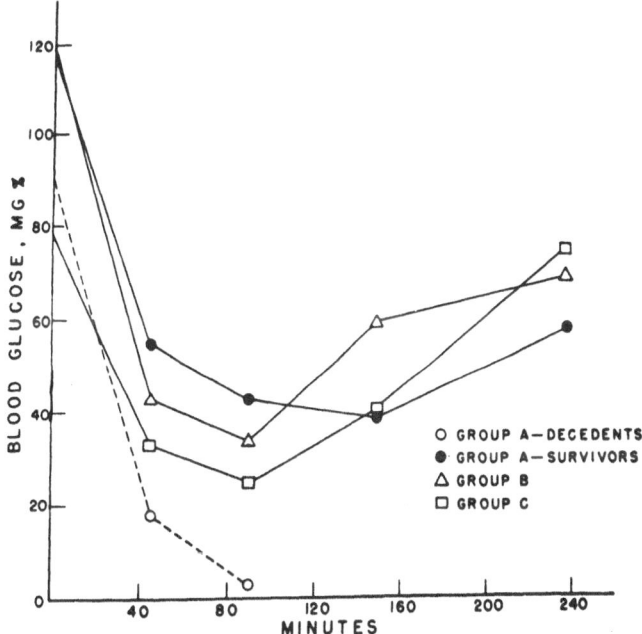

Fig. 3. Change in blood sugar concentration after administration of insulin to normal and riboflavin deficient rats. Data are represented as the mean results obtained in 20 riboflavin-deficient animals (group A), 10 rats fed a normal diet (group B), and 10 rats fed a normal diet restricted in amount (group C) to that ingested by group A. Data for riboflavin deficient animals were divided into two groups, those that remained alive and those that died during the experimental period. Animals each received a single subcutaneous injection of insulin, 0.1 unit/100 g body weight at 0 time, and blood samples were obtained at intervals for the next 4 hr. Animals were all female rats of the Long-Evans strain, weighing 45-54 g at the start of the experiments. Diets were fed for a 28-day period prior to the study. (Reprinted from Ershoff [34] with the permission of the publisher.)

either a riboflavin-deficient diet, a normal diet *ad libitum,* or a normal diet restricted in quantity to the amount ingested by the deficient animals. The results of these experiments are shown in Fig. 3. After administration of insulin, two-thirds of the deficient animals died, their blood sugar concentrations having decreased to below 20 mg%. In the remaining one-third of the deficient animals that survived, blood sugar levels before and after insulin administration were indistinguishable from those of either set of controls. The mechanism of the apparent increase in sensitivity to insulin exhibited by some but not all of the riboflavin-deficient rats was not provided by this report. It is possible that variability in the nutritional intake of the animals could account for some of the individual differences observed.

3.3 Glycogen Synthesis

In early reports,[111] liver glycogen concentrations in riboflavin-deficient animals tended to be in the low–normal range. In response to anoxia, glycogen concentrations in liver of normal animals and of pair-fed controls increased thirteenfold but in deficient animals increased only threefold. The concentration of glycogen in muscle was not affected either by riboflavin deficiency or by pair feeding.[111] More recent studies by Chatterjee *et al.*[14,17] suggest that liver glycogen concentrations in riboflavin-deficient rats may actually be greater than normal. Glycogen concentrations in deficient animals were significantly increased over levels in pair-fed controls when expressed either per gram of liver or per 100 grams body weight. The elevated levels of hepatic glycogen were attributed to increased gluconeogenesis, mediated in part by elevated alanine transaminase activity. Evidence that alanine was converted to glycogen at a greater rate than normal in riboflavin-deficient rats was provided by the subsequent demonstration of elevated specific activity of glycogen after administration of alanine-1-^{14}C.[14]

3.4. Riboflavin Metabolism in Clinical Diabetes

Studies of riboflavin metabolism in clinical diabetes were performed by Fujimoto *et al.*[46] The basal excretion of riboflavin during a 3-hr collection period was much greater in diabetics than in normal subjects. With successful treatment of the hyperglycemia, riboflavin excretion decreased toward normal. Both in normal subjects and in diabetics, administration of glucose was followed by a rise in the urinary concentration of riboflavin. To some extent, changes in the excretion of riboflavin in the severely ill diabetic patients might have been a reflection of negative nitrogen balance, a factor that by itself may increase the urinary excretion of riboflavin.[71] Administration of glucose to normal individuals also increased the excretion of lactoflavin.[107] The physiological significance of the latter finding is unknown.

In diabetic subjects not only is the basal excretion of riboflavin increased, but there is also an increase in excretion of an oral load. Lossy et al.[61] collected the urine of diabetic patients for up to 4 hr following ingestion of a multivitamin tablet containing 5 mg of riboflavin. Results of these studies are shown in Table II. In normal subjects, the 4-hr excretion of riboflavin after an administered load did not differ from that recorded in a group of miscellaneous hospital patients. In subjects with a restricted intake of B vitamins, the urinary excretion of riboflavin after a vitamin load as expected was less than normal. By contrast, in diabetic patients the excretion of riboflavin was significantly increased to nearly 50% above that in control subjects. Of the other vitamins determined in urine of diabetic subjects, thiamin was the only one increased above normal. Information concerning the ages and sex of the subjects, the urine volumes, and the basal vitamin excretion before administration of a load was not provided in this report.

Further evidence of increased excretion of riboflavin in diabetics was obtained nearly simultaneously by Pollack and Bookman.[77] They noted that in normal subjects the loss of urinary riboflavin varied directly

TABLE II. *Urinary Excretion of Riboflavin in Normal and Diabetic Subjects During a 4-Hr Period After Ingestion of a Multivitamin Dose Containing 5 mg Riboflavin*

Treatment group	Number of patients	Urinary riboflavin content, μg	Significance of difference from control subjects
(1) Control Subjects	52	1850 ± 98 [a]	—
(2) Miscellaneous hospital patients	14	1782 ± 115	N.S.
(3) Subjects receiving diets low in B vitamins	12	1195 ± 88	$p < 0.001$
(4) Patients with diabetes mellitus	22	2630 ± 11	$p < 0.001$

[a] Mean ± 1 s.e.m.
(Data are adapted from Lossy et al.[61] with the permission of the publisher.)

with the degree of negative nitrogen balance, as had been noted previously.[71] Withdrawal of insulin from the diabetic patients resulted in negative nitrogen balance and increased excretion of riboflavin, despite the fact that the dietary intake of riboflavin was kept constant. In the diabetics, riboflavinuria appeared to correlate more closely with nitrogen balance than with urinary glucose concentrations. In several diabetic patients with extremely high urinary excretion of glucose but who nevertheless remained in positive nitrogen balance, riboflavin excretion was very low. Furthermore, in obese diabetics undergoing caloric restriction, riboflavin excretion increased when nitrogen balance became negative. These experiments strongly suggest a positive correlation between nitrogen balance and riboflavin loss in clinical diabetes, but do not exclude the possibility that insulin may have a direct effect upon riboflavin metabolism. Plasma insulin concentrations have not been measured in riboflavin deficiency either in experimental animals or in man.

In additional studies of vitamin metabolism in diabetics, Field *et al.*[41] compared the urinary excretion of riboflavin and other B vitamins in hospitalized patients who exhibited degenerative complications with patients who had no such complications, and with normal controls. The basal excretion of riboflavin in normal individuals and in both groups of diabetics was similar. Furthermore, following a loading dose of 5 mg riboflavin given together with other vitamins, the incremental increase in riboflavin excretion was similar among all three groups of patients. When insulin was withdrawn from the diabetic patients for several days, there was a suggestive increase in riboflavin excretion. Although nitrogen balance was not actually determined after insulin withdrawal, it was probably negative because the patients were losing weight at the time.

Interestingly, Fukuhara[47] noted that in rabbits intravenous administration of a highly concentrated solution of glucose decreased the urinary excretion of riboflavin. It is possible that this effect may have reflected the protein-sparing nature of glucose leading to positive nitrogen balance, or might have been due to an accompanying fall in riboflavin intake during the experimental period. In rats on a high dextrose diet, the urinary excretion of riboflavin was also reduced.[63]

It is apparent that both hypoglycemia and diabetes mellitus have been observed in riboflavin deficiency, and that the blood sugar concentration may depend to some extent upon the stage of the deficiency state. The increased excretion of riboflavin in diabetes may reflect not only the blood glucose level but also the overall nutritional status of the patient. The effects of riboflavin deficiency upon insulin secretion and carbohydrate metabolism in experimental animals and in man require further clarification.

3.5. Hypoglycin Toxicity

A further relationship between riboflavin and carbohydrate metabolism concerns the hypoglycemia that occurs after ingestion of the akee nut in Jamaica. The akee nut contains a toxic substance named hypoglycin, which has been reported to inhibit fatty acid oxidation and to block gluconeogenesis.[9] Riboflavin is effective in antagonizing toxicity due to hypoglycin. When riboflavin is given to laboratory animals even after they have received the drug, hypoglycemia is prevented. When riboflavin is given prior to hypoglycin, the mitochondrial swelling otherwise produced by hypoglycin is minimized.[10,44,109] The incidence of congenital malformations produced by hypoglycin can also be reduced by administration of riboflavin.[75] Precisely how riboflavin counteracts the toxic effects of hypoglycin is unknown.

4. ADRENAL HORMONES AND ACTH

4.1. Early Studies on Adrenalectomized Animals

A relationship between the adrenal cortex and riboflavin metabolism was first indicated by Verzar and Laszt,[108] who suggested that adrenal cortical hormones facilitate the conversion of riboflavin to FMN and increase the intestinal absorption of riboflavin. They postulated that in adrenal cortical insufficiency the conversion of riboflavin to FMN is diminished, and that the administration of FMN to adrenalectomized animals would prolong their survival.

These hypotheses were subjected to subsequent testing by Bruce and Wien.[11] The effect of riboflavin, FMN, and adrenal cortical extracts on the survival time of adrenalectomized animals was determined in animals receiving normal or riboflavin-deficient diets. Animals lacking both riboflavin and the adrenal cortex died unless they received treatment with both substances.

Nevertheless, riboflavin and FMN both exerted some beneficial effects upon the body weight and survival of adrenalectomized animals. That riboflavin and FMN were similarly effective was somewhat contrary to the theory of Verzar and Laszt.[108] The effectiveness of riboflavin and FMN in prolonging the survival time of adrenalectomized animals was also studied by Nelson.[67] Daily doses of 30–120 μg FMN or 400–800 μg riboflavin failed to increase survival time significantly.

4.2 Glandular Structure and Function in Riboflavin Deficiency

The morphology of the adrenal gland in riboflavin deficiency was determined by Deane and Shaw.[27] The adrenal gland began to decrease in size only 6 weeks after the removal of riboflavin from the diet. The lipid concentration of the adrenal cortex by histological examination remained normal. Cells in the fasciculata layer of the adrenal cortex were smaller than normal in size. These findings suggested that some degree of adrenal atrophy occurred late in riboflavin deficiency but was not particularly marked.

Evaluation of adrenal cortical function in riboflavin deficiency was performed by Forker and Morgan.[42] In response to reduced oxygen tension, liver glycogen concentrations increased in normal animals but not in riboflavin deficient animals. In response to anoxia, adrenal glands of riboflavin-deficient animals did not undergo normal depletion of ascorbic acid content. Treatment of deficient animals with cortisone resulted in normal responses to anoxia. Guggenheim and Diamant[52] observed delayed excretion of a water load in riboflavin-deficient rats which could be corrected by the administration of cortisone or ACTH. These findings suggested the possibility of some degree of adrenal cortical insufficiency in riboflavin deficiency. That the failure of adrenal ascorbic acid depletion in riboflavin animals subjected to stress may not be due specifically to a deficit of riboflavin was suggested by the subsequent investigations of Slater,[97] who showed that similar impaired responses also occurred in pair-fed control animals.

A suggestive report that adrenal cortical function does not appear to be grossly impaired in riboflavin deficiency was that of Jamdar and Mookerjea.[54] These authors found that neither the ascorbic acid concentration nor the cholesterol concentration in the adrenal gland was changed by riboflavin deficiency. The adrenal gland size and the incorporation of ^{32}P into the organic and lipid fractions of the adrenal were increased slightly in riboflavin-deficient animals.[55]

Chatterjee and Ghosh suggested that riboflavin deficiency may interfere with certain effects of cortisone. Administration of cortisone and hydrocortisone produced a greater increase in the total amino acid concentration in liver, muscle, and plasma[15] and in the plasma ascorbic acid concentration[16] in pair-fed than in riboflavin-deficient animals. By contrast, ACTH provoked a comparable decrease in the eosinophil count in peripheral blood in normal and deficient animals.[43] It is apparent that a definitive statement concerning adrenal cortical function in riboflavin deficiency is not possible on the basis of these indirect studies.

The histological and functional responses of the adrenal cortex to riboflavin deficiency in baboons were studied by Foy *et al.*[45] In animals that were riboflavin deficient for relatively brief periods of time, the adrenal glands appeared to be hypertrophic and the urinary 17-hydroxy-corticoid excretion was greater than normal. In other animals sacrificed from 10 to 24 months after the onset of riboflavin deficiency, there were gross disturbances in the structure of the adrenal cortex charac-terized by hemorrhage, disorganization fibrosis, and hypoplasia. In these animals, there was a marked decrease in the urinary 17-hydroxycorticoid excretion and in the response to ACTH. The lack of statistical treatment of the data and the difficulty in making serial determinations on each of the animals limit somewhat the conclusions that can be drawn from this report.

4.3. ACTH Stimulation of Flavin Synthesis

The most direct studies of the relation of the pituitary–adrenal axis to riboflavin metabolism are those of Fazekas and Sandor.[39,40] These investigators demonstrated that the rat adrenal gland actively forms both flavin coenzymes from riboflavin. Furthermore, ACTH administration increases the rate of synthesis of FAD to 240% and that of FMN to 160% of control values. ACTH when incubated *in vitro* with surviving slices of rat adrenal gland accelerated the conversion of riboflavin to FMN and FAD. Results of some of these studies are shown in Fig. 4. Throughout the 1-hr incubation period, the synthesis of ^{14}C-FAD from ^{14}C-riboflavin increased linearly and at a rate parallel to that of corticosterone biosynthesis. ACTH increased both corticosterone and FAD biosynthesis in a generally similar fashion. Under the influence of ACTH, the biosynthesis of FMN was greatly increased after 15 min of incubation, decreased to control levels after 30 min, and rose again after 45-60 min of incubation.[39] These findings suggest that a major effect of ACTH in the adrenal may be to increase the activity of FAD pyrophosphorylase, which converts FMN to FAD. The biosynthesis of FMN, FAD, and corticosterone was increased in the presence of 3'5'-cyclic AMP, and the stimulatory effect of ACTH was blocked by cycloheximide. The previous observation[53] that the activities of several flavoprotein enzymes in the adrenal cortex are reduced after hypophysec-tomy make it likely that removal of ACTH probably would reduce the rate of adrenal flavin synthesis.

In further studies by Fazekas and Sandor,[40] the effect of ACTH on the biosynthesis of FMN and FAD was studied in liver and kidney.

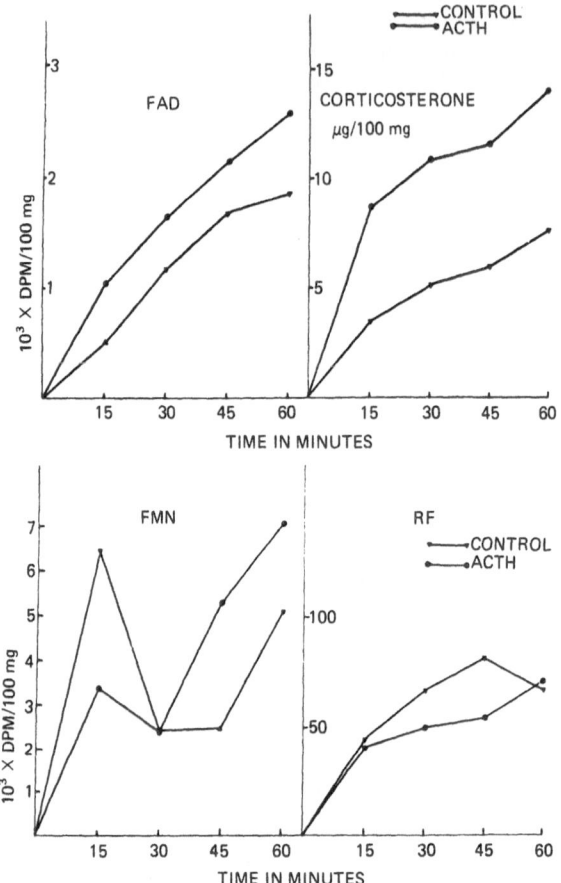

Fig. 4. Effect of ACTH *in vitro* on the biosynthesis of corticosterone, and of
¹⁴C-FAD and ¹⁴C-FMN from ¹⁴C-riboflavin by surviving rat adrenal tissue.
Samples of quartered adrenal glands from normal animals after processing were
incubated with 0.75 μCi 2-¹⁴C-riboflavin, 2 ml Krebs-Ringer bicarbonate, 3
i.u. ACTH, and various inhibitors for up to 60 min. The rates of FMN, FAD,
and corticosterone biosynthesis were determined simultaneously in flasks containing control and ACTH-treated adrenal tissue. (Reprinted from Fazekas and
Sandor[39] with the permission of the publisher.)

Results of these studies are shown in Table III. Administration of ACTH
led to an increase in the incorporation of radioactive riboflavin into
FMN but not into FAD. This finding suggests that ACTH increases
the activity of flavokinase, which catalyzes the initial conversion of
riboflavin to FMN. The lack of increase of FAD synthesis after ACTH
stimulation remains unexplained. The effects of hydrocortisone administration upon the subcellular distribution of FAD in livers of guinea

TABLE III. *Effect of Administration of ACTH upon the Biosynthesis of* ^{14}C*-FMN and* ^{14}C*-FAD from* ^{14}C*-Riboflavin in Rat Liver and Kidney in Vivo*

| | Liver | | Riboflavin |
	FAD	FMN	
Liver			
Control	17,800 ± 561	5,280 ± 221	3,430 ± 282
ACTH[a]	18,000 ± 1,310	9,920 ± 1,083[b]	3,440 ± 61
Kidney			
Control	24,500 ± 1,229	6,380 ± 365	8,660 ± 438
ACTH[a]	25,300 ± 777	10,000 ± 959[c]	8,000 ± 450

All data shown are mean ±1 s.e.m. of dpm/100 mg wet weight (five animals per group)
[a]30 I.u. ACTH injected s.c. twice daily for 2 days.
[b]Significance of difference from control = $p < 0.02$.
[c]Significance of difference from control = $p < 0.01$.
Female Wistar rats were sacrificed 1 hr after receiving a single subcutaneous injection of 5 µCi/200 g body weight of 2-^{14}C-riboflavin. Radioactivity was determined in 50-mg samples of tissue after isolation and quantitation of flavins by Sephadex G-15 column chromatography.
(Data are derived from Fazekas and Sandor[40] with the permission of the publisher.)

pigs were reported by Kuznetsova and Shestopalova.[57,58] These authors observed a decrease in the FAD concentration in nuclear but not mitochondrial or soluble fractions in hydrocortisone-treated animals. Recently, Ono *et al.*[71a,71b] have reported that in rats adrenal gland atrophy produced by dexamethasone treatment and decreased activity of adrenal gland glucose-6-phosphate dehydrogenase resulting from hypophysectomy, can both be prevented by the administration of FAD.

4.4. Clinical Studies of Riboflavin Metabolism

Clinical studies of adrenal cortical steroids in relation to riboflavin metabolism have been few in number. Rhodes and McGinty[93] observed that the administration of riboflavin and nicotinamide reduced the urinary excretion of tryptophan metabolites after injection of cortisol in several normal human subjects. It is likely that riboflavin is involved in the conversion of pyridoxine phosphate to pyridoxal phosphate, the latter coenzyme being required for several steps of tryptophan metabolism.[102]

In a group of seven patients treated with various doses of dexamethazone and triamcinolone for 8–30 days, there was no consistent alteration in the basal urinary excretion of riboflavin.[12] In view of the riboflavinuria associated with negative nitrogen balance,[71] one might have expected an increase in riboflavin excretion to occur in those patients treated with high doses of corticosteroids for a sufficient period of time. The urinary excretion of an oral load of riboflavin was also not modified by treatment with corticosteroids.

In summary, these studies suggest that some degree of functional impairment in the adrenal cortex probably occurs during riboflavin deficiency, but its nature and significance require further study. The fact that synthesis of FMN and FAD accompanies corticosteroidogenesis in the adrenal gland under the influence of ACTH suggests a possible role for riboflavin in the function of this organ, perhaps through involvement in steroid hydroxylation reactions.

5. THYROID

5.1. Early Studies Relating Riboflavin to Growth

A role for riboflavin in thyroid hormone economy was suggested by the early studies of Drill[29,30] and of Sure.[99-101] In their reports, weight loss produced by hyperthyroidism in animals could be reduced by treatment with vitamin B_2. In some instances, animals that had been treated with thyroid hormone previously could be made to regain part of the weight lost by the administration of vitamin B_2. The enhancement of weight gain appeared to be greater than that which could be accounted for by a greater intake of food alone.

The ability of riboflavin to stimulate growth in hyperthyroid animals was used by several investigators as a method of testing the biological activity of structural analogs of riboflavin. Animals were given thyroid hormone in the belief that it enhanced the development of a riboflavin-deficiency state, although there was no direct evidence that this occurred. Measurements of weight gain in hyperthyroid animals were used by Emerson and Folkers[31,32] and by Ershoff[33] to evaluate the biological activity of L-lyxoflavin.

Bertolini and Cavagna[6] reviewed the early reports on endocrine regulation of riboflavin metabolism. As part of a study of overall riboflavin economy in rats, Bessey et al.[7] measured the effects of thyroxine administration upon the whole-body concentration of riboflavin, that is, the concentration in the net carcass after removal of blood, hair, and gastrointestinal contents. In their study, animals were given thyroxine by subcutaneous injection after the animals had been kept on a riboflavin-free diet. The thyroxine-treated animals appeared to have slightly greater total body riboflavin concentration than did animals that did not receive thyroid hormone. These findings are compatible with an increase in the retention of dietary riboflavin by hyperthyroid animals and are consistent with later studies showing enhanced conversion of riboflavin into FMN and FAD.[86]

Further studies on the effects of thyroid hormone on the tissue distribution of riboflavin were performed by Rotzsch *et al.*[95] who demonstrated that the concentration of riboflavin in skeletal muscle was increased by treatment with thyroid hormone. The larger the dose of thyroid hormone, the relatively greater was the increase in riboflavin content. Physiologically active derivatives of thyroxine were also effective in raising the riboflavin concentration.

5.2. Clinical Studies of Riboflavin Metabolism in Hyperthyroidism

Clinical studies of riboflavin metabolism were performed by Barbieri and colleagues.[5] These authors noted that plasma flavin concentrations in ten patients with hyperthyroidism, whose metabolic rates ranged between +22% and +76%, were three times greater than those obtained in four normal subjects.[50] The subjects in both groups were evenly divided between male and female, but the ages of the patients were not specified. Blood samples appear to have been taken randomly, and the nutritional intake of the patients during the experimental period was not regulated. Clarke[20] also reported that in one patient with hyperthyroidism the blood riboflavin concentration was greatly increased.

Confirmatory evidence in man that increased riboflavin retention may occur in hyperthyroidism was obtained by Palagiano,[72] who measured the vitamin B_2 concentration in blood of five thyrotoxic patients and of five controls. The riboflavin concentrations per 100 g of blood were increased nearly twofold above normal in hyperthyroid subjects with no overlap of values between both groups of patients. Ten and thirty days after subtotal thyroidectomy, the riboflavin concentrations in blood were still elevated. Because results of thyroid function tests during the postoperative period were not reported, it is difficult to make an exact correlation between the plasma levels of riboflavin and the plasma levels of thyroid hormone. In further studies, Palagiano[73,74] determined the urinary excretion of riboflavin after injection of a 10-mg dose. The excretion of an administered load of riboflavin was considerably less in hyperthyroid than in normal subjects. In fact, the hyperthyroid subjects excreted less than half of the load excreted by normal subjects; 10–30 days after operation, the urinary excretion of a riboflavin load was still considerably less than that of normal individuals.

On the basis of these few reports, it is difficult to be certain of the overall status of riboflavin metabolism in clinical hyperthyroidism. There appears to be agreement that the blood levels of the vitamin are increased. The fact that increased retention of an oral dose[72] has been reported in hyperthyroidism points out the need for more definitive studies in which the nutritional intake of the patients has been carefully monitored.

5.3. Riboflavin Deficiency and Thyroid Function

An additional interrelationship between riboflavin and thyroid hormone was described by Galton and Ingbar.[49] These investigators demonstrated that in animals that were deficient in riboflavin the hepatic deiodination of thyroxine was substantially decreased. Results of some of these studies are shown in Fig. 5. The urinary iodide excretion was determined after the administration of a tracer dose of ^{131}I-thyroxine, and the percentage degradation of the hormone determined. As shown

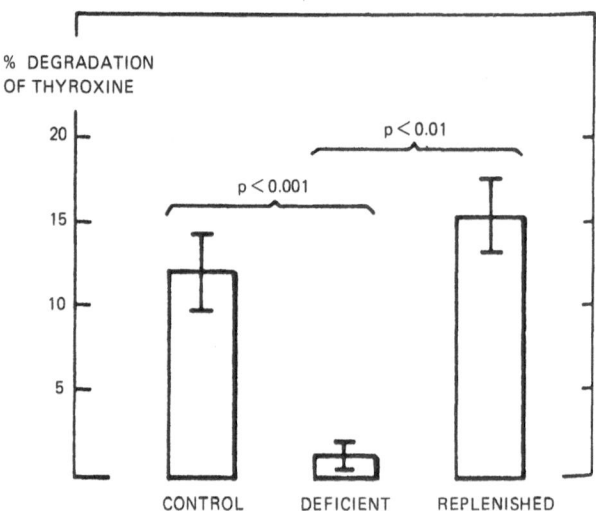

Fig. 5. Hepatic deiodination of thyroxine in normal, riboflavin-deficient, and riboflavin-deficient rats replenished with riboflavin. Data are shown as the percentage degradation of a tracer dose of ^{131}I-thyroxine given 40 hr previously. Figures are expressed as mean ± 1 s.e.m.

Studies were performed in male weanling Sprague–Dawley rats that had received normal or riboflavin-deficient diets for 8 weeks. Rats in the replenished group received a deficient diet for 7 weeks followed by a diet supplemented with vitamins for 6 days. Each group contained 5-6 rats. (Figure is reproduced from Galton and Ingbar[49] with the permission of the publisher.)

in Fig. 5, markedly reduced deiodinating activity was restored to normal by feeding deficient animals riboflavin for a 6-day period. It is relevant to these findings that Yamamoto[113] had previously shown that FMN enhances the deiodination of thyroxine by kidney and liver mitochondria. The specificity of the finding that riboflavin deficiency reduced hepatic deiodination of thyroxine was demonstrated by the fact that deficiencies of pyridoxine, niacin, vitamin A, B_6, D, or K did not affect deiodination.[49] Deiodinating ability was depressed only in slices of liver from riboflavin-deficient animals and not in extracts from kidney, muscle, or brain. In further studies, thyroxine was given for a 2-week period to riboflavin-deficient rats. Hormone treatment achieved a very slight increase in hepatic deiodinating activity, but values remained considerably lower than those obtained in normal animals.[49]

These authors were also interested in whether riboflavin deficiency alters thyroid gland function *in vivo*. They found that the 24-hr urinary excretion of ^{131}I and the serum concentration of protein bound iodine (PBI) after administration of radioactive thyroxine were nearly identical in normal and riboflavin deficient animals. More recently, Nolte *et al.*[69] reported that in riboflavin-deficient rats the serum thyroxine concentration was greatly reduced to one-eighth that of normal animals. In addition, the metabolic rates of the deficient animals were lower than normal during the early phases of deficiency. Curiously, the decrease in metabolic rate observed was much less than the decrease in serum thyroxine concentration. Treatment with thyroxine increased the metabolic rates comparably in normal and in deficient animals. In riboflavin deficiency, oxygen consumption by liver mitochondria is reduced about one-third.[13] Because flavin enzymes within the thyroid gland appear to be involved in hormone synthesis,[1,66,94] one might expect to find some impairment in hormonogenesis in riboflavin deficiency. Much more work will be required to elucidate the nature of any possible defects in thyroid function in riboflavin deficiency.

5.4. Flavin-Induced Deiodination of Thyroxine

In addition to the enzymatic degradation of thyroid hormone, FMN appears to participate in a photo-activated reaction that results in the deiodination of thyroxine and other compounds. The flavin-induced degradation of thyroxine occurs rapidly in ambient light, is greatly intensified in bright light, and is almost completely inhibited in the dark. The addition of increasing amounts of human plasma inhibits the degradative effect of flavins.[48]

The findings of Galton and Ingbar[49] on the non-enzymatic deiodination of thyroxine and triiodothyronine were extended by Reinwein and Rall.[78] These authors showed that a large number of substances including amino acids, amines, enzymes, and metal chelators influenced the rate of deiodination. Deiodination of thyroxine requires FMN, visible light, and oxygen, and it takes place most rapidly at a pH range of 6-9.

Studies of enzymatic deiodination in the thyroid gland were conducted by Rosenberg and Ahn.[94] The addition of FAD stimulated the deiodination of diiodotyrosine in homogenates of rat thyroid. This reaction was enzymatically mediated and not dependent upon light or oxygen. Deiodination was stimulated only by the fully reduced form of FAD. The enhancement of deiodination of diiodotyrosine by FAD appears to be different from the photo-activated deiodination reaction described above.

5.5 Stimulation of Flavin Synthesis by Thyroid Hormones

A direct effect of thyroid hormone upon riboflavin metabolism was demonstrated independently by Domjan and Kokai[28,56] and by Rivlin and Langdon.[88] Both groups of investigators showed that the hepatic concentration of FAD was reduced to nearly two-thirds of normal in hypothyroid rats and could be restored to normal by treatment with thyroid hormone. In animals that had been treated with excessive doses of thyroid hormone, the FAD concentration was not increased further. The first group performed their investigations in animals that were surgically thyroidectomized, and the second group employed radioactive iodine ablation of the thyroid gland. The results described by both groups were nearly identical. It is likely that the reduction in the hepatic concentration of FAD in hypothyroid animals is due, at least in part, to decreased conversion of riboflavin to FMN. Hepatic activity of flavokinase, which converts riboflavin to FMN, is reduced in half in hypothyroid animals; it is increased nearly twofold in hyperthyroid animals.[88]

The regulation of flavokinase activity by thyroid hormone appears to be complex. Treatment with actinomycin D does not block the thyroxine-induced increase of enzyme activity.[88] Results of experiments performed with this enzyme *in vitro* suggest that the thyroxine-induced increase in flavokinase activity may be due, at least in part, to a decrease in the rate of enzyme inactivation. A striking difference was observed between enzyme from normal and hyperthyroid animals in the rate at which enzyme activity was lost during incubation *in vitro*. With enzyme obtained from normal animals, nearly all flavokinase activity was lost after 90 min of incubation *in vitro*. By contrast, with enzyme from hyperthyroid animals after a similar period of incubation, only 25% of the activity had been destroyed. After passage of tissue extracts through a Sephadex G-25 column, the differential rates of inactivation of the enzyme were eliminated. These observations make it likely that the greater stability of enzyme from hyperthyroid than from normal animals is due not to an inherent property of the enzyme itself, but to the presence of increased quantities of one or more small molecules that, in turn, stabilize the enzyme protein.[83,88]

Further studies of hepatic flavin concentrations in hypothyroid animals have revealed that the level of FMN is reduced similarly to that of FAD.[90] Lanzani and Mascitelli-Coriandoli[59] had observed a decrease in the hepatic levels of FMN and free riboflavin, but not of FAD, in liver of hypothyroid rats. It is likely that thyroid hormone regulates several of the enzymes involved in the riboflavin-to-FAD pathway. Of the enzymes investigated, flavokinase undergoes the largest quantitative increase in activity after administration of thyroid hormone and is the only enzyme of the group to decrease in activity in hypothyroidism.[86,90] Thyroid hormone also provokes increases in the activities of FAD-pyrophosphorylase, which converts FMN to FAD, and of FMN-phosphatase, which degrades FMN to riboflavin.[89] Certain effects of thyroid hormone upon increasing the hepatic activities of flavoprotein enzymes may be due not only to stimulation of apoenzyme

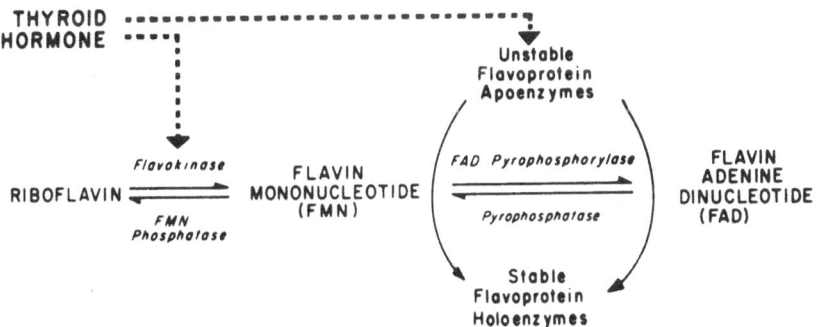

Fig. 6. Diagrammatic representation of the regulation of riboflavin metabolism by thyroid hormone. By increasing the activities of flavokinase and FAD pyrophosphorylase, thyroid hormone augments the rate of synthesis of FMN and FAD. These coenzymes combine with unstable flavoprotein apoenzyme to form stable holoenzymes. Increases in activity of flavoprotein holoenzymes produced by thyroid hormone may be due to enhancement of both apoenzyme and coenzyme synthesis. (Adapted from Rivlin[86] with the permission of the publisher.)

synthesis, but also to stimulation of synthesis of FMN and FAD that convert the unstable flavoprotein apoenzymes into stable flavoprotein holoenzymes. These relationships are shown diagrammatically in Fig. 6.

The magnitude of the changes in activity of enzymes synthesizing FMN and FAD has been compared recently with *in vivo* rates of flavin synthesis using newly devised methods of isotope dilution and ion exchange column chromatography (see Chapter 3). Results indicate that changes in the activities of riboflavin-metabolizing enzymes produced by altered thyroid function closely reflect actual changes in rates of flavin coenzyme synthesis *in vivo*.[38]

Evidence has accumulated that riboflavin deficiency and hypothyroidism have a number of biochemical similarities. These include at least three parameters in liver: (a) concentrations of FAD, FMN, and riboflavin; (b) activities of a number of FAD- and FMN-requiring enzymes; and (c) activities of enzymes that are involved in the biosynthesis and degradation of FMN and FAD.[37,85,90] The changes that occur in riboflavin deficiency are generally in the same direction as those of hypothyroidism but are of greater severity.

Further evidence of the similarity between biochemical effects of riboflavin deficiency and thyroid hormone deficiency has been provided by observations on the FAD-requiring enzyme in erythrocytes, glutathione reductase. The magnitude of the increase in activity of glutathione reductase following incubation with FAD *in vitro* has been shown to be greater in erythrocyte hemolyzate preparations from riboflavin deficient than from normal animals.[51,105] Similarly, erythrocyte hemolyzate preparations from hypothyroid animals after incubation with FAD *in vitro* have recently been shown to undergo a greater increase in activity than that from controls.[65] These observations are consistent with a state of relative riboflavin deficiency in hypothyroidism. In hyperthyroid animals, the less-than-normal increase in glutathione reductase activity observed after incubation with FAD *in vitro* suggests that the apoenzyme may be relatively saturated with FAD as a result of enhanced flavin synthesis.[65]

5.6. Enzyme Induction in Riboflavin Deficiency

A further consequence of the decreased rate of formation of FMN and FAD in riboflavin deficiency is that certain responses to thyroid hormone are diminished. Tipton *et al.*[106] demonstrated that D-amino acid oxidase activity was decreased in livers of riboflavin-deficient rats and that the administration of thyroxine did not increase enzyme activity normally in these animals. In the early stages of riboflavin deficiency thyroxine was still somewhat effective in increasing D-amino acid oxidase activity, but, in the late stages of deficiency, thyroxine produced no increase in activity at all. In later studies,[92,112] diminished responsiveness to thyroid hormone was a feature of another FAD-dependent enzyme, α-glycerophosphate dehydrogenase. The reactivity of this hepatic enzyme was increased approximately tenfold by the administration of triiodothyronine in normal animals, nearly seventy-five-fold in hypothyroid animals, but only fivefold in riboflavin-deficient animals. The diminished induction of α-glycerophosphate dehydrogenase activity by triiodothyronine appeared to follow quite closely the hepatic levels of FAD. In the riboflavin-deficient animal, the hepatic concentration of FAD could not be increased by treatment with triiodothyronine.[85] The diminished induction of mitochondrial α-glycerophosphate dehydrogenase in riboflavin-deficient rats has been recently confirmed by Nolte et al.,[69] and by Reith et al.,[80] who showed that this relationship is true also for succinic dehydrogenase. Succinic dehydrogenase activity actually decreased in riboflavin-deficient animals after the administration of triiodothyronine. Electron microscopic findings in rat heart and liver[79-81] show that riboflavin deficiency and triiodothyronine administration produce marked changes in the morphology of mitochondria. Triiodothyronine appears to stimulate biogenesis of mitochondria even in riboflavin-deficient animals. These data suggest that in riboflavin deficiency there may be some dissociation between the effects of thyroid hormone upon the induction of flavoprotein enzymes in mitochrondria and upon the alteration of mitochondrial structure. It appears likely that diminished response of these liver flavoprotein enzymes to thyroid hormone may be related to the restricted supply of FAD available for stabilizing newly synthesized enzyme protein.

Both the basal and the induced levels of mitochondrial α-glycerophosphate dehydrogenase fall progressively with increasing duration of riboflavin deficiency. Normal responsiveness to thyroid hormone can be restored by the administration of riboflavin to riboflavin-deficient animals, even if the food supply is simultaneously restricted. These data are shown in Fig. 7. During the process of refeeding, an enormous increase in body weight occurs. Even if this increase in body weight is prevented by food restriction, as shown in Fig. 7, enzyme induction is still restored to normal. This finding suggests that diminished food intake itself is not the major variable underlying the diminished responsiveness to thyroid hormone that is exhibited by riboflavin-deficient rats. Further evidence for this view has been the finding that, during

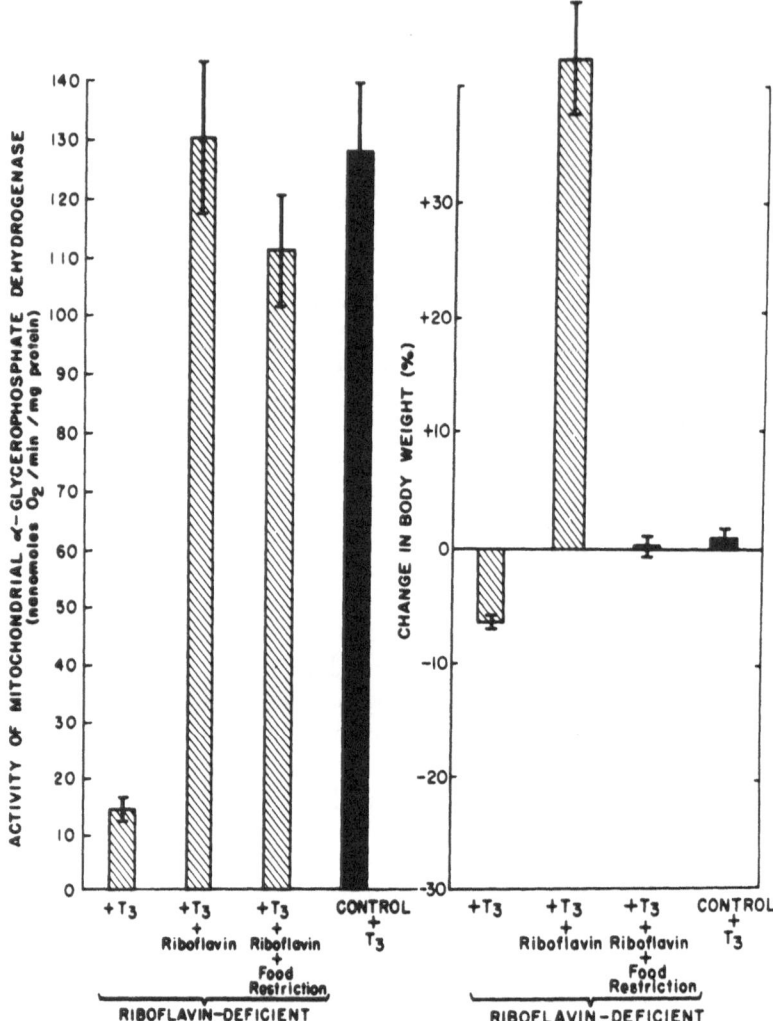

Fig. 7. Effectiveness of riboflavin refeeding of deficient rats upon the hepatic induction of mitochondrial α-glycerolphosphate dehydrogenase. Riboflavin was given by the oral and intraperitonal routes for 5-7 days to rats that had been deficient for 70 days. One group of rats refed riboflavin was permitted to eat *ad libitum* (second column), and the other group (third column) had food consumption restricted to that of animals that remained deficient. Changes in body weight during the 5- to 7-day period of refeeding are expressed as a percentage of the starting weight. Rats were sacrificed 48 hr after a single intraperitonal injection of triiodothyronine (T_3) in doses of 100 μg/100 g body weight. Results are shown as mean ± s.e.m. for 9-10 animals per group. (Derived in part from Wolf and Rivlin[112] with the permission of the publisher.)

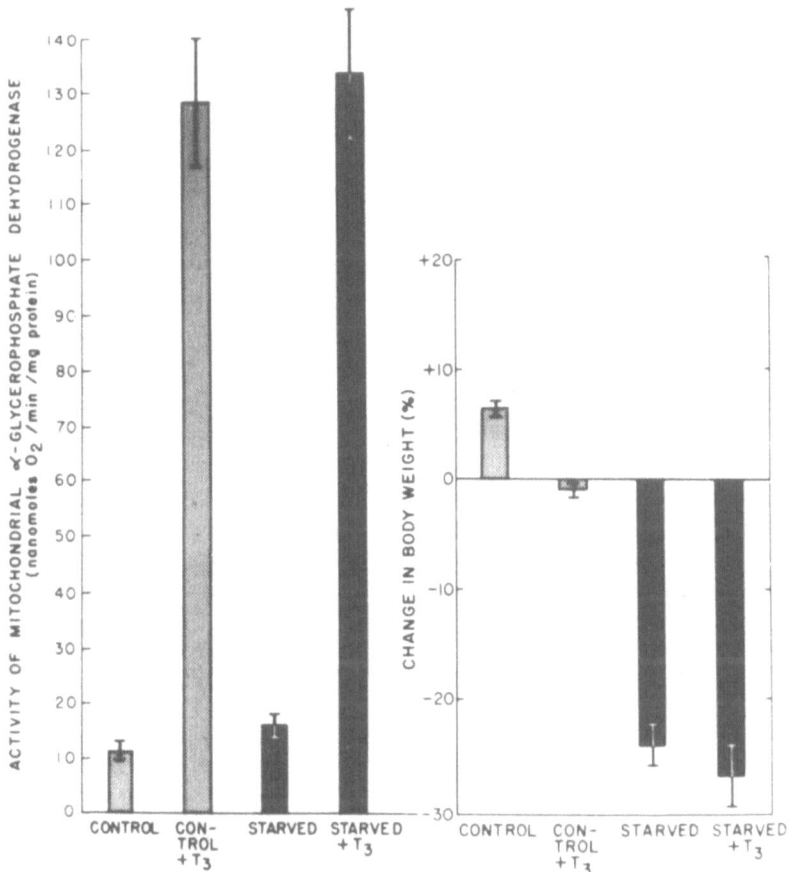

Fig. 8. Hepatic activity of mitochondrial α-glycerolphosphate dehydrogenase in control rats and in rats starved for 3-5 days. Basal activity and that induced by triiodothyronine (T$_3$) in doses of 100 μg/100 g given by i.p. injection 48 hr before sacrifice are shown for both groups. Body weight changes during the 3- to 5-day period of starvation are expressed as a percentage of the starting weight in each group. Data are expressed as the mean ±1 s.e.m. of each group of 9-13 animals. (Data are derived in part from Wolf and Rivlin[112] with the permission of the publisher.)

starvation, enzyme induction appears to be normal. As shown in Fig. 8, in animals that had been starved for 3-5 days, the induction of α-glycerophosphate dehydrogenase by triiodothyronine was nearly identical to that in normal animals. This finding is noteworthy in view of the enormous changes in body weight observed during the period of starvation.

5.7. Clinical Studies of Flavoprotein Enzymes in Thyroid Disease

Some possible relevance of this system to man has been suggested by the findings of Bray,[8] who demonstrated for the first time that triiodothyronine increases the activity of mitochondrial α-glycerophosphate dehydrogenase in human tissue. In adipose tissue from obese subjects, triiodothyronine produced a doubling of enzyme activity. As in the animal system, triiodothyronine did not affect the activity of the cytoplasmic dehydrogenase, which is not FAD-dependent. Liver and muscle biopsies in patients with thyrotoxicosis and myxedema were employed to investigate the entire spectrum of effects upon enzyme activity.[70] Two of the enzymes that increase with thyroid hormone treatment in animals, mitochondrial α-glycerophosphate dehydrogenase and succinic dehydrogenase, were not significantly increased in liver or muscle of thyrotoxic patients. In hypothyroidism, the activities of both enzymes were clearly reduced below control levels, and the differences between hypo- and hyperthyroid patients were highly significant. In another series of liver biopsies from hyperthyroid patients, activities of two FAD-dependent enzymes, glutathione reductase and TPHN cytochrome C reductase, were not increased above normal; hypothyroid patients were not studied.[68] These studies suggest that the effects of thyroid hormone upon FAD enzymes in man are perhaps less dramatic than those in experimental animals, but further studies will be required before the relevance of data obtained on experimental animals to human disorders can be determined.

In the rat pituitary gland, in contrast to other organs, thyroidectomy increases oxygen consumption and protein synthesis, and increases the activities of a number of flavoprotein enzymes.[64] It would be of interest to determine whether the rate of synthesis of FMN and FAD in the pituitary gland is also increased after thyroidectomy.

5.8. Developmental Effects of Thyroid Hormone

The hormonal regulation of riboflavin metabolism has been studied during the perinatal period. Enzymes involved in FMN and FAD biosynthesis undergo maturation earlier than do either the tissue levels of flavin coenzymes or the activities of the flavoprotein enzymes. Shortly before birth, the major increases in hepatic flavokinase and FAD-pyrophosphorylase activities occur. At the time of birth, levels similar to those of adult animals are already demonstrable.[84] In newborn animals that have been treated with subcutaneous injections of thyroxine, hepatic FAD pyrophosphorylase activity is increased above levels obtained in animals treated with saline. The magnitude of increases in enzyme activity in newborn animals are nearly identical to those observed in adult animals similarly treated with thyroid hormone.[87] In the brains of newborn animals, thyroid hormone increases FAD pyrophosphorylase activity to levels found in adult animals.[98] Thyroxine increases the activity of this enzyme in the cerebrum of the newborn but not in adult animals.[87,98] It is likely that thyroid hormone may regulate the availability of FAD for certain critical enzyme systems in the developing liver and brain.

The regulation of riboflavin metabolism during development is not restricted to mammals. Recently it was shown[36] that during thyroxine-induced metamorphosis in the bullfrog tadpole, *Rana catesbiana*, the hepatic activity of FAD pyrophosphorylase is significantly increased. After 6-11 days of immersion in thyroxine at 10^{-8} M, no increase in enzyme activity occurred. When immersion in thyroxine was continued for longer periods of time, FAD pyrophosphorylase activity was increased nearly 50%. This finding indicates that changes in the activity of an enzyme that is involved in FAD biosynthesis occur during tadpole metamorphosis induced by thyroxine. In a further extension of these findings, it was shown that structural analogues of riboflavin, each with one or more substitutions on the isoalloxazine ring, inhibit metamorphosis in tadpoles. Metamorphosis, occurring naturally or thyroxine induced, appears to be inhibited by analogues of riboflavin.[91]

These studies in sum indicate that thyroid-hormone deficiency reduces the tissue levels of FMN and FAD and diminishes the rate of conversion of riboflavin into these coenzyme derivatives. Thyroid hormone regulates riboflavin metabolism during adult life and during development. Riboflavin deficiency diminishes the effectiveness of thyroid hormone as an inducer of FAD-dependent enzymes. The overall effects of altered thyroid function upon riboflavin metabolism, particularly in man, require further elucidation.

6. SUMMARY AND CONCLUSIONS

The effects of hormones upon riboflavin metabolism are many and diverse. The estrogen-stimulated synthesis of the riboflavin-binding protein of chickens provides a fascinating example of how vitamin transport in plasma can be hormonally regulated. The influence of other hormones upon plasma binding, and the relevance of these studies to vitamin transport in higher animals, needs to be established.

That both hypoglycemia and diabetes mellitus have been observed in riboflavin deficiency indicates the complexity of the disturbances that may be occurring in carbohydrate metabolism. Until plasma insulin and glucose concentrations have been measured both in the basal state and after provocative stimuli, the role of hormonal secretion cannot be evaluated. Studies on glycogen synthesis and breakdown have largely been indirect and indicate the need for more complete investigations of intermediary metabolism in riboflavin deficiency.

With respect to the adrenal cortex, the recent demonstration that new FAD synthesis accompanies the formation of corticosterone after ACTH stimulation represents confirmation of an early theory linking the vitamin and the hormone. ACTH also increases the hepatic and adrenal synthesis of FMN. The clinical significance of these findings awaits further study.

By enhancing the conversion of riboflavin into its physiologically active coenzyme derivatives, thyroid hormones may act at an important control point in intermediary metabolism. The increased rate of coenzyme synthesis may mediate in part the increased activity of a wide variety of flavoprotein enzymes after treatment with thyroid hormones. There is a similarity between many of the biochemical effects of riboflavin and thyroid hormone deficiency. Studies to date provide evidence not only that thyroid hormones regulate riboflavin metabolism, but also that riboflavin may be required for certain effects of thyroid hormone to occur. Plasma concentrations of riboflavin tend to be increased in hyperthyroid patients, but overall effects upon riboflavin metabolism have not been defined.

The fact that riboflavin metabolism is subject to hormonal regulation may have implications for the rational use of vitamins in the therapy of human diseases. Effects must be made to define and to clarify the endogenous factors that regulate vitamin utilization.

7. REFERENCES

1. Alexander, N. M. 1972. Role of superoxide dismutase in H_2O_2 generation in thyroid glands, *Program of the Annual Meeting of the American Thyroid Association*, p. 66 (Abstr.).
2. Arscott, G. H. 1972. Effect of riboflavin in reproductive performance of adult white leghorn male chickens, *Nutr. Reports Intern.* 5:287-291.

3. Axelrod, A. E., Lipton, M. A., and Elvehjem, C. A. 1941. Riboflavin deficiency in the dog, *Amer. J. Physiol.* 133:555-561.
4. Axelrod, H. E., Gullberg, M. G., and Morgan, A. F. 1951. Carbohydrate metabolism in riboflavin-deficient dogs, *Amer. J. Physiol.* 165:604-619.
5. Barbieri, D., Marzocchi, G., and Brunelli, G. 1954. Rontgenstimolazione della tiroide ed eliminazione urinaria della tiamina, della riboflavina, della niacina, dell'acido ascorbico e dei 17-chetosteroidi, *Intern. Z. Vitamin.* 25:261-274.
6. Bertolini, A. M., and Cavagna, G. 1957. Influence of internal secretions on riboflavin metabolism, *Acta vitaminol,* 4:149-154.
7. Bessey, O. A., Lowry, O. H., Davis, E. B., and Dorn, J. L. 1958. The riboflavin economy of the rat, *J. Nutrition* 64:185-202.
8. Bray, G. A. 1969. Effect of diet and triiodothyronine on the activity of sn-glycerol-3-phosphate dehydrogenase and on the metabolism of glucose and pyruvate by adipose tissue of obese patients, *J. Clin. Invest.* 48:1413-1423.
9. Bressler, R., Corredor, C., and Brendel, K. 1969. Hypoglycin and hypoglycin-like compounds, *Pharmacol. Rev.* 21:105-130.
10. Brooks, S. E. H., and Audretsch, J. J. 1971. Hypoglycin toxicity in rats. II. Modification by riboflavin of mitochondrial changes in liver, *Amer. J. Pathol.* 62:309-320.
11. Bruce, H. M., and Wien, R. 1940. The effect of riboflavin, riboflavin phosphoric acid and the cortical hormone on the survival of adrenalectomized rats receiving normal and riboflavin-deficient diets, *J. Physiol.* 98:375-388.
12. Brummer, P., Markkanen, T. K., and Kalliomaki, J. L. 1961. Effect of corticosteriods on urinary excretion and on the intestinal absorption of thiamine, riboflavin, nicotinic acid, pantothenic acid and biotin, *Acta Med. Scand.* 170:183-186.
13. Burch, H. B., Hunter, F. E., Combs, A. M., and Schutz, B. A. 1960. Oxidative enzymes and phosphorylation in hepatic mitochondria from riboflavin-deficient rats, *J. Biol. Chem.* 235:1540-1544.
14. Chatterjee, A. K., and Ghosh, B. B. 1967. Effects of riboflavin deficiency on *in vivo* incorporation of ^{14}C from labelled alanine into liver glycogen, *Experientia* 23:633-634.
15. Chatterjee, A. K., and Ghosh, B. B. 1969. Effects of corticoids and of adrenalectomy on free amino acid nitrogen concentrations of liver, muscle and plasma in riboflavin deficiency, *Endokrinologie* 54:184-188.
16. Chatterjee, A. K., and Ghosh, B. B. 1970. Effects of cortisone and of adrenalectomy on plasma total ascorbic acid level in riboflavin deficiency. *Endokrinologie* 56:218-222.
17. Chatterjee, A. K., Jamdar, S. C., and Ghosh, B. B. 1966. Changes in alanine transaminase activity in the liver of riboflavin-deficient rats, *Experientia* 22:794-795.
18. Clagett, C. O. 1971. Genetic control of the riboflavin carrier protein, *Federation Proc.* 30:127-129.
19. Clagett, C. O., Buss, E. B., Saylor, E. M., and Girsh, S. J. 1970. The nature of the biochemical lesion in avian renal riboflavinuria: VI. Hormone induction of the riboflavin-binding protein in roosters and young chicks, *Poultry Sci.* 49:1468-1472.
20. Clarke, H. C. 1969. The relationship between whole blood riboflavin levels and results of riboflavin saturation tests in normal and pathological conditions in man, *Intern. J. Vitam. Nutr. Res.* 39:238-245.
21. Clarke, H. C. 1973. In Pregnancy: Effect of iron and folic acid on riboflavin status, *Intern. J. Vitam. Nutr. Res.* 43:438-441.
22. Colonge, A. R., and Raffy, A. 1947. Modifications histologiques des glandes endocrines et du tractus genital chez des rats soumis à un regime exclusivement depourvu de vitamine B$_2$, *Compt. rend. Soc. de Biol.,* 141:63-64.

23. Colonge, A. R., and Raffy, A. 1948. Vitamine B$_2$ et physiologie hypophysaire, *Compt. rend. Soc. de Biol.* **142**:640-642.

24. Common, R. H., Rutledge, W. A., and Bolton, W. 1947. The influence of gonadal hormones on serum riboflavin and certain other properties of blood and tissues in the domestic fowl, *J. Endocrinol.* **5**:121-130.

25. Cordona, N. A., and Payne, I. R. 1967. Absorption of riboflavin in chickens, *Poultry Sci.* **46**:1176-1179.

26. Coward, K. H., Morgan, B. G. E., and Waller, L. 1942. The influence of a deficiency of vitamin B$_1$ and of riboflavin on the reproduction of the rat, *J. Physiol.* **100**:423-431.

27. Deane, H. W., and Shaw, J. H. 1947. A cytochemical study of the responses of the adrenal cortex of the rat to thiamine, riboflavin and pyridoxine deficiencies, *J. Nutr.* **34**:1-15.

28. Domjan, G., and Kokai, K. 1966. The flavin adenine dinucleotide (FAD) content of the rat's liver in hypothyroid state and in the liver of hypothyroid animals after *in vivo* thyroxine treatment, *Acta Biol. Hung.* **16**:237-241.

29. Drill, V. A. 1938. Effect of vitamin B$_1$ and B$_2$ complex on the loss of weight produced in rats by experimental hyperthyroidism, *Proc. Soc. Exptl. Biol. & Med.* **39**:313-316.

30. Drill, V. A., and Sherwood, C. R. 1938. The effect of vitamin B$_1$ and the vitamin B$_2$ complex on the weight, food intake and estrual cycle of hyperthyroid rats, *Amer. J. Physiol.* **124**:683-691.

31. Emerson, G. A., and Folkers, K. 1951. Vitamin activity of lyxoflavin, *J. Am. Chem. Soc.* **73**:5383-5386.

32. Emerson, G. A., and Folkers, K. 1951. Tests with lyxoflavin for vitamin activity, *J. Am. Chem. Soc.* **73**:2398-2399.

33. Ershoff, B. H. 1952. Ineffectiveness of lyxoflavin as an antithyrotoxic factor for the rat, *Proc. Soc. Exptl. Biol. & Med.* **79**:469-470.

34. Ershoff, B. H. 1954. Effects of riboflavin deficiency on insulin sensitivity in the rat, *Metabolism* **3**:357-363.

35. Farrell, H. M. Jr., Buss, E. G., and Clagett, C. O. 1970. The nature of the biochemical lesion in avian renal riboflavinuria. V. Elucidation of riboflavin transport in the laying hen, *Intern. J. Biochem.* **1**:168-172.

36. Fass, S., Osnos, M., Hornibrook, R., and Rivlin, R. 1971. Effects of thyroxine on hepatic FAD pyrophosphorylase in tadpoles, *Program of the Annual Meeting of the American Thyroid Association*, p. 42 (Abstr.).

37. Fass, S., and Rivlin, R. S. 1969. Regulation of riboflavin-metabolizing enzymes in riboflavin deficiency, *Amer. J. Physiol.* **217**:988-991.

38. Fazekas, A. G., Huang, Y. P., Chaudhuri, R., and Rivlin, R. S. 1972. Enhancement of biosynthesis of flavin coenzymes *in vivo* by thyroxine, *Program of the Annual Meeting of the American Thyroid Association*, p. 63 (Abstr.).

39. Fazekas, G. A., and Sandor, T. 1971. Flavin nucleotide coenzyme biosynthesis and its relation to corticosteroidogenesis in the rat adrenal, *Endocrinology* **89**:397-407.

40. Fazekas, A. G., and Sandor, T. 1971. The *in vivo* effect of adrenocorticotropin on the biosynthesis of flavin nucleotides in rat liver and kidney, *Canad. J. Biochem.* **49**:987-989.

41. Field, J. B., Federman, D. D., McDaniel, E., and Bakerman, H. 1957. Urinary excretion patterns of some B-vitamins in diabetes. A study in patients with and without degenerative complications, *Diabetes* **6**:508-514.

42. Forker, B. R., and Morgan, A. F. 1954. Effect of adrenocortical hormone on the riboflavin-deficient rat, *J. Biol. Chem.* **209**:303-311.

43. Forker, B. R., and Morgan, A. F. 1955. Cause of pituitary-adrenal failure in the riboflavin-deficient rat, *J. Biol. Chem.* **217**:659-667.

44. Fox, H. C., and Miller, D. S. 1960. Akee toxin: a riboflavin antimetabolite? *Nature* **186**:561-562.

45. Foy, H., Kondi, A., and Verjee, A. H. M. 1972. Relation of riboflavin deficiency to corticosteroid metabolism and red cell hypoplasia in baboons, *J. Nutr.* **102**:571-582.

46. Fujimoto, T., Tanabe, H., Uchida, M., Shiba, N., Kusano, M., Sakuyama, F., Sumoya, S., and Yoshida, Y. 1960. Riboflavin metabolism in diabetics. *Bitamin* (*Kyoto*) **20**:140-150 (*Chem. Abstr.* **61**:16576, 1964).

47. Fukuhara, T. 1961. Studies on the metabolism of riboflavin in rabbits. II. The effects of intravenous injections of glucose solution on the urinary excretion of riboflavin in rabbits, *Hirosaki Med. J.* **13**:11-13, (*Biol. Abstr.* **38**:9041, 1962).

48. Galton, V. A., and Ingbar, S. H. 1962. A photoactivated flavin-induced degradation of thyroxine and related phenols, *Endocrinology* **70**:210-220.

49. Galton, V. A., and Ingbar, S. H. 1965. Effects of vitamin deficiency on the *in vitro* and *in vivo* deiodination of thyroxine in the rat, *Endocrinology* **77**:169-176.

50. Gianieri, D., and Ipata, P. L. Comportamento della cacarbossilasi e dei coenzimi flavinici nell'ipertiroidismo, *Acta vitaminol.* **11**:33-36.

51. Glatzle, E., Weber, F., and Wiss, O. 1968. Enzymatic test for the detection of a riboflavin deficiency; NADPH-dependent glutathione reductase of red blood cells and its activation by FAD *in vitro*, *Experimentia* **24**:1122, 1968.

52. Guggenheim, K., and Diamant, E. J. 1955. Effect of riboflavin and choline deficiencies on water metabolism in rats, *J. Nutr.* **57**:249-260.

53. Harding, B. W., and Nelson, D. H. 1964. Effect of hypophysectomy on several rat adrenal NADPH-generating and oxidizing systems, *Endocrinology* **75**:506-513.

54. Jamdar, S. C., and Mookerjea, S. 1962. Possible effects of riboflavin deficiency on adrenal cortical function in the rat, *Canad. J. Biochem. Physiol.* **40**:1059-1064.

55. Jamdar, S. C., and Udupa, K. B. 1967. Incorporation of ^{32}P in the adrenals of riboflavin-deficient rats, *Endokrinologie* **51**:175-178.

56. Kokai, K., and Domjan, G. 1965. Thyreoidektomia hatasa patkanymaj flavin adenin dinukleotid (FAD) tartalmara, *Biol. Kozl.* **13**:127-129.

57. Kuznetsova, L., and Shestopalova, V. M. 1972. Effect of hydrocortisone on distribution and content of riboflavin in animal tissues, *UKR. Biokhim. Zh.* **44**:500-503.

58. Kuznetsova, L., and Shestopalova, V. M. 1972. Utilization of riboflavin and its nucleotides by subcellular fractions of the liver in rats under the effect of hydrocortisone, *Vopr. Pitan.* **31**:17-20.

59. Lanzani, P., and Mascitelli-Coriandoli, E. 1965. Effecto protettivo sulla sintesi del FAD nei ratti tireotossici ad opera di una frazione estrativa del fegato suino, *Boll. Societa Ital. Biol. Sper.* **41**:666-668.

60. Lillie, R. J. 1973. Inefficacy of dietary deficiencies of vitamin A, D_3 and riboflavin on the reproductive performance of mature cockerels, *Poultry Sci.* **52**:1629-1636.

61. Lossy, F. T., Goldsmith, G. A., and Sarett, H. P. 1951. A study of test dose excretion of five B complex vitamins in man, *J. Nutr.* **45**:213-224.

62. Lust, J. E., Hagerman, D. D., and Villee, C. A. 1954. The transport of riboflavin by human placenta, *J. Clin. Invest.* **33**:38-40.

63. Magyar, I. 1948. Excretion of riboflavin in rats and phosphorylation, *Hung. Acta Med.* **1**:37-47.

64. Matsuzaki, S. 1968. Difference in effects of thyroidectomy and thyroxine supplement on hepatic and anterior pituitary enzymes in the rat, *Endocrinl. Japon.* **15**:223-228.

65. Menendez, C. E., Hacker, P., Sonnenfeld, M., McConnell, R., and Rivlin, R. S.

1974. Thyroid hormone regulation of glutathione reductase activity in rat erythrocytes and liver, *Amer. J. Physiol.* **226**:1480-1483.

66. Nagasaka, A., DeGrott, L. J., Hati, R., and Liu, C. 1971. Studies on the biosynthesis of thyroid hormone: reconstruction of a defined *in vitro* iodinating system, *Endocrinology* **88**:486-490.

67. Nelson, D. 1940. The non-effectiveness of riboflavin phosphoric acid and riboflavin in maintaining life in the adrenalectomized rat. *Amer. J. Physiol.* **129**:429 (Abstr.).

68. Nikkila, E. A., and Pitkanen, E. 1959. Liver enzyme pattern in thyrotoxicosis, *Acta Endocrinol.* **31**:573-586.

69. Nolte, J., Brdiczka, D., and Staudte, H. W. 1972. Effect of riboflavin deficiency on metabolism of the rat in hyperthyroid and euthyroid state, *Biochim. Biophys. Acta* **268**:611-619.

70. Nolte, J., Pette, D., Bachmaier, B., Keifhaber, P., Schneider, H., and Scriba, P. C. 1972. Enzyme response to thyrotoxicosis and hypothyroidism in human liver and muscle: comparative aspects, *Eur. J. Clin. Invest.* **2**:141-149.

71. Oldham, H., Lounds, E., and Porter, T. 1947. Riboflavin excretions and test dose returns of young women during periods of positive and negative nitrogen balance, *J. Nutr.* **34**:69-79.

71*a*. Ono, S., Hirano, H., and Obara, K. 1973. Preventive effect of flavin adenine dinucleotide on induction of adrenal atrophy in rat by dexamethasone, *J. Nutr. Sci. Vitaminol.* **19**:287-288.

71*b*. Ono, S., Hamajima, S., Hirano, H., and Obara, K. 1974. Effect of flavin adenine dinucleotide on the glucose-6-phosphate dehydrogenase activity of adrenal gland of hypophysectomized rats, *Japan J. Exptl. Med.* **44**:115-118.

72. Palagiano, V. 1961. La riboflavinemia nel morbo di Basedow prima e dopo l'intervento chirurgico, *Acta Chir. Italica* **17**:273-281.

73. Palagiano, V. 1962. Riboflavinuria dopo carico parenterale in soggetti ipertiroidei in relazione all'intervento chirurgico, *Acta Chir. Italica* **18**:183-192.

74. Palagiano, V., and Baldassarre, M. 1966. Sul comportamento della carbossilasi e dei coenzimi flavinici nell'ipertiroidismo in relazione l'intervento chirurgico, *Acta Chir. Italica* **22**:75-85.

75. Persaud, T. V. N. 1970. Studies on the mechanism of teratogenic action of hypoglycin, *Teratology* **3**:208 (Abstr.).

76. Platzer, E. G., and Roberts, L. S. 1970. Developmental physiology of cestodes. VI. Effect of host riboflavin deficiency on Hymenolepsis diminuta, *Exptl. Parasitol.* **28**:393-398.

77. Pollack, H., and Bookman, J. J. 1951. Riboflavin excretion as a function of protein metabolism in the normal, catabolic and diabetic human being, *J. Lab. & Clin. Med.* **38**:561-573.

78. Reinwein, D., and Rall, J. E. 1966. Nonenzymatic deiodination of thyroid hormones by flavin mononucleotide and light, *J. Biol. Chem.* **241**:1636-1643.

79. Reith, A. 1973. The influence of triiodothyronine and riboflavin deficiency on the rat liver with special reference to mitochondria. A morphologic, morphometric and cytochemical study by electron microscopy, *Lab. Invest.* **29**:216-228.

80. Reith, A., Brdiczka, D., Nolte, J., and Staudte, H. W. 1973. The inner membrane of mitochondria under influence of triiodothyronine and riboflavin deficiency in rat heart muscle and liver, *Exptl. Cell Res.* **77**:1-14.

81. Reith, A., and Fuchs, S. 1973. The heart muscle of the rat under influence of triiodothyronine and riboflavin deficiency with special reference to mitochondria.

A morphologic and morphometric study by electron microscopy, *Lab. Invest.* **29:**229-235.

82. Rhodes, M. B., Bennett, N. S., and Feeney, R. E. 1959. The flavoprotein-apoprotein system of egg white, *J. Biol. Chem.* **234:**2054-2060.
83. Rivlin, R. S. 1966. Thyroid hormone and the adolescent growth spurt: clinical and fundamental considerations, *in:* "Adolescent Nutrition and Growth" (F. Heald, ed.), pp. 235-252, Appleton-Century-Crofts, Inc., New York.
84. Rivlin, R. S. 1969. Perinatal development of enzymes synthesizing FMN and FAD, *Amer. J. Physiol.* **216:**979-982.
85. Rivlin, R. S. 1970. Regulation of flavoprotein enzymes in hypothyroidism and in riboflavin deficiency, in: "Advances in Enzyme Regulation" (G. Weber, ed.), **8:**239-250, Pergamon Press, Oxford, England.
86. Rivlin, R. S. 1970. Medical progress: riboflavin metabolism, *New Eng. J. Med.* **283:**463-472.
87. Rivlin, R. S. 1974. Regulation of riboflavin metabolism by thyroid hormone, *in:* "The Neurosciences. Third Study Program" (F. O. Schmitt and F. G. Worden, eds.), pp. 835-840, M.I.T. Press, Cambridge.
88. Rivlin, R. S., and Langdon, R. G. 1966. Regulation of hepatic FAD levels by thyroid hormone, *in:* "Advances in Enzyme Regulation" (G. Weber, ed.), **4:**45-58, Pergamon Press, Oxford, England.
89. Rivlin, R. S., and Langdon, R. G. 1969. Effects of thyroxine upon biosynthesis of flavin mononucleotide and flavin adenine dinucleotide, *Endocrinology* **84:**584-588.
90. Rivlin, R. S., Menendez, C., and Langdon, R. G. 1968. Biochemical similarities between hypothyroidism and riboflavin deficiency, *Endocrinology* **83:**461-469.
91. Rivlin, R. S., Osnos, M., and Hornibrook, R. 1972. Inhibition of thyroxine-induced tadpole metamorphosis by analogues of riboflavin, *Program of the Fourth International Congress of Endocrinology*, p. 42, 1971 (abstr.).
92. Rivlin, R. S., and Wolf, G. 1969. Diminished responsiveness to thyroid hormone in riboflavin-deficient rats, *Nature* **223:**516-517.
93. Rose, D. P., and McGinty, F. 1968. The influence of adrenocortical hormones and vitamins upon tryptophan metabolism in man, *Clin. Sci.* **35:**1-9.
94. Rosenberg, I. N., and Ahn, C. S. 1969. Enzymatic deiodination of diiodotyrosine; possible mediation by reduced flavin nucleotide, *Endocrinology* **84:**727-737.
95. Rotzsch, V. W., Aurich, H., and Franz, E. 1965. Riboflavin und Pyridoxingehalt der Skelettmuskulatur unter Schilddrusenhormonen, *Deutsch Z. Verdau Stoffwechselkr.* **25:**327-338.
96. Shaw, J. H., and Phillips, P. P. 1941. The pathology of riboflavin deficiency in the rat, *J. Nutr.* **22:**345-358.
97. Slater, G. G. 1959. Influence of galactoflavin and inanition on the adrenal ascorbic acid response to stress in rats, *Endocrinology* **65:**731-738.
98. Sturman, J. A., and Rivlin, R. S. Pathogenesis of brain dysfunction in deficiency of thiamine, riboflavin, pantothenic acid or vitamin B_6, in: "Biology of Brain Dysfunction" (G. E. Gaull, ed.), Plenum Press, New York, in press.
99. Sure, B. 1938. Influence of avitaminoses on weights of endocrine glands, *Endocrinology* **23:**575-580.
100. Sure, B., and Buchanan, K. S. 1937. Antithyrogenic action of crystalline vitamin B, *J. Nutrition* **13:**513-519.
101. Sure, B., and Ford, Z. W., Jr. 1943. Influence of hyperthyroidism on urinary excretion of thiamin and riboflavin, *Endocrinology* **32:**433-436.

102. Sylianco, C. Y. L., and Berg, C. P. 1959. The effect of riboflavin deficiency upon the metabolism of tryptophan by liver and kidney tissue, *J. Biol. Chem.* **234:**912-917.
103. Terroine, T., Buisson, F., Bertaux, O., and Hitier, Y. 1968. Activité desoxyribonucleasique et degenerescence testiculaire dans diverses avitaminoses, *Arch. Sci. Physiol.* **22:**411-427.
104. Terroine, T., and Delost, P. 1961. Influence des carences vitaminiques sur le development des organes sexuals, *Ann. Nutr. Alim.* **15:**291-335.
105. Tillotson, J. A., and Sauberlich, H. E. 1971. Effect of riboflavin depletion and repletion on the erythrocyte glutathione reductase in the rat, *J. Nutr.* **101:**1459-1466.
106. Tipton, S. R., Weldon, F., and Weiss, A. K. 1955. Effect of riboflavin or thiamine deficiency on the response of liver and kidney adenosine-triphosphatase and D-amino acid oxidase to thyroid and adrenal alterations in rats, *Amer. J. Physiol.* **180:**321-324.
107. Travia, L., and Pelosio, C. 1948. Urinary elimination of phosphorylated lactoflavin after administration of glucose and lactoflavin in normal subjects, *Boll. Soc. Ital. Biol. Sper.* **24:**737-738 (*Chem Abstr.* **43:**6707, 1949).
108. Verzar, F., and Laszt, L. 1936. Der Zusammenhang zwischen Vitamin B_2 und dem Hormon der Nebennierenrinde, *Arch. f.d. ges. Physiol,* **237:**476-482.
109. Von Holt, C., and von Holt, L. 1959. Biochemie des Hypoglycins A. I. Die Wirkung des Riboflavins auf den Hypoglycineffekt, *Biochem. Z.* **331:**422-429.
110. Warkany, J., and Schraffenberger, E. 1944. Congenital malformations induced in rats by maternal nutritional deficiency. VI. The preventive factor, *J. Nutr.* **27:**477-484.
111. Wickson, M. E., and Morgan, A. F. 1946. The effect of riboflavin deficiency upon carbohydrate metabolism in anoxia, *J. Biol. Chem.* **162:**209-220.
112. Wolf, G., and Rivlin, R. S. 1970. Inhibition of thyroid hormone induction of mitochondrial α-glycerophosphate dehydrogenase in riboflavin deficiency, *Endocrinology* **86:**1347-1353.
113. Yamamoto, K., Shimizu, S., and Ishikawa, I. 1960. Metabolism of L-thyroxine by mitochondria of various rat tissues in the presence of pyridoxal phosphate and α-ketoglutarate, diphosphopyridine nucleotide or flavin mononucleotide, *Japan. J. Physiol.* **10:**594-601.

INDEX